# AMYLOIDOSIS

Edited by **Dali Feng**

**Amyloidosis**
http://dx.doi.org/10.5772/46140
Edited by Dali Feng

## Contributors

Suguru Yamamoto, Junichiro Kazama, Hiroki Maruyama, Ichiei Narita, Jozélio de Carvalho, Tadashi Nakamura, Takeshi Kuroda, Keisuke Hagihara, Syota Kagawa, Junsuke Arimitsu, Yuki Kishida, Hesam Hashemian, Sudhir Kushwaha, Maarit Tanskanen, Fernando L Palhano, Dali Feng

**Published by InTech**
Janeza Trdine 9, 51000 Rijeka, Croatia



**Publishing Process Manager** Iva Simcic
**Technical Editor** InTech DTP team
**Cover** InTech Design team

Additional hard copies can be obtained from orders@intechopen.com

Amyloidosis, Edited by Dali Feng
p. cm.
ISBN 978-953-51-1100-9

For EU product safety concerns:
IN TECH d.o.o., Prolaz Marije Krucifikse Kozulić 3, 51000 Rijeka, Croatia,
info@intechopen.com or visit our website at intechopen.com.

# Meet the editor

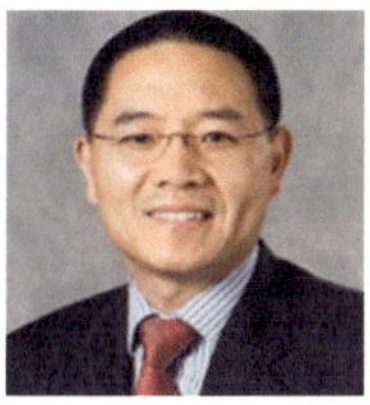

Dr. Feng received his MD from Chengde Medical College and Master Degree of Medical Science from FuWai Hospital in China. He spent six years at Beth Israel Deaconess Medical Center of Harvard Medical School investigating genetics, platelet function, and thrombosis. He finished his residency in the Boston Medical Center and cardiology fellowship at the Mayo Clinic. Dr. Feng was an assistant professor of medicine at the Mayo Clinic . Currently, Dr. Feng holds position of a cardiologist and the director of cardiac MRI, at the Metropolitan Heart and Vascular Institute in Minneapolis. His interests include cardiomyopathy, pericardial disease and cardiac imaging. Dr. Feng is an accomplished researcher with 46 original manuscripts including several seminal manuscripts published in the Circulation, ATVB, Stroke, and JACC imaging on genetic, thrombosis, cardiac amyloidosis, constrictive pericarditis and cardiac MRI. He authored or coauthored eight book chapters.

# Contents

# Preface

Amyloidosis is an uncommon disorder characterized by the deposition of extracellular fibril amyloid proteins in various organs and tissues. It is estimated that there are about 3,000 new cases annually in the United States. Amyloidosis is classified by the precursor plasma proteins that form the extracellular fibril deposits. The primary systemic type, or the AL type, is due to monoclonal immunoglobulin free light chains. The hereditary type, also known as familial type, is mostly secondary to mutant transthyretin deposition while the wild type transthyretin type or also called senile type is due to normal wild-type transthyretin deposition. The secondary type or the AA type is related to amyloid A protein, which is an acute reactive protein. Dialysis related amyloidosis is caused by the deposition of β2-microglobulin, which has been increasingly recognized. Significant advancement has been made recently, which not only provides insight into its pathophysiology but also helps to discover new therapies to fight the deadly disease.

Unfortunately, because of rarity of the disease and its protean clinical manifestations, many patients were misdiagnosed, especially at early stage of the disease. Consequently, many patients missed the opportunity window of effective therapy, in particularly the AL type. The aim of the book is to review the fascinating history and the mechanism of the disease; to help the readers become familiar with the clinical presentation; and to review the latest diagnostic and therapeutic development. Effective or even curative therapies are available, especially if accurate diagnosis and typing are made early.

I would like to thank all the authors who have contributed to the book and congratulate them on their excellent works. This volume provides a comprehensive update of our knowledge on amyloidosis of different types. It will be a useful daily reference for physician and other health care providers who take care of amyloid patients.

I would like to sincerely thank my parent and my family (Gloria, Amy, Emily and Eric) for their endless love and support. You spent more time waiting for me than being with me while I was studying, writing, and taking care of my patients. I would also like to thank my several mentors, including Drs. Liu Lisheng, Zhu Guoying, Geoffrey Toffler, James Muller, Joseph Loscalzo, Jae Oh, Rick Nishimura, Carole Warnes and Kyle Klarich. You continue to inspire me to become a better cardiologist and a better person. Finally, I greatly appreciate Dr. Cynthia Taub for her insightful suggestion, contribution and inspiration on the book.

**Dali Feng, MD, FACC.**
The Metropolitan Heart and Vascular Institute
Minneapolis, Minnesota , USA

Section 1

# History and Clinical Diagnosis and Typing

Chapter 1

# "Amyloid" — Historical Aspects

Maarit Tanskanen

Additional information is available at the end of the chapter

http://dx.doi.org/10.5772/53423

## 1. Introduction

General agreement prevails today on the contents of the term "amyloid". It refers to "a condition associated with a number of inherited and inflammatory disorders in which extracellular deposits of fibrillar proteins are responsible for tissue damage and functional compromise", as defined in the textbook of pathology [1]. One and half centuries ago, in contrast, the nature of amyloid was the very target of an academic dispute among the leading scientists, European at those days. Curiously, the term "amyloid" has prevailed although in the course of time the concept of amyloid has nearly turned upside down.

## 2. Origin of amyloid: Matthias Schleiden and botany

The term "amyloid" was brought in the scientific literature by the German botanist Matthias Schleiden (1804 - 1881). Schleiden was born in Hamburg as the son of a Hamburger physician. He first studied laws in Heidelberg and received his pHD in 1826. However, working as a lawyer felt unsatisfactory to him and he turned to study medicine in 1832, in Göttingen and Berlin. Schleiden oriented to botany, microscopy and anatomy, with a special interest in the chemical and anatomical composition of plant cell, and received his second PhD in 1839. One of Schleiden's major ideas was to apply the iodine-sulphuric acid test for starch in plants. This test was originally described in 1814 by Colin and Gaultier de Claubry to show the blue staining reaction of starch with iodine and sulphuric acid [2]. Schleiden presented his discoveries at the scientific meetings of the "Gesellschaft Naturforschender Freunde" and reported on the application of the iodine-sulphuric acid test on plants on the 20$^{th}$ February, 1838 (in: Ostwalds klassiker der exakten Wissenschaften, band 275 Verlag Harri Deutsch (Klassische Schriften zur zellenlehre. Matthias Jacob Scleiden, Theodor Schwann, Max Schulze, text in German), cited in [3]. Scleiden's original interpretation was that the reaction demonstrated the transformation of the plant material into starch [4]. Schleiden published his several botanical findings in the book form in 1842-43, with the title "Grundzige der wissenschaftlichen Botanik". It is remarkable that the 2nd and 3rd editions of the book, subtitled as "Die Botanik als inductive Wissenschaft behandelt" were also translated in English in 1849, with the name "Principles of Scientific Botany" and "Botany as an Inductive Science", reflecting the attraction that Schleiden's observations woke also outside Germany. In the above mentioned book Schleiden first time uses the term "*amyloid*" for starch, referring to"starch-like". The word itself stems from the latin word "*amylym*" for starch. Schleiden describes "amyloid" to represent "a normal amylaceous constituent in plants" [2], as shown in the straight citing from the English translation of the book [5] below.

---

"Amyloid is, when dry, a cartilaginous, but moist, gelatinous, clear, transparent body, soluble in boiling water, strong acids, and caustic alkalies, but not in ether and alcohol in a concentrated state. It is coloured blue by iodine, and the combination is soluble in water, giving it a golden-yellow colour. It is found only in the layers of the primary cell-membrane. There is no chemical analysis of this substance. It has been found at present only in the cotyledon-cells of Schotia latifolia,S. speciosa, Hymencea Courbaril, Mucuna urens, M. gigantea, and Tamarindusindica."

---

The application of the iodine-sulphuric acid test on plants was not the most remarkable among Schleiden's scientific discoveries. Based on his interest in microscopic studies he got the unique idea that plants are made of cells, and that the growth of plants depends on the production of new cells. To get to this idea Schleiden was also lucky. In Berlin he had met Theodor Schwann (1810 - 1882), another great scientist of those days who had made similar observations in animals [6]. The published observations of Schleiden (1838) and Schwann (1839) form the basis for the unified "cell theory", applicable to all living organisms. During the same time (1839) the French chemist Anselme Payen (1795 - 1878) described a substance in woods that resembled starch. This substance reacted with iodine-sulphuric acid test similarly to starch, and Payen named it "cellulose". The iodine-sulphuric acid reaction became later on a standard procedure used by botanists to demonstrate the presence of cellulose in woods [4].

It is well possible that amyloid deposits have been described even earlier, in the reports on human autopsy cases with homogenous material in liver or spleen tissue [2], probably representing amyloid. The first observation stems from the year 1639, described by Nicolaus Fontanus.

## 3. The term "amyloid" in the medical literature: Rudolf Virchow

Whereas Matthias Schleiden was the first to use the term "amyloid" in botanics, it was the German pathologist Rudolf Virchow (1804 - 1881) who applied it in the medical literature. Virchow studied medicine and anatomy in Berlin and Würzburg, and was graduated in 1843.

http://dx.doi.org/10.5772/53423

Virchow was interested in microscopic studies, similarly to Schleiden. Virchow used the word "amyloid" first time in 1854 in his publication "Über eine in Gehirn und Rückenmark des Menschen aufgefundene Substanz mit der chemischen Reaction der Cellulose", in Virchow's Archiv für Pathologische Anatomie and Physiologie und fur klinische Medicin. Berlin 6; 354-368; 1854 [7]. In this paper Virchow described the small round deposits in the nervous system (Figure 1) with the mention that those structures showed the same color reaction with iodine and sulfuric acid, i.e. a change from brown to blue, typical to starch. Therefore, Virchow was convinced that those structures were identical to starch [8]. Virchow named those structures "corpora amylacea", similarly to Schleiden (the name based on the Latin term "amylum" for starch, see previously). Later Virchow applied the iodine sulphuric acid test to other tissues infiltrated with amyloid. The representatives of the French and British Schools instead considered amyloid to be more closely related to cellulose [2]. They use the name "lardaceous" (based on the bacon-like appearance of the tissue, French School) and "waxy" (based on the homogeneity of the material, British School). They could also use the term "sago" (a sweet substance in certain palm species).

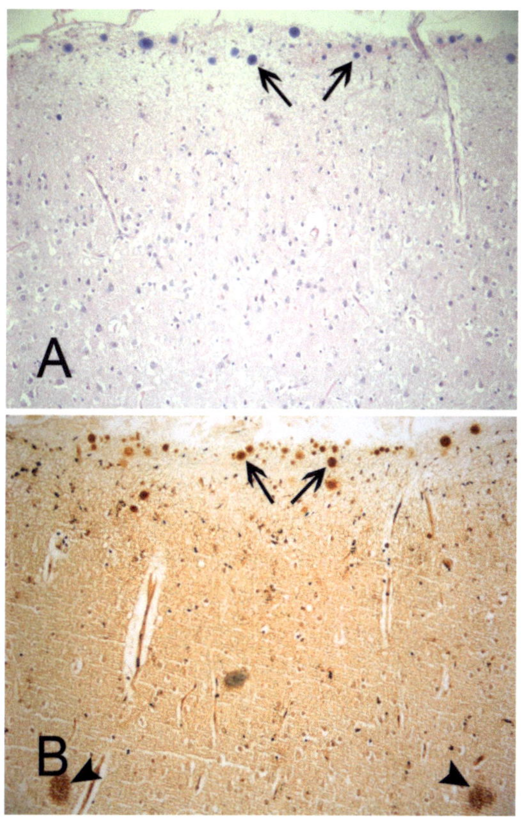


**Figure 1.** Corpora amylacea (arrows) stain blue in H&E (A) and brown in methenamine-silver (B) stain which also reveals a few senile plaques of diffuse type (B). Diffuse plaques do not contain amyloid. The patient was 104-year old female suffering from vascular dementia. Original magnification x 200.

Virchow developed an observational and experimental view on medical sciences. In this regard he resembled the French and British scientists at that time but contrasted to the more speculative German scientific tradition. As Virchow's writings received an unfavorable attention in German journals he decided to found in 1847 a journal of his own *"Archiv für pathologische Anatomie und Physiologie und für klinische Medizin"* with another German pathologist, Benno Reinhardt. The bearing idea of the new journal was not to publish papers containing "outdated, untested, dogmatic or speculative ideas". After Reinhardt's death in 1852 Virchow edited the paper alone, with the name "Virchow's Archives", a world-famous and respected journal still today.

Virchow's investigations in pathology extended to several other clinically significant issues. For instance, he discovered the mechanism of thromboembolism and developed the standard method of autopsy, as described in "The handbook on special pathology and therapeutics" in 1854. Further, in addition to Schleiden and Schwann, Virchow was the third scientist who has been nominated as an inventor of the "cell theory". He applied the concept in humans and published it in "Cellular pathology" in 1859. Yet, the probably most significant of Virchow's ideas was that he understood to combine the macroscopic and microscopic pathologies with clinical manifestations of disease [9].

Virchow was not only a pathologist. His interest and knowledge extended to anthropology, archeology, politics and social sciences [10]. For instance, Virchow established the first hospital trains bringing medicine in the battlefields, and he also was the first to understand the influence of poor hygiene on the spread of contagious illnesses. Political and social activities combined with huge scientific career brought to Virchow the status as the world-renowned physician and "Father of pathology".

## 4. The end of the 1800's: Progress in the staining methods to detect amyloid

A new insight into the biochemical character of amyloid was presented in 1859 when the prominent German chemist August Kekulé (1829 - 1896) reported on the high proportion of nitrogen in organs infiltrated with amyloid [2,11]. Kekulé assumpted that the material mainly represented "albumoid" compounds. In addition, he did not find material corresponding chemically to "amylon" or cellulose." Virchow never agreed with Kekulé, criticizing his method to analyze the whole tissue specimens (e.g. liver). After Virchow's opinion, convincing results necessitated a method to isolate the amyloid substance first [2]. Indeed, also in this he was ahead of his time. After more than one hundred years other constituents such as glycosaminoglycans and heparan sulphate [12,13] and chondroitin sulphate -containing proteoglycans [14,15] were identified as additional, albeit minor components of amyloid deposits [16].

In contrast to Virchow, Kekulé's observation on high nitrogen contents of amyloid were accepted by several scientists, including the British physician Samuel Wilks (1824 - 1919) who had collected more than 60 cases with the white, "stony", "gelatinous" or "lardaceous" visceral material, i.e. amyloid detected at the autopsy [2]. George Budd, another British internist (1808

- 1882) actually got the same result than Kekulé when analyzing the chemical composition of a pale autopsy liver [2].

There was another novel invention that Virchow did not accept: the metachromatic stains. In 1875 three scientists; the French pathologist and histologist Victor Cornil (1837 - 1908) in Paris, the Austrian anatomist Richard Heschl (1824 - 1881) in Vienna and Rudolf Jürgens in Berlin described independently the usefulness of methylviolet stain to detect amyloid. Already next year, in 1876, Soyka reported having found amyloid in the cardiac tissue with the use of this new method (Soyka J. Prag Med Wschr 1: 165, 1876; cited in Hodgkinson and Buerger [17,18]). William Ackroyd and Paul Ehrlich described methylviolet stain as "metachromatic" in 1878. Metachromatic stains challenged Virchow's iodine sulfuric acid test for decades [2] but were eventually replaced by Congo red.

## 5. Development of contemporary staining methods: Congo red dye and fluorescence microscopy

Reactivity with Congo red stain or "Congophilia with apple green birefringence" was the first criterion for amyloid [11], introduced by the Belgian Physician Paul Divry (Divry P. Etude histo-chimique des plaques seniles. J de Neurologie et de Psychiatrie 27:643-57, 1927, cited in Sipe [11]). Congo red dye itself was invented by the German chemist Paul Böttiger in 1884 (Böttiger P. Deutsches Reich's Patent 28753, August 20, 1884, cited in Frid [19]). Congo red is an aniline dye, originally created and used for staining textiles. Böttiger developed the first "direct" dye that did not require additional substances for fixation to the textile fibers. The owner of the patent, the AGFA Corporation developed the name "Congo" to the new dye after the diplomatic conference that was ongoing in Berlin just at that time (1884 - 1885). The goal of the "Congo conference" was to mediate a trade dispute between several European colonial powers in the Congo River Basin in Central Africa [2,20]. The name "Congo" referred to an exotic place that was on the tip of the lips, and proved to be effective for marketing purposes [2,20]. In addition to staining textiles Congo red was actually used to stain tissues already in 1886 [20]. However, it was not until in the year 1922 when the young German chemist Herman Bennhold discovered the capacity of Congo red to bind to amyloid (Bennhold H. Eine spezifische Amyloidfärbung mit Kongorot. Münchener Medizinische Wochenschrift (November):1537-1538, 1922; cited in Kyle [2]). In 1962 Puchtler described the renewed method for the use of Congo red in histological preparations [21].

The Puchtler modification [21] of Congo red staining is widely used in pathology as the first step in detecting amyloid in histological specimens. Of course, individual laboratories may apply their own variant of the method. Congo red staining is also applicable to frozen sections and for staining devices. In the diagnostic purposes the formalin-fixed histological samples are generally embedded in paraffin, sectioned 5-8 μm thick slices, stained with Congo red, and viewed in a light microscope under polarized light in which amyloid can be seen as red to green birefringent homogeneous material.

(Figure 2). Interestingly, the light microscope finding has been observed to vary in different types of transthyretin (TTR)-related amyloidosis and accordingly the distribution into two different histological patterns of amyloid deposition (designed as A and B) has been proposed [22]. In pattern A, seen in senile systemic amyloidosis (SSA) and in some cases with TTR-related familial amyloidosis, there is weakly congophilic, homogenous amyloid material that is patchy distributed. In pattern B, detected in a part of patients with TTR-related familial disease, strongly congophilic amyloid appears as thin streaks. Thus, the biochemical structure of amyloid fibrils can be transmitted to the microscopic finding.

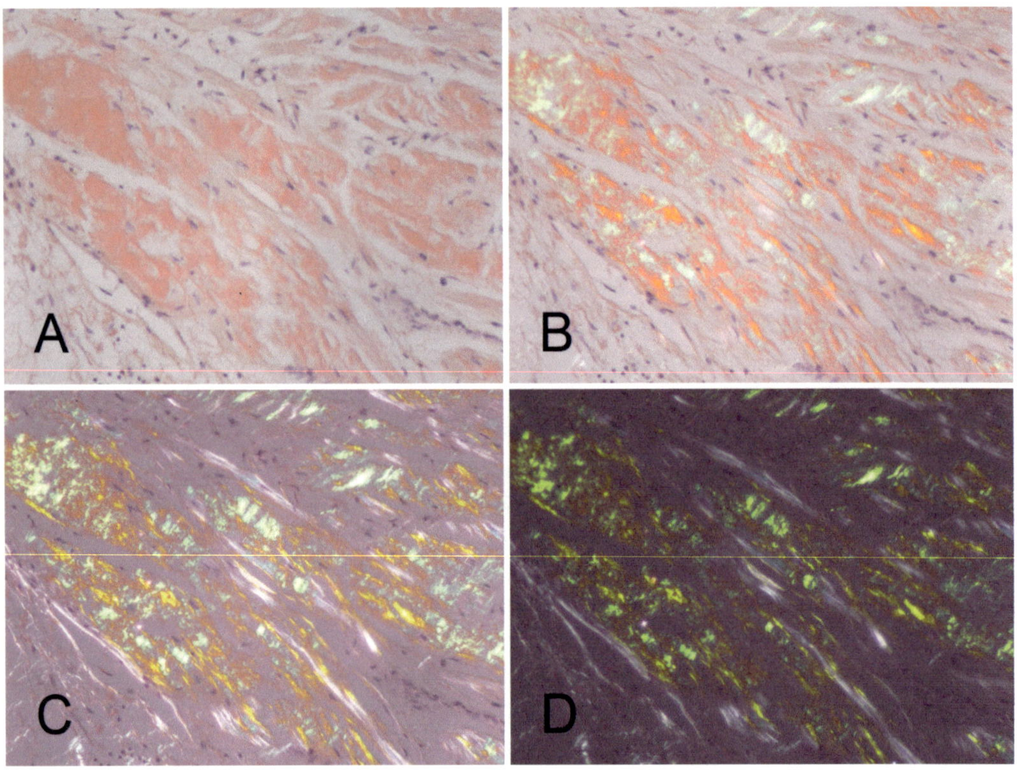


**Figure 2.** The red colour (A) of amyloid in the cardiac tissue of a patient with senile systemic amyloidosis (SSA) gradually (B,C) turns to green (D) in the polarized light. Original magnification x 400.

The chemical name of Congo red, also known as "direct red", "direct red 28", or "cotton red", is 3,3'-[(1,1′-biphenyl)-4,4′-diylbis(azo)] *bis*-(4-amino-1-naphtalene acid) disodium salt ($C_{32}H_{22}N_6O_6S_2$ 2Na). It is a symmetrical molecule with the molecular weight of 696.7 g/mol and the diameter approximately 21Å [23]. The molecule has a hydrophobic center composed of two phenyl rings that are linked via diazo bonds to two charged terminal naphtalene moieties. The terminal parts of Congo red contain sulphonic acid and amine groups. Congo red exists in chinone form in acidic solution, and in sulphonazo form in basic solution, changing the color from blue (below pH 3) to red (above pH 5). Thus, Congo red can be used as a pH indicator as well. The binding of Congo red to amyloid induces a characteristic shift in the maximal optical absorbance of the molecule from 490 nm to 540 nm. The mechanisms of interaction between Congo red and amyloid fibrils has been intensively studied [24,25] but the process is not completely understood [19]. Congo red binding has been assumed to depend on the secondary, β-pleated configuration of the fibril, possibly mediated by hydrophobic interactions of the benzidine centers as well as the electrostatically charged terminal groups [19].

Amyloid can also be visualized using the fluorescence microscope. Fluorescence microscope is a light microscope used to study the properties of organic and inorganic substances with the aid of the phenomena of fluorescence and phosphorescence. The component of interest in the specimen is labeled with a fluorescent molecule, the "fluorophore". Amyloid can be detected using thioflavin stains (Thioflavin-T or -S) which emit green fluorescence when they are bound to amyloid. Thioflavin-T (Basic Yellow 1 or CI 49005) is a benzothiazole salt, obtained by methylating dehydrothiotoluidine with methanol in the presence of hydrochloric acid. When the dye binds to β sheets it undergoes a 120 nm red shift of its excitation spectrum that may selectively be excitated at 450 nm, resulting in a fluorescence signal at 482 nm. Thioflavin-S is a mixture of compounds resulting from the methylation of dehydrothiotoluidine with sulphonic acid. The fluorescence method is specific for amyloid similarly to Congo red [26] and very sensitive. The disappearance of fluorescence during time can be regarded a disadvantage of the method, because the reaction cannot be re-examined later.

## 6. The beginning of the 1900's: Alzheimer's disease and associated pathologies

In 1907, Aloysius (Alois) Alzheimer described "senile" plaques and neurofibrillary tangles in a demented patient. Today we know that the plaques represent *extracellular* amyloid derived from amyloid beta (Aβ) protein whereas the neurofibrillary tangles represent *intracellular* amyloid formed on tau protein.

Alzheimer (1864 -1915) was German psychiatrist, born in Bavaria. He got his medical education at the universities of Tübingen and also in Berlin and Würzburg, similarly to Virchow, to receive his medical degree in 1887. Soon thereafter he began to work in a mental asylum "die Städtische Anstalt für Irre und Epileptische" in Frankfurt am Main. Alzheimer's scientific interest focused on pathology of the nervous system, especially anatomy of the cerebral cortex. He collaborated with the neuropathologist Franz Nissl (1860 - 1919) and learned Nissl's method of silver staining of the histological sections. In the year 1901 Alzheimer happened to get the 51 -year old Mrs. Auguste Deter to be his patient at the Frankfurt Asylum. Mrs. Deter had a very unusual clinical picture with loss of short-term memory and odd behavioral symptoms. In 1902 Alzheimer moved to work with his colleague, another German psychiatrist Emil Kraepelin (1856 - 1926) at the University of Heidelberg. Kraepelin had, similarly to Alzheimer, special interest in neuropathology. Both moved to Munich next year. Mrs Deter died in 1906 in Frankfurt, and Alzheimer decided to bring her brain and medical records to Munich for neuropathological study. He grasped to apply Nissl's method of silver staining on the histological sections of Mrs. Deter's brains, and thereby identified the neurofibrillary deposits in the atrophic brain. The first report of the extraordinary pathological findings was presented in the same year at the University of Tübingen, prior to the appearance of the publication in 1907 (Alzheimer A. Über eine eigenartige Erkrankung der Hirnrinde. Allgemeine Zeitschrift für Psychtiatrie und Psychisch-gerichtliche Medizin. 1907 Jan; 64:146-8).

The original histological sections on which Alzheimer based his description were rediscovered in the 1990$^{ies}$ in Munich. This gave the unique opportunity to re-evaluate his work [27]. Silver stains have been used to diagnose Alzheimer's disease (AD) during decades and the original observations made by Alzheimer's and Kraepelin are valid even today. Quite recently, techniques using the immunohistochemistry (IHC) -based techniques in the diagnosis of AD pathology have also been introduced [28]. Alzheimer's neuropathological discoveries were not restricted to AD pathology. For example, he also described the loss of nerve cells in the corpus striatum in Huntington's disease and brain changes in epilepsy [29].

Mrs. Deter suffered from a syndrome that is called today as *presenile* dementia. Presenile dementias form a group of hereditary dementia syndromes which are often autosomally dominantly inherited. It has turned out that presenile dementia syndrome is quite common in the population called Volga Germans (VG). VG stems from people who emigrated in the 1760 s from the German Hesse area around Frankfurt to the southern Volga region in Russia. During the late 19$^{th}$ and early 20$^{th}$ centuries many of the descendants of VG emigrated to US. Presenile dementia of the VG is due to the mutation N141I in the gene for presenilin (PSEN) 2 [30]. Interestingly, neuropathology of the brains of subjects with this mutation is similar to Mrs. Deter's case [27]. Therefore, especially as Mrs. Deter was living in the Hesse area in Germany, an idea was got that she would have belonged to the population of VG. Mrs. Deter's brain tissue was tested for the presence of the PSEN 2 mutation – but the result was negative [31]. Yet, this does not preclude that Mrs. Deter would have had a different mutation in PSEN 2 or a mutation in other genes such as PSEN 1 or APP.

Although the diagnosis of Mrs. Deter is still open, Alzheimer's paper was a starting point to enormous amounts of experimental and applied investigations of AD, an old age associated dementia syndrome. The disease belongs to the major causes of death in the western world, and it is estimated that about 24 million people suffer from it worldwide [32]. In spite of the huge work, the etiology of AD is still uncertain. Several hypotheses have been proposed [33], of which the "amyloid cascade hypothesis" by John Hardy and Gerald Higgins [34] has maybe got the greatest attention. The theory has recently also been criticized [35] as many therapeutic attempts based on it have failed [36].

The first descriptions of AD pathology were based on silver staining (Figure 3A) without no idea about the biochemical composition (Figure 3B) or relationship to amyloid of such structures (Figure 3C,D). Plaque amyloid however was discovered relatively soon (in 1927, see previously) by Divry after Bennhod had published his application of Congo red in tissue (in 1922, see previously). Cerebrovascular amyloid (cerebral amyloid angiopathy, CAA), detectable in 80-90% in the brains of patients with AD was first time reported by Greek Pantelakis in 1954 [37].

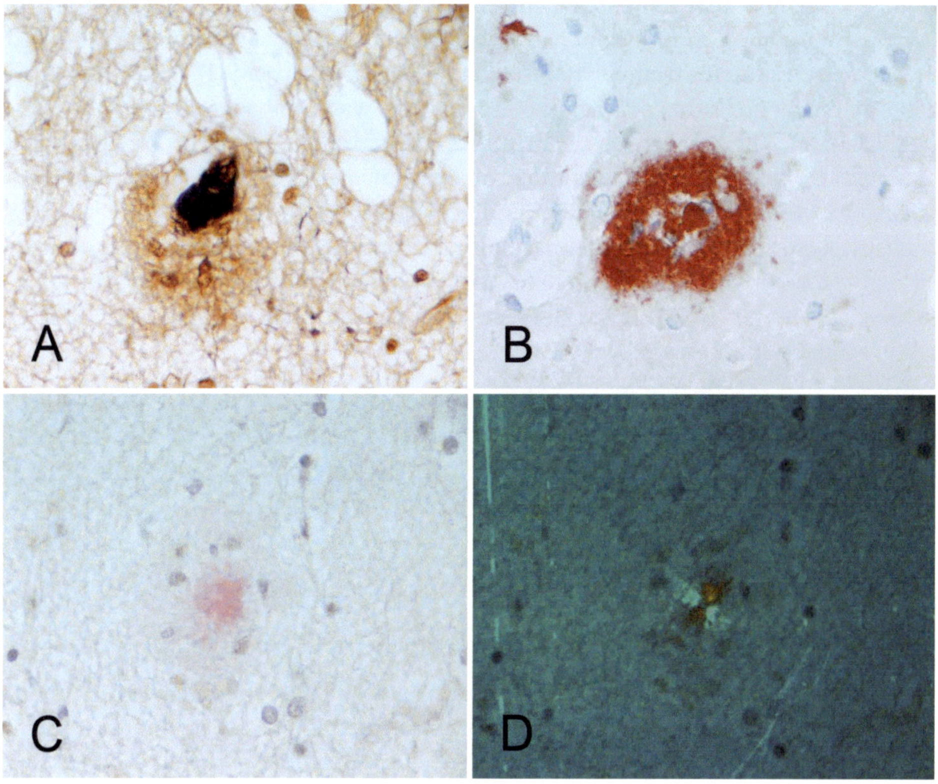


**Figure 3.** A senile plaque with amyloid core stained with methenamine-silver (A), immunohistochemistry against Aβ (B) and Congo red (C without and D with polarization) stains. Original magnification x 600.

## 7. Identification and extraction of the amyloid fibril

After the 2nd world war amyloid research stretched from Europe to include also Northern America and Japan. A substantial advance in the field took place in the late fifties. Two American researchers, Alan S Cohen from Harvard Medical School in Boston and Evan Calkins from Massachusetts General Hospital reported on the fibrillary structures in the samples of several types of amyloids in 1959 using electron microscopy (Cohen AS and Calcins E. Electron microscopic observations on a fibrous component in amyloid of diverse origins. Nature 183 1202-3, 1959; cited in Vinters [38]). Several attempts followed to isolate the fibrils from tissues and organs. Cohen and Calkins themselves described the first extraction method. It consisted of gentle physical separation and homogenization of the material in saline, followed by low-speed centrifugation. This yielded a layer of fibrils not present in the sedimentation pellets of normal tissues and demonstrated a green birefringence in polarized light after staining with Congo red [39]. The next method was published by George Glenner and Howard Bladen (NIA, Bethesda, Maryland). They had extracted amyloid fibrils using alkaline sodium glycinate in 1966 [40].

A significant step forward took place when M Pras (originally from the Tel Hashomer Hospital, Tel Aviv, Israel) and colleagues from New York University School of Medicine described the method to extract proteins from amyloid-laden tissues using water [41]. Spleen tissue from a deceased patient with "primary" (i.e. AA) amyloidosis was homogenized with physiological saline (NaCl), and the mixture was centrifuged. The sediment was next homogenized with NaCl several times to remove most of the soluble proteins and other soluble materials. Salt was then removed by homogenizing the residue in distilled water, followed by centrifugation of the suspension. Lastly, the residue was homogenized in distilled water and centrifuged four times to give a supernatant rich in protein. Adding Congo red dye and NaCl then resulted in a gelatinous precipitate with the typical green birefringence, demonstrating that the supernatant represented soluble amyloid.

The "water extraction method" of Pras has been widely used to extract almost all types of amyloid except for Aβ and prion protein amyloid [42,43]. The method was revolutionary in amyloid research as it enabled (1) identification of the β-pleated sheet configuration of amyloid proteins and (2) discovery of the biochemical structure of those proteins.

## 8. The β-pleated sheet configuration

In nature, most proteins have both α-helix and β-pleated sheet secondary structure. In the amyloid form, the proteins are mostly in the β-pleated sheet conformation though not exclusively. Factors that may influence changes in the spatial form of proteins include increased protein content, low pH, metal ions proteins that are associated with amyloid deposits but are not part of the insoluble fibrils themselves, also called " chaperones" [44]. The secondary structure of amyloid consists of the polypeptide backbone, mostly in the β-pleated sheet conformation, oriented perpendicular to the fibril axis. This β-pleated sheet structure was revealed by X-ray diffraction analysis of isolated amyloid protein fibrils by Eanes and Glenner in 1968 [45-47].

## 9. Identification of the different amyloid proteins

The major consequence of the invention of the water extraction method of Pras was the identification of the biochemical composition of several kinds of amyloids. Glenner and his colleagues soon applied the method to the "primary" (today: AL) amyloidosis [48] and found the relationship between this amyloidosis and immunoglobulin light chains. AL amyloidosis is a neoplastic disease and belongs to the clinically most significant amyloid -related conditions.

During the subsequent years, a long list of amyloid proteins was identified one after another. Inflammation-associated amyloidosis, previously called the "secondary" and today AA amyloidosis, was shown to be caused by amyloid protein A, an acute phase protein in 1972 [49]. Serum protein A was thereafter soon identified in blood [50,51]. In 1978, prealbumin (transthyretin, TTR) was found to be the protein constituent of amyloid deposits in Portuguese familial amyloid polyneuropathy (FAP) [52], the clinical condition having been described already in 1951 (Corino de Andrade, M. Preliminary note on an unusual form of peripheral neuropathy. Rev Neurol (Paris) 85: 302-6, 1951; cited in Kyle [2]). Similar diseases were found especially in Japan and Sweden in the subsequent decades. The Finnish type of familial amyloidosis, today known as AGel amyloidosis, was described in 1969 by the Finnish ophthalmologist Jouko Meretoja [53]. In 1980, TTR was characterized as the amyloid protein also in "senile cardiac amyloidosis" (SCA) [54], later renamed as senile systemic amyloidosis (SSA) [55,56]. In 1983, the Icelandic type of familial cerebral amyloid angiopathy (HCHWA-I) was found to be related to cystatin-C protein [57]. Next year, 1984, the first report on the AD-associated Aβ protein was published two Glenner and Wong who identified Aβ in the cerebrovascular tissue [58]. Colin Masters (Australian), Konrad Beyreuther (German) and colleagues described the same protein one year later, in 1985, in the plaques (Figure 3B). Japanese Fumitage Gejyo described beta 2 - microglobulin as the amyloid fibril protein in the dialysis-related amyloid arthropathy in the same year [60]. Tau protein of the neurofibrillary tangles was identified in 1986 in the laboratory of Henryk Wisniewsky in New York by Inge Grundke-Iqbal and colleagues [61].

The nature of islet amyloid polypeptide (IAPP) was discovered by Swedish pathologist Per Westermark from University of Uppsala and his colleagues in 1986 [62,63]. In 1988, apolipoprotein A1 (APOA1) was characterized as the amyloid protein in the hereditary amyloid disease in Iowa, USA [64]. In 1990, two groups discovered independently that amyloid fibril protein in the Finnish (AGel) amyloidosis was related to gelsolin [65,66] and identified the causative Asn-187 mutation in the gene for gelsolin [67,68]. The first description of a genetic cause for a hereditary amyloid disease was already published several years earlier, as the Japanese Satoru Tawara and colleagues identified the point mutation in the gene coding for TTR leading to the substitution of methionine instead of valine at position 30 in TTR-related FAP in 1983 [69]. Development of the polymerase chain reaction (PCR) –based techniques have accelerated the identification of mutations in the genes of the amyloidogenic proteins, and today more than one hundred different mutations have been described in the TTR gene. Most of the mutations lead to clinical disease with the deposition of amyloid in different organs.

In the past two decades three different proteins were characterized describing three novel different familial amyloid diseases with a preference for renal manifestation: fibrinogen A-α chain [70], lysozyme [71] and apolipoprotein AII [72]. The last identified amyloid fibril protein, also presenting with renal amyloidosis especially in Mexican Americans, was leucocyte chemotactic factor 2 [73].

## 10. Prion diseases

Characterization of the prion protein (PrP) in 1982 [74] opened up a new perspective in the amyloid reseach. Scrapie, a prion disease in sheeps and cows, was described in Spanish merino sheeps already in 1732 [75] but it took two and a half centuries to detect the causative agent. Scrapie belongs to prion diseases, also referred to "transmissible protein misfolding disorders" [76]. The highest degree in the conformational shift from α-helix to β-sheet structure occurs in the genetically determined form (Gerstmann-Straussler- Scheinken disease) and in PrP - associated CAA [77].

Prion diseases occur in several mammalian species and can be sporadic, hereditary, or acquired. The disease exists in nine different types in humans. The first known descriptions of human prion disease appeared independently in 1920 and 1921 by Creuzfeld and (Creutzfeldt HG: Über eine eigenartige herdformige erkrankung des Zentralnervensystems. Z gesamte Neurol Psychiatr 1920, 57: 1-19) and Jacob (Jacob A: Über eigenartige Erkrankungen des Zentralnervensystems mit bemerkenswertem anatomischen Befunde. (Spastische Pseudoskleros- Encephalomyelopathie mit disseminierten Degenerationsherden). Z Gesamte Neurol Psychiatr 1921, 64: 147-228.), cited in Imram [76]). This has formed the basis for the contemporary name of the disease: "sporadic Creutzfeldt –Jacob's disease".

Two Australian anthropologists, Ronald and Catherine Berndt, were the first to describe the peculiar disease occurring in the Fore linguistic group of people in the Australian Pretectorate of New Guinea, today Papua-New Guinea. Vincent Zigas, the district medical officer started to study the disease in 1957 with the young American virologist and pediatrician Carleton Gajdusek who was interested in infectious diseases. The clinical picture of the disease, as described in the article: "Degenerative Disease of the Central Nervous System in New Guinea — The Endemic Occurrence of Kuru in the Native Population" [78], cited in Libersky [79], consisted of headache and pain, cerebellar ataxia, tremors, shivering and choreiform or athetoid movements. The disease, named as "kuru", occurred exclusively in that Fore linguistic group people and was due to the ritualistic cannibalism ("transumption"). Kuru was neuropathologically characterized with neuronal degeneration, myelin degeneration, astroglial and microglial proliferation and plaque formations [80]. Interestingly, another human prion disease presenting with similar plaques occurred in Western Europe four decades later. The disease, first reported in UK in 1996 by British investigators and called as "variant CJD" [81] however manifested differently. The typical features of variant CJD include agitation, aggression, apathy and paranoid delusions [81]. BSE (Bovine spongiform encephalopathy) prions were soon shown to be causally linked with variant CJD [82].

The American scientist Stanley Prusiner purified the prion protein (PrP Scr) from sheep in 1982 [83]. The name "prion" was based on the letters of the word *Pro*te*in*aceus. Prusiner assumed that PrP would act solely in the protein level without influence of any genetic material, as it had been proposed several years previously [84]. This and several other several issues are still open, such as if there are factors rendering cells capable of replicating prions and propagating them to the nervous system, and if PrP is fully infective without any cofactors [85]. Gajdusek (in 1976) and Prusiner (in 1997) were honored with Nobel Prize in Medicine for their work in prion diseases.

## 11. Nomenclature

The modern nomenclature of different types of amyloids (Table 1) is based on the amyloid fibril protein. An originally informal amyloid nomenclature committee was established in 1974

| Amyloid protein | Precursor protein | Type | Syndrome (Involved tissue) |
| --- | --- | --- | --- |
| AA | (Apo)serum AA | S | Reactive, previously: "secondary" |
| AANF | Atrial natriuretic factor | L | (Cardiac atria) |
| AApoAI | Apolipoprotein AI | S, L | Familial (aorta, meniscus) |
| AApoAII | Apolipoprotein AII | S | Familial |
| AApoAIV | Apolipoprotein AIV | S | Sporadic, aging |
| ABri | ABriPP | S | Familial dementia, British |
| ACal | (Pro)calcitonin | L | C-cell thyroid tumors |
| ACys | Cystatin C | S | Familial |
| ADan | ADanPP | L | Familial dementia, Danish |
| AFib | Fibrinogen α-chain | S | Familial |
| AGel | Gelsolin | S | Familial, previously: "Finnish" |
| AH | Immunoglobulin heavy chain | S; L | Myeloma-associated, previously: "primary" |
| AIAPP | Islet amyloid polypeptide | L | Insulinomas, aging, previously: "amylin" (Islets of Langerhans) |
| AIns | Insulin | L | Iatrogenic |
| AKer | Kerato-epithelin | L | Familial (cornea) |
| AL | Immunoglobulin light chain | S; L | Myeloma-associated, previously: "primary" |
| ALac | Lactoferrin | L | (Cornea) |
| ALect2 | Leukocyte chemotactic factor 2 | S | Mainly kidney |
| ALys | Lyspzyme | S | Familial |
| AMed | Lactadherin | L | Aortic and arterial media, aging |
| AOAAP | Odontogenic ameloblast-associated protein | L | Odonogenic tumors |
| APro | Prolactin | L | Prolactinomas, aging (pituitary gland) |
| APrP | Prion protein | L | Spongiform encephalopathies (brain) |
| ASemI | Semenogelin I | L | (Vesicula seminalis) |
| ATTR | Transthyretin | S,L? | Familial, SSA (localized: tenosynovium) |
| Aβ | Aβ protein precursor (AβPP) | L | Aging, AD, CAA |
| Aβ2M | β2-microglobulin | S; L? | Hemodialysis-associated (localized: joints) |

S = systemic; L = localized; SSA = senile systemic amyloidosis; AD = Alzheimer's disease; CAA = cerebral amyloid angiopathy.

**Table 1.** Human amyloid fibril proteins and their precursors.

in Helsinki, Finland, in connection with the 1st International Symposium on Amyloidosis. The 1st official nomenclature committee was founded at the 3rd international symposium on amyloidosis in Povoa de Varzim, Portugal (1979). Thereafter the committee (the Nomenclature Committee of the International Society of Amyloidosis) has met several times to create the official nomenclature lists for each types of amyloid. The last meeting took place in 2010 in Rome, Italy (2010), in conjunction with the 12th International Symposium on Amyloidosis [86]. The reports of the meetings are published in "Amyloid", the official journal of amyloid diseases.

To be included in the official nomenclature list, the amyloid fibril protein fibril must have been unambiguosly characterized and described in a peer-reviewed journal. The present nomenclature list contains 27 fibril proteins capable to cause human disease. Nine of them have been tested in animals. There are also at least and six proteins appearing as *intracellular* inclusions, with all or some properties of amyloid [86].

## 12. The clinical diagnosis of amyloidosis

The diagnosis of the depositon of amyloid in diverse clinical conditions has traditionally needed a tissue sample stained with Congo red or thioflavin compounds, followed by the definition of the fibril protein using the IHC-based techniques. These techniques, using commercially available antibodies are quite well applicable in most of the clinically significant amyloid diseases.

The usage of radiological techniques to detect amyloid deposits started in 1988 when Philip Hawkins (London) reported on the usage of in vivo radiological techniques using the $^{123}I$ labeled serum amyloid P component (SAP) in mice [87]. Two years later the same technique was applied successfully in humans [88]. Recently, antibodies to human SAP molecule were even shown to have potential therapeutic properties in both mice and humans [89], based on the ability of the antibodies to trigger a giant-cell reaction to eliminate visceral amyloid deposits. Another milestone in the radiological diagnostics of amyloid diseases was the discovery by Klunk and colleagues (University of Pittsburgh, US) of the $^{11}C$-labeled PET tracer "Pittsburgh compound B" (PiB) to bind selectively to fibrillar Aβ [90]. This made it possible to reveal amyloid pathology *noninvasively* in subjects with AD pathology. Yet, the half-time ($T_{1/2}$) of $^{11}C$ is very short (about 20 min) and therefore not applicable in clinical use. The recent invention of a comparable $^{18}F$-labeled tracer with much longer $T_{1/2}$ (110 min) is expected to expand the applicability of PET in a larger number of patients. Of the potential $^{18}F$-labeled tracers tested, $^{18}F$-AV-45[91] seems to be the most promising [92].

## 13. Conclusion

The concept of amyloid has transformed several times during the nearly two century long research history of the issue. It is now clear that the cerebral corpora amylacea that inspired

Virchow so greatly are mostly composed of glycogen-like substances with sulfate and phosphate groups. In this regard, Virchow actually was right. On the other hand, it has also turned out that those structures do not represent amyloid. Therefore, it can be asked why the term "amyloid" still has prevailed. The most apparent explanation is Virchow's standing as one of the most valued scientists of his time and probably also the iodine staining that was used for a long time as the diagnostic test for amyloid [93].

Amyloid research has traditionally related to the diagnosis and clinical manifestations of the deposition of amyloid in the tissues and organs in diverse disease conditions. Applications in other branches of science such as biotechnology may outline the future prospects in the amyloid field [94].

## Author details

Maarit Tanskanen

Address all correspondence to: maarit.tanskanen@helsinki.fi

Department of Pathology, Haartman Institute, University of Helsinki and HUSLAB, Helsinki, Finland

## References

[1] Kumar V, Abbas AK, Fausto N, Mitchell RN. Robbins Basic Pathology, 8th edition. Philadelphia, USA: Saunders; 2007. p166.

[2] Kyle RA. Amyloidosis: a convoluted story. Br J Haematol 2001;114(3) 529-538. Doi:bjh2999 [pii].

[3] Matthias Jacob Scleiden, Theodor Schwann, Max Schulze. Klassische Schriften zur Zellenlehre. In: Ostwalds klassiker der exakten Wissenschaften, band 275: Verlag Harri Deutsch. Available from http//books.google/fi/books/about/Klassische_Schriften_zur_Zellenlehre.html?=h9_WFhLD8uYC&redir_esc=y.

[4] Aterman K. A historical note on the iodine-sulphuric acid reaction of amyloid. Histochemistry 1976;49(2) 131-143.

[5] Dr. J. M. Schleiden. Scientific botany. First book: chemistry of Plants, Chapter II of the organic elements, section I of the assimilated bodies, p9. Available from htpp:archive.org/details/priciplesofscie00schlrich.

[6] Vasil IK. A history of plant biotechnology: from the Cell Theory of Schleiden and Schwann to biotech crops. Plant Cell Rep 2008;27(9) 1423-1440. Doi:10.1007/s00299-008-0571-4.

[7] Virchow R. Über eine in Gehirn und Rückenmark des Menschen aufgefundene Substanz mit der chemischen Reaction der Cellulose. Virchow's Archiv fur pathologische Anatomie und für klinische Medicin, Berlin 1854;6:135-138.

[8] Virchow R. Über den Gang der amyloiden Degeneration. Virchow's Archiv für pathologische Anatomie und Physiologie und für klinische Medicin, Berlin 1854;8:364-368.

[9] Tan SY, Brown J. Rudolph Virchow (1821-1902): "pope of pathology". Singapore Med J 2006;47(7) 567-568.

[10] Brown TM, Fee E. Rudolf Carl Virchow: medical scientist, social reformer, role model. Am J Public Health 2006;96(12) 2104-2105. Doi:10.2105/AJPH.2005.078436.

[11] Sipe JD, Cohen AS. Review: history of the amyloid fibril. J Struct Biol 2000;130(2-3) 88-98. Doi:10.1006/jsbi.2000.4221.

[12] Snow AD, Willmer J, Kisilevsky R. Sulfated glycosaminoglycans: a common constituent of all amyloids? Lab Invest 1987;56(1) 120-123.

[13] Snow AD, Sekiguchi R, Nochlin D, Fraser P, Kimata K, Mizutani A et al. An important role of heparan sulfate proteoglycan (Perlecan) in a model system for the deposition and persistence of fibrillar A beta-amyloid in rat brain. Neuron 1994;12(1) 219-234.

[14] Niewold TA, Flores Landeira JM, van den Heuvel LP, Ultee A, Tooten PC, Veerkamp JH. Characterization of proteoglycans and glycosaminoglycans in bovine renal AA-type amyloidosis. Virchows Arch B Cell Pathol Incl Mol Pathol 1991;60(5) 321-328.

[15] Magnus JH, Stenstad T, Kolset SO, Husby G. Glycosaminoglycans in extracts of cardiac amyloid fibrils from familial amyloid cardiomyopathy of Danish origin related to variant transthyretin Met 111. Scand J Immunol 1991;34(1) 63-69.

[16] Gruys E. Protein folding pathology in domestic animals. J Zhejiang Univ Sci 2004;5(10) 1226-1238. Doi:10.1631/jzus.2004.1226.

[17] Hodkinson HM, Pomerance A. The clinical significance of senile cardiac amyloidosis: a prospective clinico-pathological study. Q J Med 1977;46(183) 381-387.

[18] L BUERGER, H BRAUNSTEIN. Senile cardiac amyloidosis. Am J Med 1960;28: 357-367.

[19] Frid P, Anisimov SV, Popovic N. Congo red and protein aggregation in neurodegenerative diseases. Brain Res Rev 2007;53(1) 135-160. Doi:10.1016/j.brainresrev. 2006.08.001.

[20] SteensmaDP. "Congo" red: out of Africa? Arch Pathol Lab Med 2001;125(2) 250-252.

[21] Puchtler H, Sweat F, Levine M. On the binding of Congo red by amyloid. J. Histochem. Cytochem 1962;10: 355-364.

[22] Bergstrom J, Gustavsson A, Hellman U, Sletten K, Murphy CL, Weiss DT et al. Amyloid deposits in transthyretin-derived amyloidosis: cleaved transthyretin is associated with distinct amyloid morphology. J Pathol 2005;206(2) 224-232. Doi:10.1002/path.1759.

[23] Romhanyi G. Selective differentiation between amyloid and connective tissue structures based on the collagen specific topo-optical staining reaction with Congo red. Virchows Arch A Pathol Pathol Anat 1971;354(3) 209-222.

[24] Klunk WE, Pettegrew JW, Abraham DJ. Quantitative evaluation of Congo red binding to amyloid-like proteins with a beta-pleated sheet conformation. J Histochem Cytochem 1989;37(8) 1273-1281.

[25] Turnell WG, Finch JT. Binding of the dye Congo red to the amyloid protein pig insulin reveals a novel homology amongst amyloid-forming peptide sequences. J Mol Biol 1992;227(4) 1205-1223.

[26] Revesz T, Ghiso J, Lashley T, Plant G, Rostagno A, Frangione B et al. Cerebral amyloid angiopathies: a pathologic, biochemical, and genetic view. J Neuropathol Exp Neurol 2003;62(9) 885-898.

[27] Graeber MB, Kosel S, Egensperger R, Banati RB, Muller U, Bise K et al. Rediscovery of the case described by Alois Alzheimer in 1911: historical, histological and molecular genetic analysis. Neurogenetics 1997;1(1) 73-80.

[28] Braak H, Alafuzoff I, Arzberger T, Kretzschmar H, Del Tredici K. Staging of Alzheimer disease-associated neurofibrillary pathology using paraffin sections and immunocytochemistry. Acta Neuropathol 2006;112(4) 389-404. Doi:10.1007/s00401-006-0127-z.

[29] Vishal S, Sourabh A, Harkirat S. Alois Alzheimer (1864-1915) and the Alzheimer syndrome. J Med Biogr 2011;19(1) 32-33. Doi:10.1258/jmb.2010.010037.

[30] Bird TD, Lampe TH, Nemens EJ, Miner GW, Sumi SM, Schellenberg GD. Familial Alzheimer's disease in American descendants of the Volga Germans: probable genetic founder effect. Ann Neurol 1988;23(1) 25-31. Doi:10.1002/ana.410230106.

[31] Muller U, Winter P, Graeber MB. Alois Alzheimer's case, Auguste D., did not carry the N141I mutation in PSEN2 characteristic of Alzheimer disease in Volga Germans. Arch Neurol 2011;68(9) 1-author reply 1211. Doi:10.1001/archneurol.2011.218.

[32] Ballard C, Gauthier S, Corbett A, Brayne C, Aarsland D, Jones E. Alzheimer's disease. Lancet 2011;377(9770) 1019-1031. Doi:10.1016/S0140-6736(10)61349-9.

[33] Querfurth HW, LaFerlaFM. Alzheimer's disease. N Engl J Med 2010;362: 329-344. Doi:10.1056/NEJMra0909142.

[34] Hardy JA, Higgins GA. Alzheimer's disease: the amyloid cascade hypothesis. Science 1992;256(5054) 184-185.

[35] Castellani RJ, Smith MA. Compounding artefacts with uncertainty, and an amyloid cascade hypothesis that is 'too big to fail'. J Pathol 2011;224(2) 147-152. Doi:10.1002/path.2885; 10.1002/path.2885.

[36] The amyloid cascade hypothesis has misled the pharmaceutical industry. Biochem Soc Trans 2011;39(4) 920-923. Doi:10.1042/BST0390920.

[37] PANTELAKIS S. A particular type of senile angiopathy of the central nervous system: congophilic angiopathy, topography and frequency. Monatsschr Psychiatr Neurol 1954;128(4) 219-256.

[38] Vinters HW, Wang ZZ, Secor DL. Brain parenchymal and microvascular amyloid in Alzheimer's disease. Brain Pathol 1996;6(2) 179-195.

[39] COHEN AS, CALKINS E. The Isolation of Amyloid Fibrils and a Study of the Effect of Collagenase and Hyaluronidase. J Cell Biol 1964;21: 481-486.

[40] Glenner GG, Bladen HA. Purification and reconstitution of the periodic fibril and unit structure of human amyloid. Science 1966;154(3746) 271-272.

[41] Pras M, Schubert M, Zucker-Franklin D, Rimon A, Franklin EC. The characterization of soluble amyloid prepared in water. J Clin Invest 1968;47(4) 924-933.

[42] Selkoe DJ, Abraham CR. Isolation of paired helical filaments and amyloid fibers from human brain. Methods Enzymol 1986;134: 388-404.

[43] Prusiner SB, DeArmond SJ. Prion diseases of the central nervous system. Monogr Pathol 1990; 32: 86-122.

[44] Ghiso J, Frangione B. Amyloidosis and Alzheimer's disease. Adv Drug Deliv Rev 2002;54(12) 1539-1551.

[45] Eanes ED, Glenner GG. X-ray diffraction studies on amyloid filaments. J Histochem Cytochem 1968;16(11) 673-677.

[46] Bonar L, Cohen AS, Skinner MM. Characterization of the amyloid fibril as a cross-beta protein. Proc Soc Exp Biol Med 1969;131(4) 1373-1375.

[47] Sunde M, Blake C. The structure of amyloid fibrils by electron microscopy and X-ray diffraction. Adv Protein Chem 1997;50: 123-159.

[48] Glenner GG, Terry W, Harada M, Isersky C, Page D. Amyloid fibril proteins: proof of homology with immunoglobulin light chains by sequence analyses. Science 1971;172(988) 1150-1151.

[49] Bendit EPt, Eriksen N. Chemical similarity among amyloid substances associated with long standing inflammation. Lab Invest 1971;26(6) 615-625.

[50] Levin M, Pras M, EC Franklin EC. Immunologic studies of the major nonimmunoglobulin protein of amyloid. I. Identification and partial characterization of a related serum component. J Exp Med 1973;138(2) 373-380.

[51] Husby G, Natvig JB. A serum component related to nonimmunoglobulin amyloid protein AS, a possible precursor of the fibrils. J Clin Invest 1974;53(4) 1054-1061. Doi: 10.1172/JCI107642.

[52] Costa PP, Figueira AS, Bravo FR. Amyloid fibril protein related to prealbumin in familial amyloidotic polyneuropathy. Proc Natl Acad Sci U S A 1978;75(9) 4499-4503.

[53] Meretoja J. Familial systemic paramyloidosis with lattice dystrophy of the cornea, progressive cranial neuropathy, skin changes and various internal symptoms. A previously unrecognized heritable syndrome. Ann Clin Res 1969;1(4) 314-324.

[54] Sletten K, Westermark P, Natvig JB. Senile cardiac amyloid is related to prealbumin. Scand J Immunol 1980;12(6) 503-506.

[55] Cornwell GG 3rd, Murdoch WL, Kyle RA, Westermark P, Pitkanen P. Frequency and distribution of senile cardiovascular amyloid. A clinicopathologic correlation. Am J Med 1983;75(4) 618-623.

[56] Gustavsson A, Jahr H, Tobiassen R, Jacobson DR, Sletten K, Westermark P. Amyloid fibril composition and transthyretin gene structure in senile systemic amyloidosis. Lab Invest 1995;73(5) 703-708.

[57] Cohen DH, Feiner H, Jensson O, Frangione B. Amyloid fibril in hereditary cerebral hemorrhage with amyloidosis (HCHWA) is related to the gastroentero-pancreatic neuroendocrine protein, gamma trace. J Exp Med 1983;158(2) 623-628.

[58] Glenner GG, Wong CW. Alzheimer's disease: initial report of the purification and characterization of a novel cerebrovascular amyloid protein. Biochem Biophys Res Commun 1984;120(3) 885-890.

[59] Masters CL, Simms G, Weinman NA, Multhaup G, McDonald BL, Beyreuther K. Amyloid plaque core protein in Alzheimer disease and Down syndrome. Proc Natl Acad Sci U S A 1985;82(12) 4245-4249.

[60] Gejyo F, Yamada T, Odani S, Nakagawa Y, Arakawa M, Kunitomo T et al. A new form of amyloid protein associated with chronic hemodialysis was identified as beta 2-microglobulin. Biochem Biophys Res Commun 1985;129(3) 701-706.

[61] Grundke-Iqbal I, Iqbal K, Quinlan M, Tung YC, Zaidi MS, Wisniewski HM. Microtubule-associated protein tau. A component of Alzheimer paired helical filaments. J Biol Chem 1986;261(13) 6084-6089.

[62] Westermark P, Wernstedt C, Wilander E, Sletten K. A novel peptide in the calcitonin gene related peptide family as an amyloid fibril protein in the endocrine pancreas. Biochem Biophys Res Commun 1986;140(3) 827-831.

[63] Westermark P. Amyloid in the islets of Langerhans: thoughts and some historical aspects. Ups J Med Sci 2011;116(2) 81-89. Doi:10.3109/03009734.2011.573884.

[64] Nichols WC, Dwulet FE, Liepnieks J, Benson MD. Variant apolipoprotein AI as a major constituent of a human hereditary amyloid. Biochem Biophys Res Commun 1988;156(2) 762-768. Doi:S0006-291X(88)80909-4 [pii].

[65] Haltia M, Prelli F, Ghiso J, Kiuru S, Somer H, Palo J et al. Amyloid protein in familial amyloidosis (Finnish type) is homologous to gelsolin, an actin-binding protein. Biochem Biophys Res Commun 1990;167(3) 927-932.

[66] Maury CP, Alli K, Baumann M. Finnish hereditary amyloidosis. Amino acid sequence homology between the amyloid fibril protein and human plasma gelsoline. FEBS Lett 1990;260(1) 85-87.

[67] Ghiso J, Haltia M, Prelli F, Novello J, Frangione B. Gelsolin variant (Asn-187) in familial amyloidosis, Finnish type. Biochem J 1990;272(3) 827-830.

[68] Maury CP, Kere J, Tolvanen R, de la Chapelle A. Finnish hereditary amyloidosis is caused by a single nucleotide substitution in the gelsolin gene. FEBS Lett 1990;276(1-2) 75-77.

[69] Tawara S, Nakazato M, Kangawa K, Matsuo H, Araki S. Identification of amyloid prealbumin variant in familial amyloidotic polyneuropathy (Japanese type). Biochem Biophys Res Commun 1990;116(3) 880-888. Doi:S0006-291X(83)80224-1 [pii].

[70] Benson MD, Liepnieks J, Uemichi T, Wheeler G, Correa R. Hereditary renal amyloidosis associated with a mutant fibrinogen alpha-chain. Nat Genet 1993;3(3) 252-255. Doi:10.1038/ng0393-252 [doi].

[71] Pepys MB, Hawkins PN, Booth DR, Vigushin DM, Tennent GA, Soutar AK et al. Human lysozyme gene mutations cause hereditary systemic amyloidosis. Nature 1993;362(6420) 553-557. Doi:10.1038/362553a0 [doi].

[72] Benson MD, Liepnieks JJ, Yazaki M, Yamashita T, Hamidi Asl K, Guenther Bet al. A new human hereditary amyloidosis: the result of a stop-codon mutation in the apolipoprotein AII gene. Genomics (2001;72(3) 272-277. Doi:10.1006/geno.2000.6499 [doi]; S0888-7543(00)96499-1 [pii].

[73] Benson MD, James S, Scott K, Liepnieks JJ, Kluve-Beckerman B. Leukocyte chemotactic factor 2: A novel renal amyloid protein. Kidney Int 2008;74(2) 218-222. Doi: 10.1038/ki.2008.152.

[74] Prusiner SB. Novel proteinaceous infectious particles cause scrapie. Science 1982;216(4542) 136-144.

[75] Poser CM. Notes on the history of the prion diseases. Part I. Clin Neurol Neurosurg 2002;104(1) 1-9.

[76] Imran M, Mahmood S. An overview of human prion diseases. Virol J 2011;8: 559. Doi:10.1186/1743-422X-8-559.

[77] Ghetti B, Piccardo P, Frangione B, Bugiani O, Giaccone G, Young K et al. Prion protein amyloidosis. Brain Pathol 1996;6(2) 127-145.

[78] GAJDUSEK DC, ZIGAS V. Degenerative disease of the central nervous system in New Guinea; the endemic occurrence of kuru in the native population. N Engl J Med 1957;257(20) 974-978. Doi:10.1056/NEJM195711142572005.

[79] Liberski PP. Historical overview of prion diseases: a view from afar. Folia Neuropathol 2012;50(1) 1-12.

[80] GAJDUSEK DC, ZIGAS V. Kuru; clinical, pathological and epidemiological study of an acute progressive degenerative disease of the central nervous system among natives of the Eastern Highlands of New Guinea. Am J Med 1959;26(3) 442-469.

[81] Will RG, Ironside JW, Zeidler M, Cousens SN, Estibeiro K, Alperovitch A et al. A new variant of Creutzfeldt-Jakob disease in the UK. Lancet 1996;347(9006) 921-925.

[82] Bruce ME, Will GR, Ironside JW, McConnell I, Drummond D, Suttie A et al. Transmissions to mice indicate that 'new variant' CJD is caused by the BSE agent. Nature 1997;389(6650) 498-501. Doi:10.1038/39057.

[83] Bolton DC, McKinley MP, Prusiner SB. Identification of a protein that purifies with the scrapie prion. Science 1982;218(4579) 1309-1311.

[84] Griffith JS. Self-replication and scrapie. Nature 1967;215(5105) 1043-1044.

[85] Aguzzi A, Falsig J. Prion propagation, toxicity and degradation. Nat Neurosci 2012;15(7) 936-939. Doi:10.1038/nn.3120; 10.1038/nn.3120.

[86] Sipe JD, Benson MD, Buxbaum JN, Ikeda S, Merlini G, Saraiva MJ et al. Amyloid fibril protein nomenclature: 2010 recommendations from the nomenclature committee of the International Society of Amyloidosis. Amyloid 2010;17(3-4) 101-104. Doi: 10.3109/13506129.2010.526812.

[87] Hawkins PN, Myers MJ, Lavender JP, Pepys MB. Diagnostic radionuclide imaging of amyloid: biological targeting by circulating human serum amyloid P component. Lancet 1988;1(8600) 1413-1418.

[88] Hawkins PN, Lavender JP, Pepys MB. Evaluation of systemic amyloidosis by scintigraphy with 123I-labeled serum amyloid P component. N Engl J Med 1990;323(8) 508-513. Doi:10.1056/NEJM199008233230803.

[89] Bodin K, Ellmerich S, Kahan MC, Tennent GA, Loesch A, Gilbertson JA et al. Antibodies to human serum amyloid P component eliminate visceral amyloid deposits. Nature 2010;468(7320) 93-97. Doi:10.1038/nature09494.

[90] Klunk WE, Wang Y, Huang GF, Debnath ML, Holt DP, Mathis CA. Uncharged thioflavin-T derivatives bind to amyloid-beta protein with high affinity and readily enter the brain. Life Sci 2001;69(13) 1471-1484.

[91] Choi SR, Golding G, Zhuang Z, Zhang W, Lim N, Hefti F et al. Preclinical properties of 18F-AV-45: a PET agent for Abeta plaques in the brain. J Nucl Med 2009;50(11) 1887-1894. Doi:10.2967/jnumed.109.065284.

[92] Furst AJ, Kerchner GA. From Alois to Amyvid: Seeing Alzheimer disease. Neurology 2012. Doi:10.1212/WNL.0b013e3182662084.

[93] Doyle L. Lardaceous disease: some early reports by British authors (1722-1879). J R Soc Med 1988;81(12) 729-731.

[94] Sweers KK, Bennink ML, Subramaniam V. Nanomechanical properties of single amyloid fibrils. J Phys Condens Matter 2012;24(24) 243101. Doi: 10.1088/0953-8984/24/24/243101.

Chapter 2

# Diagnosis of Amyloidosis

Cezar Augusto Muniz Caldas and
Jozélio Freire de Carvalho

Additional information is available at the end of the chapter

http://dx.doi.org/10.5772/52901

## 1. Introduction

Despite a strong clinical suspicion of amyloidosis, the diagnosis must be confirmed by tissue biopsy. Histological examination of biopsy specimens demonstrates an amorphous, eosinophilic substance that stains pink with the Congo red, and displays characteristic apple-green birefringence by polarized microscopy [1]. The histological analysis is the only method for establishing the diagnosis of amyloidosis [2,3]. The deposition of amyloid occurs in extracellular matrix, and often in a perivascular distribution with some degree of heterogeneity [1-3].

Although in the systemic amyloidosis the biopsies can be obtained from any organ affected, the blood vessel fragility associated with amyloid deposition carries a risk of bleeding [2,3]. Thus, in the clinical routine, biopsies from non-symptomatic sites are more commonly used [2,3]. In the past, rectal and gingival biopsies were considered the gold standard for the diagnosis of amyloidosis, but actually, abdominal fat pad aspiration has been the preferred due its simplicity, low cost, minimal complications, and good accuracy [1,4].

## 2. Abdominal fat pad aspiration or biopsy

Westermark and Stenkvist in 1973 described a method to remove pieces of subcutaneous abdominal fat for diagnosis of amyloidosis[3].Although some variants has been described, normally the aspiration is done using an 18-23 gauge needle, with 2-5 aspirations [3,5]. The sensitivity reported range from 55-75% and specificity is over than 90% [2,6]. Guy and Jones, analyzing the performance of the abdominal fat pad aspiration in 45 patients with systemic amyloidosis found sensitivity of 58%, specificity of 100%, positive predictive value of 100% and negative predictive value of 85%, confirming the accuracy of the methodology [7].

The clinician and pathologist must be familiarized with the methodology, histological pitfalls and the possibility of false negative, as possible in preferential deposition in terms of organ involvement of amyloid depending of its subtype, as the transthyretin type, with its predilection to deposit in the heart [1,3]. Another situation that can result in false negative, for example, is when the disease is an early stage with amyloid deposits in plaques [8].

## 3. Rectal biopsy and others gastrointestinal tract sites

The rectal biopsy was the most used diagnostic method in the past. Actually it has been replaced by abdominal fat pad aspiration, because this is more feasible in the clinical practice with low cost and lack of complications. Analysis of deep fragments including the submucosa, obtained during a rectoscopic examination, the sensitivity ranges from 75-85% [3,9].

Other sites of gastrointestinal tract can be biopsied. Tada studied 42 patients with gastrointestinal amyloidosis and found amyloid deposition especially in the duodenum and jejunum [10]. Okuda Y et al had similar results assessing rheumatoid arthritis patients, where the proportion of amyloid deposition was 76.5% for duodenal cap and 88.6% for second portion of the duodenum, suggesting a good efficacy of duodenal biopsy in this population [11].

Labial and gingival biopsy has been shownuseful in the amyloidosis diagnosis, but the lateris less sensitivity [3]. Several studies have confirmed the usefulness of labial biopsy, such as Fatihi et al that evaluated labial biopsy in patients with renal amyloidosis and found amyloid deposits in 80% of accessory gland biopsy and 75% of rectal biopsy [12]. Lechapt-Zalcmanet al performed labial salivary biopsy in 32 patients with polyneuropathy of unknown origin and detected amyloid deposits in 7 (transthyretin in five and AL in two), proposing this technique as routine in investigation of axonal polyneuropathies [13]. Hachula et al detected amyloid deposits in 26 of the 30 patients with systemic amyloidosis using labial salivary gland biopsy, emphasizing the importance of this procedure, even in the absence of oral symptoms [14].

## 4. Others biopsy sites

Because there is risk of life-threatening bleeding, biopsy from others sites is used only whether abdominal fat pad aspiration, rectal or labial salivary gland biopsy fail to establish the diagnosis [3].

The kidney is the most frequently involved organ in systemic amyloidosis and although kidney biopsy is fundamental for diagnosis, this procedure has been contraindicated in some situations, for example, bleeding diathesis, and can be complicated by perirenal hematoma or arteriovenous fistula [15]. Before performing a kidney biopsy, less invasive biopsy procedures from easily accessible tissues should be considered. Yilmaz M et al studying 78 patients with chronic kidney disease found the frequency of amyloid deposition was 100% in the duodenum, 83% in the rectum, and 29% in the gingiva, without complications related to endoscopy or biopsies [15].

Since the cardiac involvement is the major prognostic determinant in systemic amyloidosis [16], the evidence of cardiac lesion is crucial to therapeutic decisions. The gold standard test for diagnosing cardiac amyloidosis is the endomyocardial biopsy, however, it is not performed routinely due risk of complications, although infrequent, such as ventricular wall perforation, cardiac tamponade, pneumothorax, and arrhythmias [17]. Therefore, the cardiac amyloidosis is normally established by echocardiographic evidence of amyloidosis and histologic confirmation of amyloid on noncardiac tissue [17]. The changes observed in the echocardiography are those of restrictive cardiomyopathy with concentric ventricular hypertrophy, especially in the interventricular septum and posterior wall of the left ventricle [3]. Low voltage on electrocardiography and interventricularseptal thickness of > 19.8mm on echocardiography together have a sensitivity of 72% and specificity of 91% for cardiac amyloidosis [18].

## 5. Determining the type of amyloid protein

Effective medical treatment needs an accurate diagnosis with demonstration of amyloid deposition in the tissues and accurate molecular classification of amyloidosis [1,19,20]. For example, in AL amyloidosis, derived from immunoglobulin light chain, the cornerstone of treatment is the aggressive treatment of the underlying neoplastic process, and in AA amyloidosis, the target of treatment is the underlying inflammatory disease [20-23].

Immunohistochemistry is currently the standard methodology for amyloid typing in routine clinical practice; it has been able to identify amyloid deposits through binding antibodies directed against most of the amyloid molecules identified to date. In patients with systemic amyloidosis, studies with antibodies to AA and to the immunoglobulin light chains are usually sufficient [2,20]. Some pitfalls are present in the clinical practice, and in some cases, misdiagnoses may occur, especially when immunohistochemical staining is performed in the absence of standardized antibodies and appropriate positive controls [24].

The majority of cases of AA can be reliably typed in frozen and/or paraffin sections, but immunohistochemical typing of AL is still challenging, due commercial antibodies are raised against the constant regions of the respective immunoglobulin light chains, and whether a subset of AL, in which amyloid fibrils are derived from a truncated light chain (ie, containing only variable regions), will be expected to be nonreactive with commercial antibodies [25-27].

Another important pitfall is the presence of background stainin the tissue, which in paraffin sections in particular can be significant due the "locking-in" of serum proteins during fixation [20]. The use of frozen specimens and immunofluorescence stains considerably increases the reliability and reproducibility of labeling with antibodies to immunoglobulin light chain, due provide a cleaner background [20,28]. Picken emphasizes that the interpretation of immunohistochemistry performed in paraffin sections and immunofluorescence in frozen sections is not a simple matter and also depends on the experience and expertise of the operator [20].

Since early diagnosis is a very important step to appropriate treatment of transthyretin (TTR) amyloidosis, and this amyloidogenic protein causes two different forms of the disease (hereditary amyloidogenic TTR [ATTR] amyloidosis and senile systemic amyloidosis [SSA]), we should accurately distinguish them. For instance, to detect Val30Met mutation in TTR gene, which is the most frequent pathogenic mutation in hereditary ATTR amyloidosis, some researchers use real-time PCR genotyping assay, considering reliable, rapid, cost-effective, and suitable analysis, however, to achieve accurate results the application of both genetic and proteomic methods is preferable to compensate the disadvantages and possible pitfalls in each of the techniques used [19]. Using proteomics techniques, amyloid typing can be successful in small samples, including biopsies [29,30]. Several TTR variants can be detected in serum specimens using mass spectrometry or sophisticated electrophoresis techniques [31,32], however, this methodologies, and others new technologies, such as laser microdissection, are frequently available only at specialized centers.

## 6. Assessing the extension of involvement in systemic amyloidosis

The amyloid typing must be followed by distinction between localized and systemic amyloidosis [20]. While the treatment of localized forms is mainly conservative, the treatment of systemic forms has been more aggressive, and the prognosis is directly related with the disease extension, and the organs affected [2,20]. To determine the extension of the disease, some investigations are necessary, and it is presented in Table 1.

| Organ | Performed routinely | Performed as clinically indicated |
|---|---|---|
| Kidneys | Proteinuria, serum creatinine, ultrasonography | Renal vein Doppler ultrasound |
| Heart | Chest radiography, ECG, echocardiography, MRI, NT-proBNP/troponin | $^{99m}$Tc-pyrophosphate scan, 24-h Holter |
| Gastrointestinal tract | Serum protein electrophoresis | Gastrointestinal endoscopy, oesophagealmanometry |
| Liver | Liver enzymes | Ultrasonography |
| Spleen | Ultrasonography, blood cell counts | Howell-Jolly bodies in blood smears |
| Nerves | - | EMG |
| Respiratory system | Chest radiography | Blood gas analysis, bronchoscopy, CT scan of the chest |
| Endocrine glands | ACTH test, TSH | - |
| Eyes | Fundoscopy | Slit-lamp examination |
| Haemostasis | PT, X factor | - |

ECG – electrocardiography; MRI – magnetic resonance imaging; NT-proBNP – N-terminal pro-brain natriuretic peptide; EMG – electromyography; ACTH – adrenocorticotropic hormone; TSH – thyroid stimulating hormone; PT – prothrombin.

**Table 1.** Determining site and extent of amyloidosis [3,17]

http://dx.doi.org/10.5772/52901

# 7. Conclusion

The clinical suspicion must be confirmed with histological examination, and the amyloid typing is crucial to determine the correct treatment. Although the apparently simplicity of the abdominal fat pad aspiration has facilitated the diagnosis of amyloidosis, the physicians should be aware to pitfalls, especially in the amyloid typing, requiring an expert pathologist to correct analysis.

# Author details

Cezar Augusto Muniz Caldas[1] and Jozélio Freire de Carvalho[2]

*Address all correspondence to: jotafc@gmail.com

1 Internal Medicine Department, Universidade Federal do Pará - UFPA, and Curso de Medicina do Centro Universitário do Estado do Pará - CESUPA, Belém-PA, Brazil

2 Rheumatology Division, Hospital Universitário Prof. Edgard Santos, Federal University of Bahia, School of Medicine, Salvador-BA, Brazil

# References

[1] Halloush RA, Lavrovskaya E, Mody DR et al. Diagnosis and typing of systemic amyloidosis: The role of abdominal fat pad fine needle aspiration biopsy. Cytojournal 2010;15(6):24.

[2] Hachulla E, Grateau G. Diagnostic tools for amyloidosis. Joint Bone Spine2002;69(6): 538-45.

[3] Hachulla E, Beyne-Rauzy O, Soubrier M et al. Systemic consequences of the inflammatory process. In: Bijlsma JWJ. (ed.) Eular Compendium on Rheumatic Diseases. Affinity: 2009. p388-407.

[4] Westermark P, Benson L, Juul J, Sletten K. Use of subcutaneous abdominal fat biopsy specimen for detailed typing of amyloid fibril protein-AL by amino acid sequence analysis.J ClinPathol1989;42(8):817-9.

[5] Westermark P, Stenkvist B.A new method for the diagnosis of systemic amyloidosis.Arch Intern Med1973;132(4):522-3.

[6] Ansari-Lari MA, Ali SZ. Fine-needle aspiration of abdominal fat pad for amyloid detection: a clinically useful test? DiagnCytopathol2004;30(3): 178-81.

[7] Guy CD, Jones CK.Abdominal fat pad aspiration biopsy for tissue confirmation of systemic amyloidosis: specificity, positive predictive value, and diagnostic pitfalls.DiagnCytopathol2001;24(3): 181-5.

[8] Buxbaum JN. Amiloidoses. In: Goldman L, Ausiello D. (ed.) Cecil Medicina. Elsevier: 2009. p2397-401.

[9] Kyle RA, Spencer RJ, Dahlin DC.Value of rectal biopsy in the diagnosis of primary systemic amyloidosis.Am J Med Sci1966;251(5):501-6.

[10] Tada S. Diagnosis of gastrointestinal amyloidosis with special reference to the relationship with amyloid fibril protein.Fukuoka IgakuZasshi1991;82(12):624-47.

[11] Okuda Y, Takasugi K, Oyama T et al. Amyloidosis in rheumatoid arthritis--clinical study of 124 histologically proven cases. Ryumachi 1994;34(6): 939-46.

[12] Fatihi E, Ramdani B, Fadel H et al. Prevalence of subcutaneous, labial and rectal amyloid lesions in patients with histologically confirmed renal amyloidosis. Nephrologie 2000;21(1): 19-21.

[13] Lechapt-Zalcman E, Authier FJ, Creange A et al. Labial salivary gland biopsy for diagnosis of amyloid polyneuropathy. Muscle Nerve 1999;22(1): 105-7.

[14] Hachulla E, Janin A, Flipo RM et al. Labial salivary gland biopsy is a reliable test for the diagnosis of primary and secondary amyloidosis. A prospective clinical and immunohistologic study in 59 patients.Arthritis Rheum 1993;36(5):691-7.

[15] Yilmaz M, Unsal A, Sokmen M et al. Duodenal biopsy for diagnosis of renal involvement in amyloidosis.ClinNephrol2012;77(2): 114-8.

[16] Gertz MA, Kyle RA, Greipp PR. Response rates and survival in primary systemic amyloidosis.Blood1991;77(2): 257-62.

[17] Kapoor P, Thenappan T, Singh E et al.Cardiac amyloidosis: a practical approach to diagnosis and management.Am J Med2011;124(11): 1006-15

[18] Rahman JE, Helou EF, Gelzer-Bell R et al. Noninvasive diagnosis of biopsy-proven cardiac amyloidosis. J Am CollCardiol2004;43(3): 410-5.

[19] Ando Y, Ueda M. Diagnosis and therapeutic approaches to transthyretin amyloidosis.Curr Med Chem2012;19(15): 2312-23.

[20] Picken MM.Amyloidosis-where are we now and where are we heading?Arch Pathol Lab Med2010;134(4):545-51.

[21] Sanchorawala V, Skinner M, Quillen K et al.Long-term outcome of patients with AL amyloidosis treated with high-dose melphalan and stem-cell transplantation.Blood2007;110(10):3561-3.

[22] Obici L, Merlini G.AA amyloidosis: basic knowledge, unmet needs and future treatments.Swiss Med Wkly2012;142:0.

[23] Nakamura T.AmyloidA amyloidosis secondary to rheumatoid arthritis: pathophysiology and treatments.ClinExpRheumatol2011;29(5):850-7.

[24] Linke RP, Oos R, Wiegel NM, Nathrath WB. Classification of amyloidosis: misdiagnosing by way of incomplete immunohistochemistry and how to prevent it.ActaHistochem2006;108(3):197-208.

[25] Picken MM.New insights into systemic amyloidosis: the importance of diagnosis of specific type.Curr Opin Nephrol Hypertens2007;16(3): 196-203.

[26] Novak L, Cook WJ, Herrera GA, Sanders PW. AL-amyloidosis is underdiagnosed in renal biopsies. Nephrol Dial Transplant2004;19(12): 3050-3.

[27] Satoskar AA, Burdge K, Cowden DJ et al. Typing of amyloidosis in renal biopsies: diagnostic pitfalls.Arch Pathol Lab Med2007;131(6):917-22.

[28] Droz D, Nochy D. Amyloid substance and amyloidosis.Ann Pathol1995;15(1):11-20.

[29] Murphy CL, Wang S, Williams T et al. Characterization of systemic amyloid deposits by mass spectrometry.Methods Enzymol2006;412: 48-62.

[30] Lavatelli F, Perlman DH, Spencer B et al.Amyloidogenic and associated proteins in systemic amyloidosis proteome of adipose tissue.Mol Cell Proteomics2008;7(8): 1570-83.

[31] Connors LH, Ericsson T, Skare J et al. A simple screening test for variant transthyretins associated with familial transthyretin amyloidosis using isoelectric focusing. BiochimBiophysActa1998;1407(3): 185-92.

[32] Ranløv I, Ando Y, Ohlsson PI et al. Rapid screening for amyloid-related variant forms of transthyretin is possible by electrospray ionization mass spectrometry. Eur J Clin Invest1997;27(11): 956-9.

Chapter 3

# Cardiac Amyloidosis: Typing, Diagnosis, Prognosis and Management

Glenn K. Lee, DaLi Feng, Martha Grogan, Cynthia Taub, Angela Dispenzieri and Kyle W. Klarich

Additional information is available at the end of the chapter

http://dx.doi.org/10.5772/53763

## 1. Introduction

Amyloidosis is uncommon, with age-adjusted incidences of between 6.1 and 10.5 per million person-years,[1] and an estimated 1275 to 3200 new cases occurring annually in the United States.[1, 2] The contemporary understanding of amyloidosis points to a group of complex systemic disorders involving the extracellular deposition of misfolded proteinaceous material in many organs, most commonly the kidneys, heart, liver, central and peripheral nervous systems.[2-4] The normal function of tissues is altered, and end-organ dysfunction usually ensues. Cardiac amyloidosis can be isolated to the heart, but it often coexists with disease elsewhere in the body.[4, 5] Cardiac manifestations may predominate the clinical presentation or may be subclinical and detected on routine investigation of a patient presenting with non-cardiac complaints.[5] The presence and relative prominence of cardiac involvement in the clinical picture is dependent on the type of amyloidosis and severity of amyloid infiltration in the tissue.[5]

## 2. Classification of amyloidosis

Amyloidosis refers to a group of unrelated diseases involving the extracellular deposition of proteinaceous material that demonstrates apple-green birefringence under polarized light on staining with Congo red.[5] In all forms of amyloidosis, abnormal and unstable protein is produced in response to a variety of stimuli and precipitates as amyloid in the extracellular matrix.[2, 3] The contemporary classification of amyloidosis is primarily based on the biochemistry of the disease process from the precursor amyloid proteins, and comprises several major subgroups. Table 1 describes the typical characteristics of each type of amyloidosis.

| Type of amyloidosis | Precursor protein | Spectrum of organ involvement | Frequency of cardiac involvement | Median survival, months | Diagnostic testing | Treatment |
|---|---|---|---|---|---|---|
| Immunoglobulin amyloidosis (AL) | Immunoglobulin light chain | Heart, kidneys, liver, peripheral/ autonomic nervous systems, soft tissue, gastrointestinal system | Up to 50% have clinical cardiac involvement | 13 (4 months if heart failure present at diagnosis) | SPEP, UPEP, bone marrow biopsy tissue analysis revealing plasma cell dyscrasia, κ and λ light chain antiserum staining | Anti-plasma cell chemotherapy, autologous stem cell replacement, sequential heart and stem cell transplant |
| Familial amyloidosis (ATTR) | Mutant transthyretin | Peripheral/autonomic nervous systems, heart | Variable, depending on exact mutation | 70 | ATTR antiserum staining, serum TTR isoelectric focusing, restriction fragment length polymorphism analysis | Liver transplantation, combined liver and heart transplantation in certain cases, new pharmacological strategies to stabilize TTR |
| Senile systemic amyloidosis | Wild-type transthyretin | Heart (predominant, usually atrial) | Common | 75 | ATTR antiserum staining | Supportive, new pharmacological strategies to stabilize TTR |
| Reactive amyloidosis (SAA) | Serum amyloid A | Kidney, heart | Uncommon, <10% | 24.5 | Target organ biopsy specimen analysis, AA antiserum staining | Treat the underlying inflammatory process |
| Hemodialysis-associated amyloidosis | β2-microglobulin | Musculoskeletal system, rare in heart | Unknown, asymptomatic | Unclear clinical significance | Synovial and bone biopsy specimen analysis, β2-microglobulin antiserum, serum β2-microglobulin concentration | Renal transplantation |
| Isolated atrial amyloidosis | Atrial natriuretic peptide | Heart | Limited to heart | Unclear clinical significance | Atrial natriuretic peptide antiserum staining | None required |

**Table 1.** Types of amyloidosis affecting the heart.

### 2.1. Immunoglobulin light chain amyloidosis (AL)

AL amyloidosis is a monoclonal plasma cell disorder in which the precursor protein is an immunoglobulin light chain or light chain fragment. It may occur as a primary disease or in association with multiple myeloma or other plasma cell dyscrasias.[3, 6], 7] The median number of clonal plasma cells in AL amyloidosis is between 5% and 10%.[2] The extent of clonal plasma cell marrow infiltration is an important prognositic indicator, presumably because it reflects the degree of pathogenic light chain synthesis.[8] In primary amyloidosis, there is 2:1 preponderance for $\lambda$ over $\kappa$ light chain synthesis.[9] While in itself uncommon, with an incidence of 8.9 per million,[1] AL amyloidosis is the commonest type of amyloidosis, accounting for about 85% of all newly diagnosed cases.[3, 10] The clinical picture of AL amyloidosis is the most varied, since it commonly affects a large number of organ systems including the heart, kidney, liver, peripheral and autonomic nervous systems, soft tissue and gastrointestinal systems.[3, 5] The heart is affected in over 50% of cases,[11] and symptomatic cardiac involvement portends a worse prognosis.[11, 12] Conversely, involvement limited to the heart constitutes <5% of patients with AL amyloidosis.[11] Cardiac involvement with resultant heart failure or arrhythmia accounts for >50% of the mortality in patients with AL amyloidosis.[12] Furthermore, thromboembolism also contributes significantly to morbidity and mortality. Intracardiac thrombosis was found in 51% and 35% of subjects with AL amyloidosis in the Mayo amyloid autopsy study and in a group of patients undergoing follow up echocardiographic imaging respectively.[13, 14]

### 2.2. Familial amyloidosis (ATTR)

Familial amyloidosis is a hereditary autosomal dominant disorder involving amyloidogenic mutations in most commonly the transthyretin gene.[15] The age of onset of familial amyloidosis appears to vary with ethnicity. Interestingly, about 10% of gene carriers remain asymptomatic (although the disease manifestation can be age dependent with variable penetrance),[16-18] suggesting that the pathogenesis of these diseases may involve other genetic or environmental factors. Familial amyloidosis usually affects the peripheral and autonomic nervous systems and the heart.[5] While usually more slowly progressive than AL amyloidosis, the familial type may also cause clinically significant heart failure. Significant cardiac disease is associated with mutations at positions 30, 60 and 84 of the transthyretin gene.[17] A mutation involving isoleucine at position 122 which involves solely the heart has been described in elderly African-American persons.[19, 20] This form of amyloid is probably underdiagnosed since nearly 4% of newborn African Americans harbor this mutation.[19] The TranstHyretin Amyloidosis Outcome Survey (THAOS) registry is a global observational survey set up with the aim of furthering our understanding of hereditary amyloidosis.

### 2.3. Senile systemic amyloidosis

Senile systemic amyloidosis is primarily a disease of the elderly, most commonly affecting men over the age of 70. It accounts for approximately 25% of patients over 80 years with amyloidosis.[21, 22] It is caused by wild-type transthyretin.[5, 21] Cardiac, particularly atrial, involvement is common,[23, 24] and may be associated with clinically significant heart failure, atrial fibrillation and conduction abnormalities.[25, 26]

### 2.4. Reactive amyloidosis (SAA)

Reactive amyloidosis is characterized by the deposition of serum amyloid A protein (SAA), an acute phase reactant produced in response to chronic inflammatory processes such as chronic infections, rheumatologic disease and familial periodic fever syndromes.[27, 29] With efficacious treatment of chronic infections in patients in the developed world, the incidence of reactive amyloidosis has fallen.[29] The kidney is commonly involved, [5] and cardiac involvement, if present, is rarely clinically significant.[30, 31]

### 2.5. Hemodialysis-associated amyloidosis (Aβ2M)

Hemodialysis-associated amyloidosis occurs in chronic renal failure patients undergoing hemodialysis.[12] β2-microglobulin is the precursor protein.[32, 33] Musculoskeletal involvement is common, and the clinical effect from cardiac deposition is minimal and typically clinically insignificant.[34, 35]

### 2.6. Isolated atrial amyloidosis (AANF)

Isolated atrial amyloidosis is predominantly seen in those >80 years and in females,[23] but also occurs in younger patients with valvular abnormalities or chronic atrial fibrillation. [36-38] The precursor protein is atrial natriuretic peptide.[39-41] Involvement is usually limited to the subendocardial region of the heart, and its clinical significance is unclear.[42]

## 3. Pathophysiology of cardiac amyloidosis

In cardiac amyloidosis, the clinical presentation is typically heart failure with initially preserved ejection fraction and restrictive diastolic physiology. This has led to its classification as a "restrictive" cardiomyopathy.[3, 5, 9, 43] This is defined by a high filling pressure that can lead classically to heart failure with preserved ejection fraction. Cardiac contractile function and electrical conduction can be impaired with amyloid infiltration.[9] At a cellular level, amyloid infiltration results in abnormal cellular metabolism, calcium transport and receptor regulation. [3] Adrenergic input is disrupted and the neurohormonal milieu is altered in cardiac amyloidosis.[44] Amyloid deposition induces oxidant stress[45] and modulates interstitial matrix composition and tissue remodeling,[46] leading to further depression of myocyte contractility. Furthermore, there is evidence of a direct toxic role of the monoclonal light chain extracted from the urine of AL patients on myocardial diastolic function in the mouse hearts; infusion of the monoclonal light chain caused a significant elevation in the LV end diastolic pressure in this animal model.[47] Involvement of the coronary microvasculature may also result in coronary flow abnormalities; this is seen in 90% of patients with AL amyloidosis.[48] This global involvement leads to diffuse ischemia and microinfarction,

http://dx.doi.org/10.5772/53763

further compromising cardiac contractility.[49] The resultant perivascular amyloid infiltration commonly involves the conduction system, leading to conduction abnormalities.[50, 51]

# 4. Clinical presentation – When should physicians suspect amyloidosis?

Depending on the spectrum of organ involvement, a patient can present with a multitude of symptoms and signs which are often nonspecific and variable, especially in the early stages of disease.[12] This is particularly so in AL amyloidosis, in which many systems can be affected. Common constitutional complaints include weakness, fatigue, peripheral edema and weight loss.[9] Hepatomegaly is common and results from either direct hepatic infiltration or congestion secondary to cardiac failure.[52, 53] Renal involvement may cause profound proteinuria and the nephrotic syndrome.[5, 9] Easy bruising and periorbital purpura results from clotting factor deficiencies and fragile venules; the latter is virtually pathognomonic of the AL type disease.[54, 55] Soft tissue involvement may result in carpal tunnel syndrome[5, 9] and macroglossia,[56] while peripheral and/or autonomic neuropathy may be the hallmark of neurological involvement.[5, 9, 12] The presence of complaints involving multiple organ systems without any other known cause should trigger a search for multisystem disease, one of which being amyloidosis. Early diagnosis improves outcomes, given the irreversible damage caused by amyloidosis and that patients with advanced disease are often not candidates for definitive treatment options (some of which may be curative),[43] but this requires a high index of suspicion and a systematic algorithm for evaluation.[4, 9]

Cardiac findings are predominantly due to diastolic dysfunction, also known as heart failure with preserved ejection fraction.[3, 5, 9] The initial presentation is often that of progressive exertional dyspnea followed by worsening heart failure, pulmonary congestion, pleural effusions, edema, and ascites.[11] Valvular insufficiency or stenosis due to endocardial involvement may result in a murmur,[9, 43, 57] and atrial fibrillation is common, although all manner of arrhythmias have been reported.[57, 58] Coronary flow abnormalities due to microvascular involvement may present as angina chest pain;[59] rarely, this may be the only presenting complaint.[59-63] Patients may have syncope and lightheadedness, particularly postural, caused by autonomic dysfunction and arrhythmias in the face of declining cardiac functional reserve.[64] The heart should be screened in all patients with known or suspected amyloidosis even in the absence of cardiac symptoms, as involvement of the heart portends a poor prognosis and affects treatment strategies.[3]

# 5. Diagnosis and evaluation of cardiac amyloidosis

Histologic examination remains the definitive diagnostic modality in cardiac amyloidosis.[9, 65] While not definitive, certain non-invasive imaging and laboratory findings may guide further diagnostic testing and management and assess the severity of the disease for prognostic purposes.[9, 43] Often, the diagnosis of cardiac amyloidosis and perhaps the type of amyloidosis can be reasonably ascertained by employing one or more non-invasive imaging and laboratory modalities.

### 5.1. Echocardiography

Echocardiography remains the most widely utilized noninvasive modality in the diagnosis of cardiac amyloidosis, in part because of its widespread availability and relatively low cost.[5, 66] In cases with characteristic echocardiographic findings, signs and symptoms of heart failure, and a positive biopsy of another organ, cardiac involvement is almost certain. However, echocardiography cannot determine the type of amyloidosis and in some patients with early disease the findings may be subtle.[43]

Echocardiography may show mild diastolic dysfunction [9] as the only clue in early amyloid heart disease, but this is non-specific and may often be mistaken for more common conditions such as hypertensive or hypertrophic cardiomyopathy. Recently, it has been found that tissue Doppler imaging could identify abnormalities in both early and late-stage cardiac amyloidosis, affording the possibility for early diagnosis and disease-modifying intervention.[66, 67] Tissue Doppler imaging can also be helpful in differentiating restrictive cardiomyopathy from constrictive pericarditis.[68, 69] Diastolic dysfunction is the predominant pathology in cardiac amyloidosis; the classic picture of a thick and stiff ventricle elevates diastolic filling pressures causing restrictive hemodynamics and atrial dilatation.[70, 71] Decreased ejection fraction typically occurs only in late-stage disease as a result of loss of myocardial contractile function through myocyte necrosis and local interstitial amyloid infiltration;[5, 72-75] despite preserved ejection fraction, systolic function is not normal in cardiac amyloidosis. Techniques of myocardial deformation imaging have shown that abnormal strain and strain rate imaging occur in most cases of cardiac amyloidosis.[76-79] Amyloid cardiomyopathy seems to be associated with a marked dissociation between short and long-axis systolic function; tissue Doppler or strain rate imaging may show severe impairment in long-axis contraction even when the left ventricular ejection fraction remains within the normal range.

The typical features of cardiac amyloidosis such as left ventricular wall thickening[66, 72-74, 80, 81] with myocardial hyperechogenicity,[74, 81-84] biatrial enlargement,[74, 75, 81] thickened atrial septum[81] and valve leaflets,[75, 81] as well as pericardial effusion [75, 81] are usually seen at a more advanced stage of the disease (Figure 1). A thickened left ventricular wall in the absence of high electrocardiographic voltages is suggestive of infiltrative cardiac disease. Deposition in the atria is usually extensive and may cause atrial mechanical failure and atrial standstill, i.e. atrial electro-mechanical dissociation even in patients who are in normal sinus rhythm. Atrial involvement may also result in atrial arrhythmias; in fact, atrial fibrillation can significantly affect the cardiac output from an already impaired ventricle.[85, 86] Heart failure can be further worsened by valvular insufficiency caused by subendocardial infiltration. [9] Rarely, pericardial involvement occurs in severe disease leading to pericardial effusion or constriction.[48] In some cases, pulmonary hypertension and cor pulmonale may occur in patients with amyloidosis.[87] Although usually caused by concomitant and frequently more severe cardiac amyloidosis with left ventricular failure,[88] pulmonary hypertension may be the result of advanced pulmonary amyloid infiltration.[87]

http://dx.doi.org/10.5772/53763

While pulmonary involvement is a harbinger of adverse outcome, it is often difficult to determine the exact extent to which pulmonary amyloid deposition contributes to symptoms or outcome because cardiac deposition commonly coexists.[89]

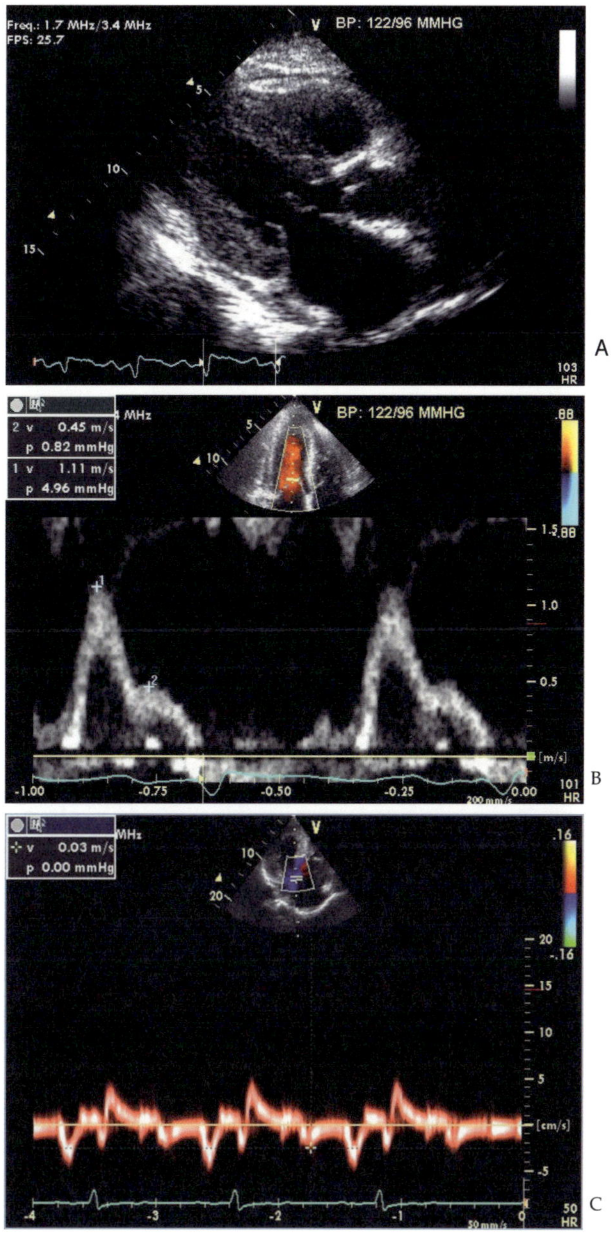


**Figure 1.** (A) Two-dimensional echocardiographic, (B) transmitral Doppler and (C) tissue Doppler images classical of AL amyloidosis.

Several other findings on echocardiography may have prognostic significance in cardiac amyloidosis, such as left ventricular ejection time,[90] wall motion abnormalities,[91, 92] dyssynchrony,[93] as well as increased right ventricular Tei index (which reflects right ventricular dysfunction).[94] Myocardial contrast echocardiography can reveal microvascular dysfunction, and may be a useful adjunct in echocardiographic assessment for the early diagnosis of cardiac amyloidosis, although it is not typically utilized in day to day practice. [95] Transesophageal echocardiography (TEE) may be useful in characterizing atrial thrombi and assessing left atrial appendage dysfunction,[96] a common finding in cardiac amyloidosis even in the absence of atrial fibrillation (Figure 2).[96, 97] Risk factors for intracardiac thrombosis include: AL type amyloidosis, atrial fibrillation, and diastolic dysfunction. Increased right ventricular wall thickness is a marker of increased risk in intracardiac thrombosis, probably due to the presence of advanced infiltrative cardiomyopathy.[14] Timely assessment for intracardiac thrombosis in high-risk patients is important for anticoagulation considerations.[13, 14, 98] Patients with amyloidosis should not be cardioverted without adequate anticoagulation and in some institutions, TEE imaging is routinely performed prior to cardioversion even in the presence of adequate anticoagulation.

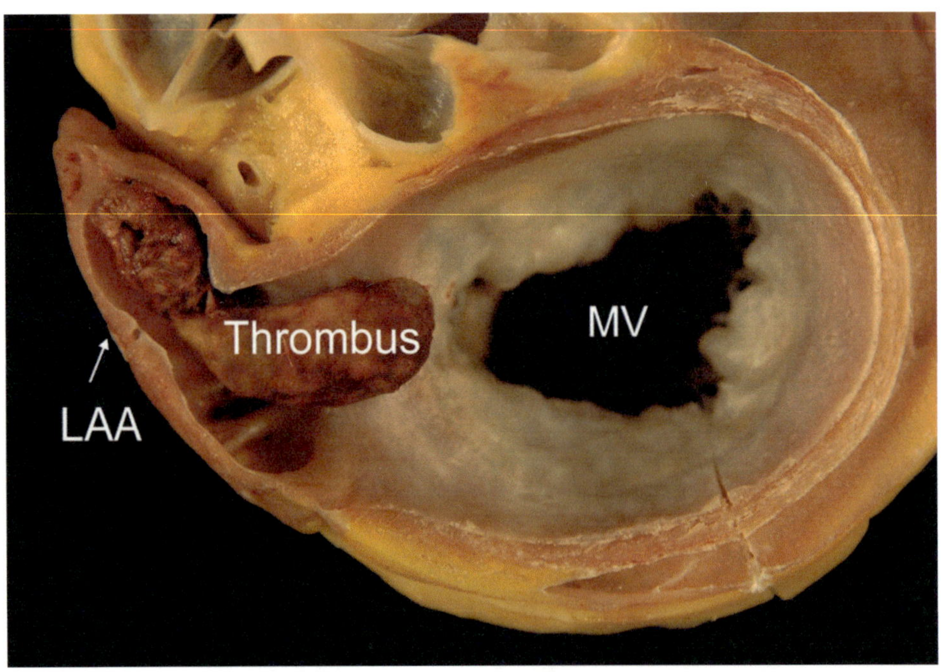


**Figure 2.** Left atrial appendage (LAA) thrombus in a patient with cardiac amyloidosis; the patient was known to be in sinus rhythm. (With permission from Feng et al. *Circulation.* Nov 20 2007;116(21):2420-2426.)

Besides its diagnostic value, echocardiography is a useful adjunct during the endomyocardial biopsy procedure. It complements, and in some institutions has replaced, fluoroscopy as a method of bioptome guidance because of its superior resolution of the tricuspid valve anatomy, endocardial surface, and thin right ventricular free wall and apex.[99]

### 5.2. Electrocardiography

Electrocardiography (ECG) provides useful and complementary information in patients with cardiac amyloidosis. The classic findings of low voltages and pseudoinfarct patterns (Figure 3) are common occurrences,[11, 58, 100] and both findings may occur in 25% to 50% of patients.[43] Poor R wave progression is also often seen.[3, 101] Low voltage correlated with the presence of a pericardial effusion but not with decreased ejection fraction.[43] The combination of low voltage and an interventricular septum thickness >1.98 cm is very specific for cardiac amyloidosis.[74] The finding of low voltage in a patient with echocardiographic evidence of increased wall thickness should raise the clinical suspicion of infiltrative cardiomyopathy, but the reverse is not necessarily true – normal voltage does not exclude amyloidosis.[58] ECG criteria for left ventricular hypertrophy, especially limb lead ECG left ventricular hypertrophy, however, is rarely present in patients with cardiac biopsy proven amyloidosis.[58]

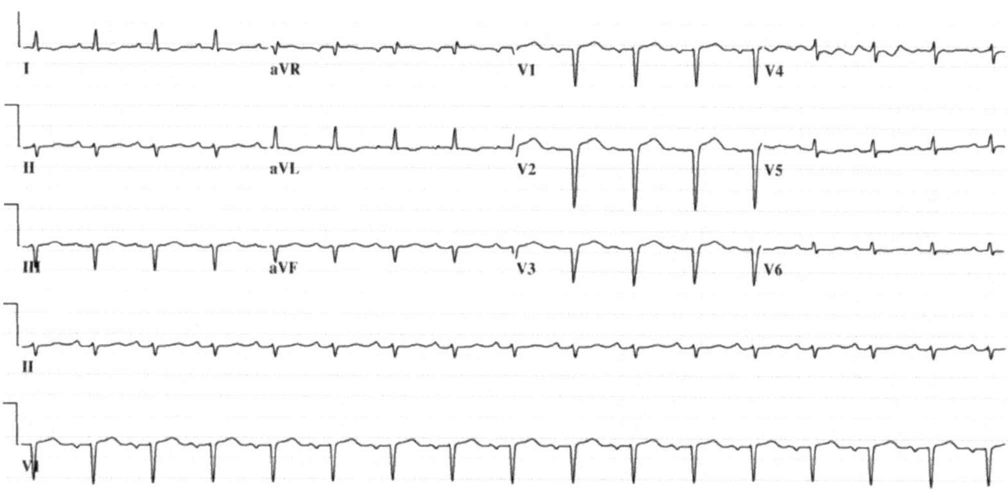


**Figure 3.** ECG changes classical of cardiac amyloidosis with sinus tachycardia, low voltage and pseudoinfarct patterns.

The conduction system can often be affected in cardiac amyloidosis.[11] Atrial fibrillation and flutter are the commonest arrhythmias seen,[58] but atrioventricular and bundle branch blocks may occur.[65] Sinus tachycardia seen in advanced cardiac amyloidosis is probably due to the restrictive filling leading to cardiac output adjustments based solely on heart rate; in one study this was a marker of increased risk for intracardiac thrombosis.[14] Prolonged QT intervals and junctional rhythms may be present. [9] Advanced ventricular arrhythmias such as sustained ventricular tachycardia are rarely seen (although frequent PVCs, couplets or triplets are common), which is likely due to poorly tolerance of the arrhythmia in the advanced cardiac amyloid patients who would die suddenly from sustain VT.[58, 102] Sudden death in severe cardiac amyloidosis is commonly attributed to electromechanical dissociation; a pattern similar to severe cardiac diseases of other etiologies.[64]

The largest reported ECG series consists of 127 patients with AL amyloidosis and biopsy proven cardiac involvement seen at the Mayo Clinic. The two most common abnormalities were low voltage and a pseudoinfarct pattern, which were seen in 46 and 47 percent of cases. Other findings included first degree AV block in 21 percent, nonspecific intraventricular conduction delay in 16 percent, second or third degree AV block in 3 percent, atrial fibrillation or flutter in 20 percent, and ventricular tachycardia in 5 percent. ECG criteria for left ventricular hypertrophy were present in 16 percent, but some of these patients had a history of hypertension. The left ventricular hypertrophy criteria were limited almost exclusively to precordial leads, sometimes with low-voltage limb leads.[58] In patients with AL amyloidosis, signal-averaged ECG may demonstrate delayed myocardial activation or "late potentials"; this is an independent predictor of sudden death.[43, 100] Reduced heart rate variability predicts mortality in the short-term in both AL and familial amyloidosis, and probably represents autonomic dysfunction.[103, 104]

Many of the ECG findings in cardiac amyloidosis are nonspecific, and other causes of such should be ruled out.[65] On the other hand, ECGs, especially if done serially, allows for early diagnosis and intervention in cardiac amyloidosis. Physicians should understand the characteristics and symptoms of amyloidosis, and be aware of subtle changes in the ECG, especially abnormalities that suggest disorders in the conduction system (such as prolonged PR interval, widened QRS, atrioventricular blocks, and bundle branch blocks) or decreased electromotive force (such as progressive R wave decrease).[105]

### 5.3. Cardiac magnetic resonance imaging

Cardiac magnetic resonance imaging (CMR) is emerging as a useful tool in the diagnosis of cardiac amyloidosis. Its strength lies in its high three-dimensional spatial resolution and signal-to-noise ratio, permitting reproducible measurements of cardiac chamber volumes and mass, as well as left ventricular and atrial septal wall thickness.[106] Additionally, it can characterize pericardial and pleural fluid.[106] Late gadolinium enhancement (LGE) is the cornerstone of detecting myocardial amyloid infiltrates and is seen in almost all cases.[107] Compared with normal myocardium which has no LGE because of little gadolinium accumulation on delayed imaging, contrast accumulates in the extracellular space in cardiac amyloidosis which is expanded by amyloid infiltration, resulting in LGE. [108] The predominant pattern of LGE seen in cardiac amyloidosis is global transmural (Figure 4) or subendocardial; [108, 109] other patterns including focal patchy LGE and difficulty nulling can also be seen.

http://dx.doi.org/10.5772/53763

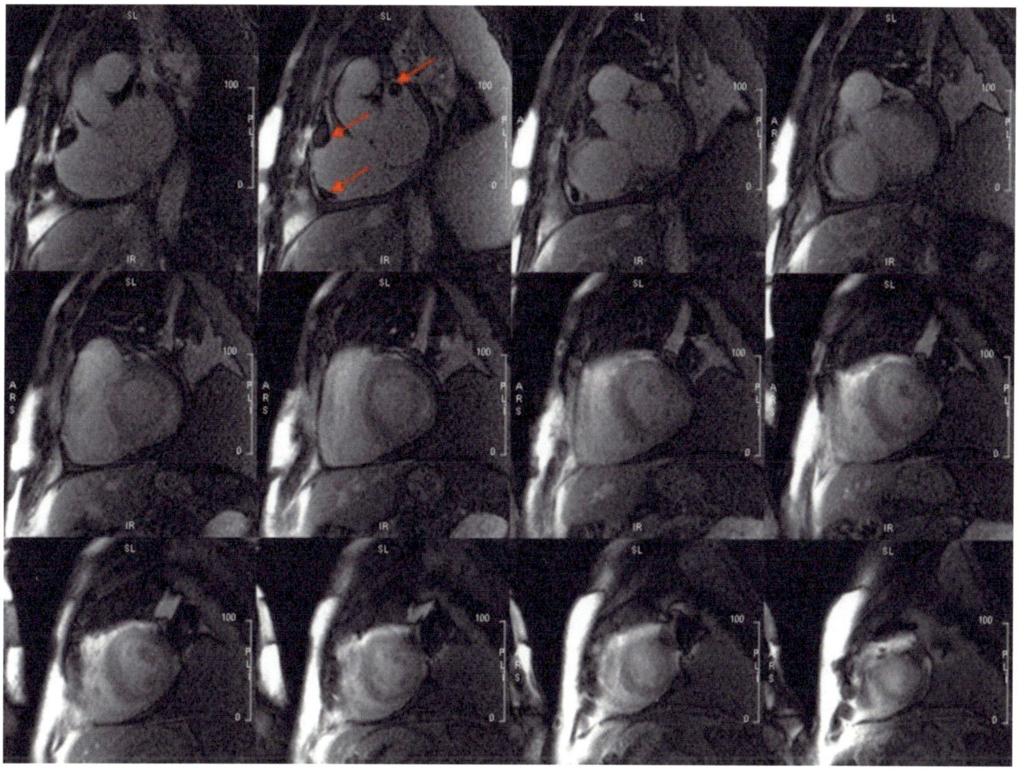

**Figure 4.** CMR findings of global transmural LGE classical of cardiac amyloidosis; this patient had histologically proven AL amyloidosis. Furthermore, three intracardiac thrombi (red arrows) were detected in the left atrial appendage, right atrial appendage and at the right atrial free wall close to tricuspid annulus.

Maceira et al [108] first studied LGE in CMR in 29 patients with cardiac amyloidosis. They found that CMR shows a characteristic pattern of global subendocardial LGE coupled with abnormal myocardial and blood-pool gadolinium kinetics. In 22 of these, myocardial gadolinium kinetics with T1 mapping was compared with that in 16 hypertensive controls. Subendocardial T1 in amyloid patients was shorter than in controls (at 4 minutes: 427±73 vs. 579±75 ms; $p<0.01$), and was correlated with markers of increased myocardial amyloid load such as left ventricular mass, wall thickness, interatrial septal thickness and diastolic function. Global subendocardial LGE was found in 20 amyloid patients (69%); these patients had greater left ventricular mass than unenhanced patients. Histological quantification showed substantial interstitial expansion with amyloid (30.5%) but only minor fibrosis (1.3%). Amyloid deposition was predominantly subendocardial (42%), compared with midwall (29%) and subepicardial (18%). The LGE findings agree with the transmural histological distribution of amyloid protein and the cardiac amyloid load. Using the difference between the T1 of subendomyocardium and blood, a cutoff value of 191 ms at 4 minutes had 90% sensitivity, 87% specificity and 88% of accuracy for the correct diagnosis of cardiac amyloidosis. There was 97% concordance in diagnosis of cardiac amyloidosis by combining the presence of late gadolinium enhancement and an optimized T1 threshold between myocardium and blood.

Mayo investigators further evaluated the mechanism of LGE in CMR in identifying cardiac involvement in a population of known amyloidosis patients and to investigate associations between LGE and clinical, morphological, functional, and biochemical features.[107] Gadolinium-enhanced CMR was performed in 120 patients with amyloidosis of which 100 had AL amyloidosis, 11 had familial amyloidosis and 9 had senile amyloidosis. Cardiac autopsy and/or histology was available in 35 patients. The remaining 85 patients were divided into those with and without echocardiographic evidence of cardiac amyloidosis. Abnormal LGE was present in 34 (97%) patients with histologically proven cardiac amyloidosis. Global transmural or subendocardial LGE (83%) was most common while suboptimal myocardial nulling (8%) and patchy focal LGE (6%) were also observed (Figure 5). Global LGE was associated with a higher burden of interstitial amyloid quantified from histology. LGE distribution matched the deposition pattern of interstitial amyloid at autopsy. Importantly, the study found that LGE was present in 47% of patients without evidence of cardiac amyloidosis by echocardiography. LGE presence and pattern was associated with New York Heart Association class, ECG voltages, left ventricular mass index and thickness, right ventricular thickness, troponin-T, and B-type natriuretic peptide levels. The global LGE patterns were associated with the worst clinical, ECG, echocardiographic and biomarker abnormalities compared to other types of LGE (focal or suboptimal nulling).

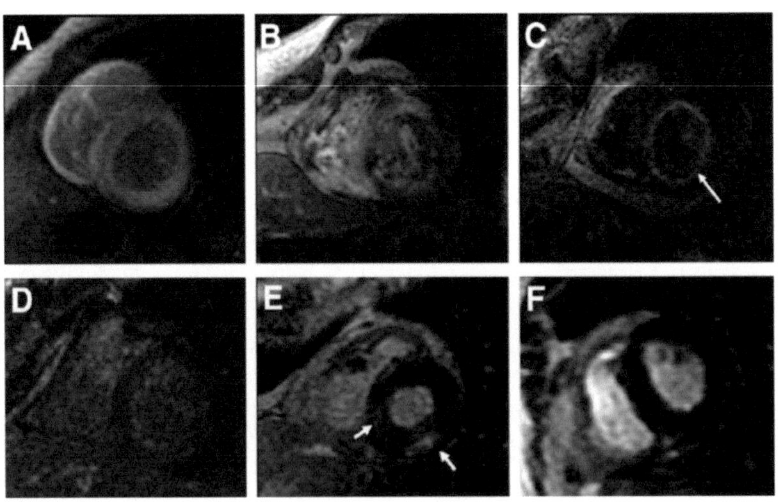


**Figure 5.** The different patterns of LGE on CMR in patients with cardiac amyloidosis. (With permission from Syed et al. *JACC Cardiovasc Imaging.* 2010;3:155-164.)

CMR relaxometry is a novel approach in the diagnosis of cardiac amyloidosis, showing elevated relaxation times in patients with the disease. A T1 relaxation time cutoff value of

≥1273 milliseconds was found to be both sensitive and specific for the diagnosis of cardiac amyloidosis.[110]

Based on these studies, it is apparent that gadolinium-enhanced CMR is the most accurate imaging modality to diagnose cardiac amyloidosis. LGE is common in cardiac amyloidosis and it is due to interstitial expansion from amyloid deposition and kinetic change of gadolinium in the blood pool and myocardium/interstitia. This modality may potentially detect early cardiac involvement in patients with amyloidosis and normal left ventricular wall thickness.[43, 107] It also affords global assessment of the heart, eliminating the sampling error that endomyocardial biopsy may potentially carry.[111] Furthermore, it may be useful in detecting subclinical early cardiac involvement;[43] indeed studies have shown that even early cardiac involvement carried a significant mortality risk, in particular cardiac mortality.[112, 113] Serial CMR studies may have the potential to chart the progression or regression of the disease over time after the initiation of treatment.[114] However, despite the high sensitivity and specificity of CMR in the diagnosis of cardiac amyloidosis, similar patterns, while uncommon, have been occasionally reported in systemic sclerosis and post-heart transplant patients. The autopsy study by Syed et al suggests that rarely, gadolinium-enhanced CMR may be falsely negative because the amyloid infiltrate is mild.[107]

CMR may be a reasonable adjuvant or even an alternative to endomyocardial biopsy, especially in patients with a tissue diagnosis from a remote site and who are high-risk for invasive investigation. However, it is important to notice that the diagnosis of cardiac amyloidosis is confirmed by demonstrating amyloid deposits on endomyocardial biopsy. Cardiac amyloidosis may be presumably, but not conclusively, established in patients with appropriate cardiac imaging findings with demonstration of amyloid deposits on histological examination of a biopsy from other tissues (e.g., abdominal fat pad, rectum, or kidney).

There are several limitations in the use of this modality. Firstly, it is incompatible with patients with implanted devices such as pacemakers or implantable cardioverter-defibrillators. Nevertheless, pacemakers compatible with magnetic resonance imaging were recently approved by the United States Food and Drug Administration for clinical use in the 1.5 tesla magnetic resonance imaging scanner. Secondly, gadolinium contrast administration is contraindicated in patients whose creatinine clearance is less than 30 mL/minute given the risk of nephrogenic systemic fibrosis.[115] Many patients with cardiac amyloidosis have indications for heart failure device therapy (e.g. pacemakers, implantable cardioverter-defibrillators) as well as renal impairment as a result of amyloid deposition in the kidneys, both of which may preclude them from undergoing CMR.

### 5.4. Nuclear scintigraphy

Several single-photon emission computed tomography tracers have been evaluated in the diagnosis of cardiac amyloidosis.[116] There is evidence that [123]I-metaiodobenzylguanidine may be an indirect measure of cardiac amyloid deposition. The finding of intense uptake in the heart on [99]mTc-pyrophosphate scintigraphy, which was indicative of cardiac amyloidosis, was insufficiently sensitive to warrant routine use in the diagnosis of the disease. While not routinely performed for diagnosing cardiac amyloidosis given its variable sensitivity, a new technique, [99]mTc-3,3-diphosphono-1,2-propanodicarboxylic acid scintigraphy, may be able to differentiate familial transthyretin-associated amyloidosis from AL amyloidosis, a clinically-relevant distinction; however, further study into this new technique is needed.[117]

### 5.5. Fat aspirate and endomyocardial biopsy for tissue diagnosis

Even with current imaging technology, amyloidosis remains a histological diagnosis (Figure 6). The presence of serum or urine monoclonal paraprotein is suggestive of AL amyloidosis, but on its own does not firmly establish the diagnosis because low serum concentrations of a monoclonal protein (possibly from an unrelated monoclonal gammopathy of undetermined significance) can incorrectly suggest AL amyloid in some familial cardiac amyloidosis confirmed later by cardiac biopsy.[118] For the diagnosis of systemic disease, less invasive tissue sampling methods are available.[9] Biopsies may be taken from the abdominal subcutaneous fat, with sensitivities of >80% for the latter in AL.[119-121]. Abdominal subcutaneous fat aspiration is easily obtained with minimal risk and is now preferred over rectal biopsy. Endomyocardial biopsy should be considered if the diagnosis of amyloidosis cannot be made with noninvasive techniques and the suspicion of cardiac amyloidosis remains high, or in cases of isolated cardiac amyloidosis, for example in the isoleucine 122 form of familial amyloidosis and senile systemic amyloidosis.[9] The sensitivity of four endomyocardial biopsy samples for the disease is nearly 100%.[111] Mass spectrometry of the tissue biopsy is used to determine the type of amyloidosis.

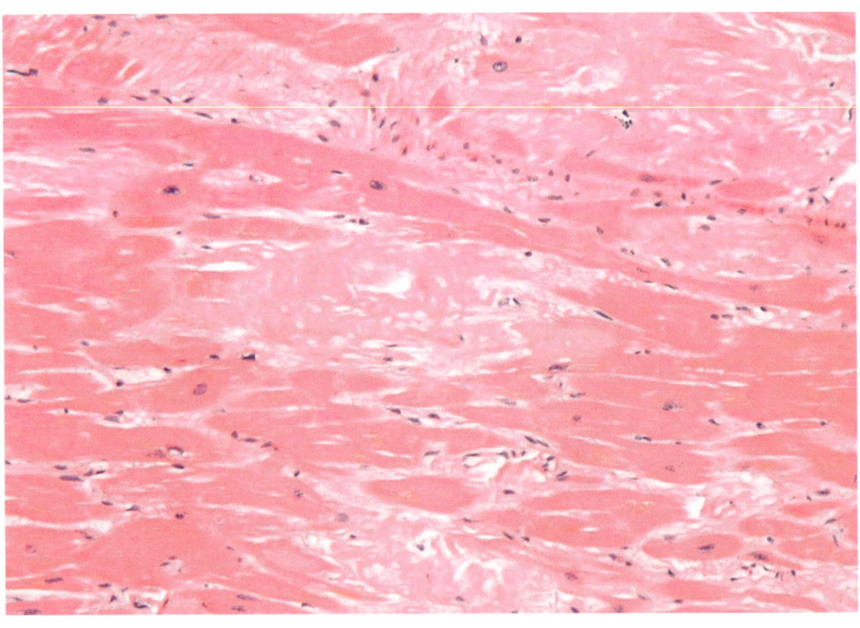

**Figure 6.** Histologic findings classical of cardiac amyloidosis. Hematoxylin and eosin staining of an amyloid-infiltrated left ventricular myocardium is shown here. The amyloid protein stained an amorphic light pink color (arrows).

### 5.6. Biochemical markers and prognostication

Cardiac biomarkers may be elevated in cardiac amyloidosis, often disproportionate to the clinical presentation.[122] Amyloid-induced myonecrosis and small vessel ischemia causes raised cardiac troponins,[123] while diastolic dysfunction and upregulation of natriuretic peptide genes in diseased ventricles result in elevated B-type natriuretic peptide levels.[124]

Cardiac troponins and N-terminal-pro-B-type natriuretic peptide are important prognostic indicators in cardiac amyloidosis, and also allow for monitoring progression of disease or efficacy of therapy.[43, 77, 125-127] One study showed a significantly decreased median survival in patients with troponin elevation; this may even predict survival better than symptomatic congestive heart failure and two-dimensional echocardiographic findings.[128] A 30% decrease in N-terminal-pro-B-type natriuretic peptide after effective chemotherapy correlates with increased event-free survival even without objective echocardiographic findings.[129] A combination of high-sensitivity cardiac troponin T at presentation and N-terminal-pro-B-type natriuretic peptide changes after chemotherapy had superior predictive value for survival.[130] Serum uric acid is a novel independent prognostic factor in AL amyloidosis. The median overall survival was lower in patients with uric acid levels ≥8 mg/dL.[131] A combination of uric acid, troponin T and N-terminal-pro-B-type natriuretic peptide provides a strong predictive model for early mortality.[132]

The serum immunoglobulin free light chain assay enables quantification of aberrant circulating amyloidogenic fibril protein precursors.[129] It enables serial monitoring of amyloidogenic light chain production during chemotherapy.[133] A fall in aberrant free light chain production by half following chemotherapy was associated with reductions in N-terminal-pro-B-type natriuretic peptide but not in left ventricular wall thickness, and was associated with clinical improvement.[129] Further highly reproducible and quantifiable imaging studies such as CMR may assist in defining associations between cardiac function and alterations in light chain load.[43]

## 6. Management of cardiac amyloidosis

Although the management of cardiac amyloidosis is challenging, evolution of treatment options have improved prognosis. It is essential to determine the type of amyloidosis to guide treatment.[43] In general, the management aims can be broadly divided into the general supportive care of cardiac and extracardiac manifestations of the disease, as well as type-specific targeted therapy.[5, 43] Table 2 shows a general algorithm for the investigation and management of cardiac amyloidosis.

**Step 1 – Identification of clinical scenarios suspicious for cardiac amyloidosis**

*Any one of the features below could trigger clinical suspicion – NOT all are required*

•Dyspnea with exertion or heart failure of unknown etiology, often with thickening of the LV and/or RV walls, especially if associated with low voltages on ECG

•Unexplained fatigue and weight loss

•Associated hepatomegaly, nephrotic-range proteinuria, peripheral or autonomic neuropathy, carpal tunnel syndrome, family history of amyloidosis

•Periorbital purpura (rare but almost pathognomonic) and macroglossia

**Step 2 – Cardiac diagnostic assessment**

•Detailed echocardiographic examination including diastolic function analysis, tissue Doppler, strain imaging, assessment of RV wall thickness

•Cardiac MRI with late gadolinium enhancement

•Cardiac biomarkers: troponin T and NT-proBNP

**Step 3 – Further evaluation for the diagnosis of amyloidosis**

•Screening biopsy of abdominal subcutaneous fat aspirate or rectal mucosa with Congo red staining

•Screen serum and urine for monoclonal protein, serum free light chain assay

•If clinical suspicion remains high despite the above being negative, consider endomyocardial biopsy (or other involved organ) with Congo red staining

**Step 4 – Determination of the amyloid fibril type (if the diagnosis of amyloidosis is made)**

*Tissue diagnosis and correct typing of amyloid is critical*

•Mass spectrometry based proteomic analysis of tissue containing amyloid to determine specific type of amyloid protein

**Step 5 – Do specific testing based on type of amyloidosis**

•Bone marrow aspirate and biopsy if diagnosis is AL amyloidosis or myeloma with associated amyloidosis

•For TTR-related amyloidosis, genetic testing to distinguish between age-related and hereditary variant TTR types

•For other hereditary amyloidoses, appropriate genetic testing for family counseling

**Step 6 – Type-specific treatment**

•AL amyloidosis: quantify light chains (as baseline for follow-up), exclude concomitant myeloma, troponin and NT-proBNP measurements for staging (if not done), supportive therapy, and determine which chemotherapy (including possible autologous stem cell transplant) and/or whether, sequential cardiac and autologous stem cell transplant is appropriate

•Familial amyloidosis: supportive therapy; assess for liver transplant with or without heart transplant

•Reactive amyloidosis: treating the underlying chronic inflammatory state and anti-cytokines therapy (IL-6, TNFα)

•Senile systemic amyloidosis: supportive therapy and possibly tafamidis in the future

AL, immunoglobulin light chain; ECG, electrocardiogram; LV, left ventricular; NT-proBNP, N-terminal prohormone brain natriuretic peptide; RV, right ventricular; TTR, transthyretin

**Table 2.** Evaluating a patient with suspected cardiac amyloidosis.

### 6.1. General supportive care

The traditional teaching that amyloidosis with cardiac involvement is universally fatal has dramatically changed in the last decade, largely due to chemotherapy and stem cell transplant therapies. However, important supportive care measures are necessary to achieve these outcomes.

Cardiac manifestations of amyloidosis primarily include heart failure and cardiac arrhythmias. The mainstay of heart failure treatment in cardiac amyloidosis is diuresis; patients with hypoalbuminemia due to concomitant nephrotic syndrome require high doses. It is essential to monitor fluid balance meticulously with daily weighing and diuretic dose adjustment.[5, 43] For a variety of reasons, beta-blockers, [9] renin-angiotensin system inhibitors,[5, 43] digoxin [134, 135] and calcium channel blockers[136]-[138] should be avoided where possible. In markedly impaired diastolic filling and reduced stroke volume, tachycardia is a compensatory mechanism that maintains cardiac output. Consequently, high doses of beta-adrenergic receptor blocking agents are often poorly tolerated. Calcium channel blockers and digitalis are considered contraindicated in cardiac amyloid disease due to potential binding of amyloid fibrils and potentiation of drug toxicity. Evidence for the use of vasodilator or inotropic agents in cardiac amyloidosis is lacking, but renal-dose dopamine may be helpful in the treatment of anasarca if renal function is unimpaired.[5] Recurrent large pleural effusions may represent pleural amyloid and may require thoracentesis and occasionally, pleurodesis.[139] Placement of a pleural catheter can helpful for palliation of recurrent pleural effusions. Anticoagulation should be administered for standard indications such as intracardiac thrombus and atrial fibrillation, and an embolic event even in the absence of atrial fibrillation should trigger a search for intracardiac thrombosis.[14, 43, 97, 140] Appropriate selection of patients suitable for thromboembolic prophylaxis is difficult given the high anticoagulation-associated bleeding risk due to vascular fragility and coagulopathy in amyloidosis.

Patient with cardiac amyloidosis are predisposed to many different types of arrhythmias, [57, 58] most commonly atrial fibrillation.[58] Given the atrial dilation from increased ventricular end-diastolic pressures as well as atrial amyloid infiltration, restoration of sinus rhythm is challenging and frequently unsuccessful in the long term.[14] It is reasonable, however, to attempt sinus rhythm restoration with DC cardioversion in highly symptomatic and medication refractory cases, provided no atrial thrombus is present by TEE. Atrial fibrillation recurs in most patients, and as such a rate-control and anticoagulation strategy is warranted in most circumstances. Patients with AL amyloidosis with concomitant AF are at an extremely high risk of thromboembolism, and the thromboembolic risk in transthyretin-related amyloidosis is also elevated above that of non-amyloid AF patients. Proper anticoagulation therapy reduces thromboembolic risk.[14] Amiodarone can be useful as both a rate controlling and rhythm maintaining agent. Amiodarone is presumed safe in cardiac amyloidosis although systemic study is lacking. Patients must be monitored for the known toxicities, and the drug should be avoided in the presence of significant conduction disease (e.g., left bundle branch block) without pacemaker placement. Dronedarone as well as many other antiarrhythmic medications (typically of classes IA, IC and III) have not been well studied in cardiac amyloidosis. However, based on studies in patients with structural heart disease and heart failure, they should be considered as contraindicated in advanced amyloid patients at this time. Sudden death is often due to electromechanical dissociation; however, ventricular tachyarrhythmias are not infrequent.[102] The role of implantable cardioverter-defibrillator for primary prevention of sudden cardiac death in cardiac amyloid remains unclear and controversial. Strategies to reduce the elevated defibrillation thresholds in cardiac amyloidosis such as a subcutaneous array lead system may improve the efficacy of implantable cardioverter-defibrillator therapy.[141] The standard indications for pacing generally apply to cardiac amyloidosis,[142] but the threshold to introduce pacing is often lower in view of the propensity for the concomitant autonomic neuropathy and hypoalbuminemia to worsen any preexisting amyloidosis-related hemodynamic compromise.[43] Dual-chamber pacing may be particularly useful for optimizing the atrial filling component in this restrictive cardiomyopathy.[43] However, there is no evidence that the symptomatic improvement from pacing translates into increased survival.[143] The generally accepted indications for cardiac resynchronization therapy apply in cardiac amyloidosis.[144] There are currently no prospective randomized controlled trials evaluating the use of continuous intra-axial cardiac flow pumps and left ventricular assist devices, but one patient received the former in a feasibility study with subsequent symptom relief.[145]

### 6.2. Targeting the underlying amyloid pathology

This is an area of management that is specific to the type of amyloidosis, but the general aim is to decrease the formation new amyloid proteins and possibly facilitate the regression of existing deposits.[5, 43] Recent advancements in both our ability to diagnose the type of amyloidosis and the treatment options for the various types have greatly improved outcome.[43]

*AL amyloidosis*. The mainstay of treatment in this type of amyloidosis is targeting the pathogenic light chain-producing clonal plasma cells with chemotherapy.[146-152] This minimizes amyloid production (potentially reversing the disease process), preserves organ function and enhances survival.[153, 154] Indeed, immunoassays for free light chains are useful in monitoring the disease process and responses to treatment, and halving the aberrant monoclonal light chain on a sustained basis improves survival.[154] Reducing the circulating amyloidogenic precursor may result in some improvement in cardiac function even as the cardiac amyloid load found on echocardiography remains fairly constant.[129] These findings supports the direct toxic role of the aberrant monoclonal light chain on myocardial function that was shown in an animal model.[47] Moreover, similar findings were observed in other organs. For example, serial kidney biopsies in patients with AL amyloidosis before and after clinically successful treatments reveal unchanging amyloid burden despite significant improvement in proteinuria.[155, 156]

For patients who are fit for chemotherapy, several treatment regimens exist. The historic regimen of melphalan and prednisolone had responses that were few and much delayed;[157] more rapid responses are seen with intermediate-intensity regimens like melphalan and dexamethasone.[43] High-dose chemotherapy with autologous stem cell replacement has been attempted, but significant cardiac involvement precludes it given the high peri-treatment mortality.[5, 153] Many patients are diagnosed at a stage at which such an aggressive therapeutic modality is too toxic; early studies in which patients were not carefully selected for high-dose chemotherapy with autologous stem cell transplant had transplant-related mortality of nearly 50%.[5, 158] The presence of symptomatic and structural features of cardiac amyloidosis strongly predicts poor outcomes from autologous stem cell replacement,[159, 160] and the presence of clinical findings consistent with advanced disease, multiorgan involvement and poor functional status should preclude autologous stem cell therapy.[160, 161] Newer and investigational approaches include thalidomide or lenolidamide mono- or combination therapy,[151, 162, 163] rituximab to target CD20-positive plasma cell clones,[164] and the proteasome inhibitor bortezomib.[165-167] Heart transplantation is infrequently performed due to concerns about extracardiac disease progression as well as amyloid deposition in the transplant heart. Indeed heart transplant survival rates were lower in cardiac amyloidosis compared with other indications.[168, 169] Sequential heart and stem cell transplant is promising in young patients with cardiac failure and preserved extracardiac organ function, with a 1-year survival of between 75% and 83%.[170-173] While there are several predictors of prognosis, it is at present difficult to select patients for the appropriate treatment regimen.[5, 43] In some patients high-intensity regimens may be excessive, but in others the disease remains refractory even to the most intense of regimens.[43] Therefore highly-individualized management of cardiac amyloidosis is essential.[43]

*Familial amyloidosis.* Because plasma transthyretin is mainly synthesized in the liver, definitive treatment for familial amyloidosis requires liver transplantation to arrest the synthesis of amyloidogenic proteins, as well as transplantation of failed organs.[174] Outcomes are generally favorable in young and fit patients with the methionine 30 mutation. However, in older patients of the non-methionine 30 variants, paradoxical acceleration of disease progression has been reported, necessitating combined heart and liver transplants.[175-177] There is some evidence that transthyretin can be stabilized by certain nonsteroidal agents like diflunisal; clinical trials are necessary to investigate their efficacy in preventing disease progression.[178] These agents, however, may precipitate or aggravate congestive heart failure by fluid retention, and other agents are actively being sought.[179] One promising therapeutic candidate is tafamidis, a small-molecule transthyretin stabilizer which prevents transthyretin from forming amyloid fibrils. Tafamidis has demonstrated efficacy for the treatment of ATTR polyneuropathy, and has therefore been granted orphan drug status in the United States. Tafamidis is currently undergoing Phase II trials for the treatment of ATTR cardiomyopathy.[180]

*Reactive amyloidosis.* Definitive treatment involves treating the underlying inflammatory process and decreasing the serum amyloid A concentration, improving survival.[181] Inflammatory syndromes such as rheumatoid arthritis, Crohn's disease, seronegative spondyloarthropathies, and several periodic fever syndromes can be effectively treated with tumor necrosis factor and interleukin-1 inhibitors.[182] Familial Mediterranean fever can be treated with colchicine,[183] while excision of interleukin-6-secreting masses is an effective treatment for Castleman's disease.[184] A randomized controlled trial showed that eprodisate slows the decline of renal function in reactive amyloidosis, [185] and may have possible applicability to other types of amyloidosis.[186]

Currently, there is no known treatment that specifically targets senile amyloid, but research into this field is quickly evolving. Investigational approaches undergoing intensive research include targeted therapies that stabilize the soluble form of amyloidogenic proteins and reverse preexisting deposits. A new therapy based on epigallocatechin gallate, a compound that binds to denatured protein thereby inhibiting the formation of insoluble amyloid, has been proposed.[65] These potential new therapies offer exciting prospects for improvements in treatment.[43, 65]

## 7. Conclusion

Amyloidosis describes a heterogeneous group of several uncommon diseases by aberrant protein deposition in tissues throughout the body. Cardiac amyloidosis refers to clinically significant cardiac involvement, causing restrictive cardiomyopathy and its resultant effects, the most severe being congestive heart failure and arrhythmias. It is often underdiagnosed. However, recent advances in imaging have allowed us to accurately diagnose the condition and better characterize the degree of cardiac involvement. Cardiac biomarkers are useful in monitoring disease progression and response to therapy. The treatment of cardiac amyloidosis is rapidly evolving, and encompasses general supportive care of cardiac and extracardiac manifestations of the disease, and in addition, the management of the underlying amyloid disease process. Importance must be attached to early diagnosis of the disease, particularly in AL amyloidosis, because patients diagnosed late are often too ill to undergo disease-modifying chemotherapy. Novel therapies are actively being investigated and may present exciting new frontiers in the treatment of the disease.

## Author details

Glenn K. Lee[1], DaLi Feng[2], Martha Grogan[3], Cynthia Taub[4], Angela Dispenzieri[3] and Kyle W. Klarich[3]

1 Department of Medicine, National University Health System, Singapore

2 Metropolitan Heart and Vascular Institute, Minneapolis, MN, USA

3 Division of Cardiovascular Diseases, Mayo Clinic, Rochester, MN, USA

4 Division of Cardiology, Montefiore Medical Center, New York, NY, USA

## References

[1] Kyle RA, Linos A, Beard CM, et al. Incidence and natural history of primary systemic amyloidosis in Olmsted County, Minnesota, 1950 through 1989. Blood. Apr 1 1992;79(7):1817-1822.

[2] Falk RH, Comenzo RL, Skinner M. The systemic amyloidoses. N Engl J Med. Sep 25 1997;337(13):898-909.

[3] Hassan W, Al-Sergani H, Mourad W, Tabbaa R. Amyloid heart disease. New frontiers and insights in pathophysiology, diagnosis, and management. Tex Heart Inst J. 2005;32(2):178-184.

[4] Desai HV, Aronow WS, Peterson SJ, Frishman WH. Cardiac amyloidosis: approaches to diagnosis and management. Cardiol Rev. Jan-Feb 2010;18(1):1-11.

[5] Falk RH. Diagnosis and management of the cardiac amyloidoses. Circulation. Sep 27 2005;112(13):2047-2060.

[6] Merlini G, Palladini G. Amyloidosis: is a cure possible? Ann Oncol. Jun 2008;19 Suppl 4:iv63-66.

[7] Telio D, Bailey D, Chen C, Crump M, Reece D, Kukreti V. Two distinct syndromes of lymphoma-associated AL amyloidosis: a case series and review of the literature. Am J Hematol. Oct 2010;85(10):805-808.

[8] Perfetti V, Colli Vignarelli M, Anesi E, et al. The degrees of plasma cell clonality and marrow infiltration adversely influence the prognosis of AL amyloidosis patients. Haematologica. Mar 1999;84(3):218-221.

[9] Shah KB, Inoue Y, Mehra MR. Amyloidosis and the heart: a comprehensive review. Arch Intern Med. Sep 25 2006;166(17):1805-1813.

[10] Chee CE, Lacy MQ, Dogan A, Zeldenrust SR, Gertz MA. Pitfalls in the diagnosis of primary amyloidosis. Clin Lymphoma Myeloma Leuk. Jun 2010;10(3):177-180.

[11] Dubrey SW, Cha K, Anderson J, et al. The clinical features of immunoglobulin light-chain (AL) amyloidosis with heart involvement. QJM. Feb 1998;91(2):141-157.

[12] Kyle RA, Gertz MA. Primary systemic amyloidosis: clinical and laboratory features in 474 cases. Semin Hematol. Jan 1995;32(1):45-59.

[13] Feng D, Edwards WD, Oh JK, et al. Intracardiac thrombosis and embolism in patients with cardiac amyloidosis. Circulation. Nov 20 2007;116(21):2420-2426.

[14] Feng D, Syed IS, Martinez M, et al. Intracardiac thrombosis and anticoagulation therapy in cardiac amyloidosis. Circulation. May 12 2009;119(18):2490-2497.

[15] Merlini G, Westermark P. The systemic amyloidoses: clearer understanding of the molecular mechanisms offers hope for more effective therapies. J Intern Med. Feb 2004;255(2):159-178.

[16] Holmgren G, Holmberg E, Lindstrom A, et al. Diagnosis of familial amyloidotic polyneuropathy in Sweden by RFLP analysis. Clin Genet. Mar 1988;33(3):176-180.

[17] Jacobson DR, Buxbaum JN. Genetic aspects of amyloidosis. Adv Hum Genet. 1991;20:69-123, 309-111.

[18] Skare J, Yazici H, Erken E, et al. Homozygosity for the met30 transthyretin gene in a Turkish kindred with familial amyloidotic polyneuropathy. Hum Genet. Nov 1990;86(1):89-90.

[19] Jacobson DR, Pastore R, Pool S, et al. Revised transthyretin Ile 122 allele frequency in African-Americans. Hum Genet. Aug 1996;98(2):236-238.

[20] Jacobson DR, Pastore RD, Yaghoubian R, et al. Variant-sequence transthyretin (isoleucine 122) in late-onset cardiac amyloidosis in black Americans. N Engl J Med. Feb 13 1997;336(7):466-473.

[21] Westermark P, Sletten K, Johansson B, Cornwell GG, 3rd. Fibril in senile systemic amyloidosis is derived from normal transthyretin. Proc Natl Acad Sci U S A. Apr 1990;87(7):2843-2845.

[22] Cornwell GG, 3rd, Murdoch WL, Kyle RA, Westermark P, Pitkanen P. Frequency and distribution of senile cardiovascular amyloid. A clinicopathologic correlation. Am J Med. Oct 1983;75(4):618-623.

[23] Kawamura S, Takahashi M, Ishihara T, Uchino F. Incidence and distribution of isolated atrial amyloid: histologic and immunohistochemical studies of 100 aging hearts. Pathol Int. May 1995;45(5):335-342.

[24] Olson LJ, Gertz MA, Edwards WD, et al. Senile cardiac amyloidosis with myocardial dysfunction. Diagnosis by endomyocardial biopsy and immunohistochemistry. N Engl J Med. Sep 17 1987;317(12):738-742.

[25] Kyle RA, Spittell PC, Gertz MA, et al. The premortem recognition of systemic senile amyloidosis with cardiac involvement. Am J Med. Oct 1996;101(4):395-400.

[26] Pitkanen P, Westermark P, Cornwell GG, 3rd. Senile systemic amyloidosis. Am J Pathol. Dec 1984;117(3):391-399.

[27] Dubrey SW, Davidoff R, Skinner M, Bergethon P, Lewis D, Falk RH. Progression of ventricular wall thickening after liver transplantation for familial amyloidosis. Transplantation. Jul 15 1997;64(1):74-80.

[28] Kluve-Beckerman B, Dwulet FE, Benson MD. Human serum amyloid A. Three hepatic mRNAs and the corresponding proteins in one person. J Clin Invest. Nov 1988;82(5):1670-1675.

[29] Husby G. Amyloidosis and rheumatoid arthritis. Clin Exp Rheumatol. Apr-Jun 1985;3(2):173-180.

[30] Dubrey SW, Cha K, Simms RW, Skinner M, Falk RH. Electrocardiography and Doppler echocardiography in secondary (AA) amyloidosis. Am J Cardiol. Feb 1 1996;77(4):313-315.

[31] Gertz MA, Kyle RA. Secondary systemic amyloidosis: response and survival in 64 patients. Medicine (Baltimore). Jul 1991;70(4):246-256.

[32] Gejyo F, Yamada T, Odani S, et al. A new form of amyloid protein associated with chronic hemodialysis was identified as beta 2-microglobulin. Biochem Biophys Res Commun. Jun 28 1985;129(3):701-706.

[33] Gorevic PD, Casey TT, Stone WJ, DiRaimondo CR, Prelli FC, Frangione B. Beta-2 microglobulin is an amyloidogenic protein in man. J Clin Invest. Dec 1985;76(6): 2425-2429.

[34] Noel LH, Zingraff J, Bardin T, Atienza C, Kuntz D, Drueke T. Tissue distribution of dialysis amyloidosis. Clin Nephrol. Apr 1987;27(4):175-178.

[35] Gal R, Korzets A, Schwartz A, Rath-Wolfson L, Gafter U. Systemic distribution of beta 2-microglobulin-derived amyloidosis in patients who undergo long-term hemodialysis. Report of seven cases and review of the literature. Arch Pathol Lab Med. Jul 1994;118(7):718-721.

[36] Leone O, Boriani G, Chiappini B, et al. Amyloid deposition as a cause of atrial remodelling in persistent valvular atrial fibrillation. Eur Heart J. Jul 2004;25(14): 1237-1241.

[37] Looi LM. Isolated atrial amyloidosis: a clinicopathologic study indicating increased prevalence in chronic heart disease. Hum Pathol. Jun 1993;24(6):602-607.

[38] Rocken C, Peters B, Juenemann G, et al. Atrial amyloidosis: an arrhythmogenic substrate for persistent atrial fibrillation. Circulation. Oct 15 2002;106(16):2091-2097.

[39] Johansson B, Wernstedt C, Westermark P. Atrial natriuretic peptide deposited as atrial amyloid fibrils. Biochem Biophys Res Commun. Nov 13 1987;148(3):1087-1092.

[40] Kaye GC, Butler MG, d'Ardenne AJ, Edmondson SJ, Camm AJ, Slavin G. Isolated atrial amyloid contains atrial natriuretic peptide: a report of six cases. Br Heart J. Oct 1986;56(4):317-320.

[41] Levin ER, Gardner DG, Samson WK. Natriuretic peptides. N Engl J Med. Jul 30 1998;339(5):321-328.

[42] Westermark P, Johansson B, Natvig JB. Senile cardiac amyloidosis: evidence of two different amyloid substances in the ageing heart. Scand J Immunol. 1979;10(4): 303-308.

[43] Selvanayagam JB, Hawkins PN, Paul B, Myerson SG, Neubauer S. Evaluation and management of the cardiac amyloidosis. J Am Coll Cardiol. Nov 27 2007;50(22): 2101-2110.

[44] Volpi A, Cavalli A, Maggioni AP, Matturri L, Rossi L. Cardiac amyloidosis involving the conduction system and the aortocoronary neuroreceptors. Clinicopathologic correlates. Chest. Oct 1986;90(4):619-621.

[45] Brenner DA, Jain M, Pimentel DR, et al. Human amyloidogenic light chains directly impair cardiomyocyte function through an increase in cellular oxidant stress. Circ Res. Apr 30 2004;94(8):1008-1010.

[46] Muller D, Roessner A, Rocken C. Distribution pattern of matrix metalloproteinases 1, 2, 3, and 9, tissue inhibitors of matrix metalloproteinases 1 and 2, and alpha 2-macroglobulin in cases of generalized AA- and AL amyloidosis. Virchows Arch. Nov 2000;437(5):521-527.

[47] Liao R, Jain M, Teller P, et al. Infusion of light chains from patients with cardiac amyloidosis causes diastolic dysfunction in isolated mouse hearts. Circulation. Oct 2 2001;104(14):1594-1597.

[48] Smith TJ, Kyle RA, Lie JT. Clinical significance of histopathologic patterns of cardiac amyloidosis. Mayo Clin Proc. Aug 1984;59(8):547-555.

[49] Smith RR, Hutchins GM. Ischemic heart disease secondary to amyloidosis of intramyocardial arteries. Am J Cardiol. Sep 1979;44(3):413-417.

[50] James TN. Pathology of the cardiac conduction system in amyloidosis. Ann Intern Med. Jul 1966;65(1):28-36.

[51] Ridolfi RL, Bulkley BH, Hutchins GM. The conduction system in cardiac amyloidosis. Clinical and pathologic features of 23 patients. Am J Med. May 1977;62(5): 677-686.

[52] Gillmore JD, Lovat LB, Hawkins PN. Amyloidosis and the liver. J Hepatol. 1999;30 Suppl 1:17-33.

[53] Chopra S, Rubinow A, Koff RS, Cohen AS. Hepatic amyloidosis. A histopathologic analysis of primary (AL) and secondary (AA) forms. Am J Pathol. May 1984;115(2): 186-193.

[54] Daoud MS, Lust JA, Kyle RA, Pittelkow MR. Monoclonal gammopathies and associated skin disorders. J Am Acad Dermatol. Apr 1999;40(4):507-535; quiz 536-508.

[55] Rubinow A, Cohen AS. Skin involvement in generalized amyloidosis. A study of clinically involved and uninvolved skin in 50 patients with primary and secondary amyloidosis. Ann Intern Med. Jun 1978;88(6):781-785.

[56] Burroughs EI, Aronson AE, Duffy JR, Kyle RA. Speech disorders in systemic amyloidosis. Br J Disord Commun. Aug 1991;26(2):201-206.

[57] McCarthy RE, 3rd, Kasper EK. A review of the amyloidoses that infiltrate the heart. Clin Cardiol. Aug 1998;21(8):547-552.

[58] Murtagh B, Hammill SC, Gertz MA, Kyle RA, Tajik AJ, Grogan M. Electrocardiographic findings in primary systemic amyloidosis and biopsy-proven cardiac involvement. Am J Cardiol. Feb 15 2005;95(4):535-537.

[59] Mueller PS, Edwards WD, Gertz MA. Symptomatic ischemic heart disease resulting from obstructive intramural coronary amyloidosis. Am J Med. Aug 15 2000;109(3): 181-188.

[60] Ishikawa Y, Ishii T, Masuda S, et al. Myocardial ischemia due to vascular systemic amyloidosis: a quantitative analysis of autopsy findings on stenosis of the intramural coronary arteries. Pathol Int. Mar 1996;46(3):189-194.

[61] Narang R, Chopra P, Wasir HS. Cardiac amyloidosis presenting as ischemic heart disease. A case report and review of literature. Cardiology. 1993;82(4):294-300.

[62] Saffitz JE, Sazama K, Roberts WC. Amyloidosis limited to small arteries causing angina pectoris and sudden death. Am J Cardiol. Apr 1983;51(7):1234-1235.

[63] Schafer S, Schardt C, Burkhard-Meier U, Klein RM, Heintzen MP, Strauer BE. Angina pectoris and progressive fatigue in a 61-year-old man. Circulation. Dec 15 1996;94(12):3376-3381.

[64] Chamarthi B, Dubrey SW, Cha K, Skinner M, Falk RH. Features and prognosis of exertional syncope in light-chain associated AL cardiac amyloidosis. Am J Cardiol. Nov 1 1997;80(9):1242-1245.

[65] Halwani O, Delgado DH. Cardiac amyloidosis: an approach to diagnosis and management. Expert Rev Cardiovasc Ther. Jul 2010;8(7):1007-1013.

[66] Cueto-Garcia L, Tajik AJ, Kyle RA, et al. Serial echocardiographic observations in patients with primary systemic amyloidosis: an introduction to the concept of early (asymptomatic) amyloid infiltration of the heart. Mayo Clin Proc. Sep 1984;59(9): 589-597.

[67] Koyama J, Ray-Sequin PA, Davidoff R, Falk RH. Usefulness of pulsed tissue Doppler imaging for evaluating systolic and diastolic left ventricular function in patients with AL (primary) amyloidosis. Am J Cardiol. May 1 2002;89(9):1067-1071.

[68] Ha JW, Ommen SR, Tajik AJ, et al. Differentiation of constrictive pericarditis from restrictive cardiomyopathy using mitral annular velocity by tissue Doppler echocardiography. Am J Cardiol. Aug 1 2004;94(3):316-319.

[69] Butz T, Piper C, Langer C, et al. Diagnostic superiority of a combined assessment of the systolic and early diastolic mitral annular velocities by tissue Doppler imaging for the differentiation of restrictive cardiomyopathy from constrictive pericarditis. Clin Res Cardiol. Apr 2010;99(4):207-215.

[70] Chew C, Ziady GM, Raphael MJ, Oakley CM. The functional defect in amyloid heart disease. The "stiff heart" syndrome. Am J Cardiol. Oct 6 1975;36(4):438-444.

[71] Swanton RH, Brooksby IA, Davies MJ, Coltart DJ, Jenkins BS, Webb-Peploe MM. Systolic and diastolic ventricular function in cardiac amyloidosis. Studies in six cases diagnosed with endomyocardial biopsy. Am J Cardiol. May 4 1977;39(5):658-664.

[72] Klein AL, Hatle LK, Taliercio CP, et al. Serial Doppler echocardiographic follow-up of left ventricular diastolic function in cardiac amyloidosis. J Am Coll Cardiol. Nov 1990;16(5):1135-1141.

[73] Nishikawa H, Nishiyama S, Nishimura S, et al. Echocardiographic findings in nine patients with cardiac amyloidosis: their correlation with necropsy findings. J Cardiol. Mar 1988;18(1):121-133.

[74] Rahman JE, Helou EF, Gelzer-Bell R, et al. Noninvasive diagnosis of biopsy-proven cardiac amyloidosis. J Am Coll Cardiol. Feb 4 2004;43(3):410-415.

[75] Simons M, Isner JM. Assessment of relative sensitivities of noninvasive tests for cardiac amyloidosis in documented cardiac amyloidosis. Am J Cardiol. Feb 1 1992;69(4): 425-427.

[76] Bellavia D, Pellikka PA, Abraham TP, et al. Evidence of impaired left ventricular systolic function by Doppler myocardial imaging in patients with systemic amyloidosis and no evidence of cardiac involvement by standard two-dimensional and Doppler echocardiography. Am J Cardiol. Apr 1 2008;101(7):1039-1045.

[77] Bellavia D, Pellikka PA, Al-Zahrani GB, et al. Independent predictors of survival in primary systemic (Al) amyloidosis, including cardiac biomarkers and left ventricular strain imaging: an observational cohort study. J Am Soc Echocardiogr. Jun 2010;23(6): 643-652.

[78] Koyama J, Falk RH. Prognostic significance of strain Doppler imaging in light-chain amyloidosis. JACC Cardiovasc Imaging. Apr 2010;3(4):333-342.

[79] Koyama J, Ray-Sequin PA, Falk RH. Longitudinal myocardial function assessed by tissue velocity, strain, and strain rate tissue Doppler echocardiography in patients with AL (primary) cardiac amyloidosis. Circulation. May 20 2003;107(19):2446-2452.

[80] Hamer JP, Janssen S, van Rijswijk MH, Lie KI. Amyloid cardiomyopathy in systemic non-hereditary amyloidosis. Clinical, echocardiographic and electrocardiographic findings in 30 patients with AA and 24 patients with AL amyloidosis. Eur Heart J. May 1992;13(5):623-627.

[81] Siqueira-Filho AG, Cunha CL, Tajik AJ, Seward JB, Schattenberg TT, Giuliani ER. M-mode and two-dimensional echocardiographic features in cardiac amyloidosis. Circulation. Jan 1981;63(1):188-196.

[82] Bhandari AK, Nanda NC. Myocardial texture characterization by two-dimensional echocardiography. Am J Cardiol. Mar 1 1983;51(5):817-825.

[83] Child JS, Levisman JA, Abbasi AS, MacAlpin RN. Echocardiographic manifestations of infiltrative cardiomyopathy. A report of seven cases due to amyloid. Chest. Dec 1976;70(6):726-731.

[84] Falk RH, Plehn JF, Deering T, et al. Sensitivity and specificity of the echocardiographic features of cardiac amyloidosis. Am J Cardiol. Feb 15 1987;59(5):418-422.

[85] Maeda S, Tanaka T, Hayashi T. Familial atrial standstill caused by amyloidosis. Br Heart J. Apr 1988;59(4):498-500.

[86] Plehn JF, Southworth J, Cornwell GG, 3rd. Brief report: atrial systolic failure in primary amyloidosis. N Engl J Med. Nov 26 1992;327(22):1570-1573.

[87] Dingli D, Utz JP, Gertz MA. Pulmonary hypertension in patients with amyloidosis. Chest. Nov 2001;120(5):1735-1738.

[88] Smith RR, Hutchins GM, Moore GW, Humphrey RL. Type and distribution of pulmonary parenchymal and vascular amyloid. Correlation with cardiac amyloid. Am J Med. Jan 1979;66(1):96-104.

[89] Utz JP, Swensen SJ, Gertz MA. Pulmonary amyloidosis. The Mayo Clinic experience from 1980 to 1993. Ann Intern Med. Feb 15 1996;124(4):407-413.

[90] Migrino RQ, Mareedu RK, Eastwood D, Bowers M, Harmann L, Hari P. Left ventricular ejection time on echocardiography predicts long-term mortality in light chain amyloidosis. J Am Soc Echocardiogr. Dec 2009;22(12):1396-1402.

[91] Belkin RN, Kupersmith AC, Khalique O, et al. A Novel Two-Dimensional Echocardiographic Finding in Cardiac Amyloidosis. Echocardiography. Jun 24 2010.

[92] Porciani MC, Cappelli F, Perfetto F, et al. Rotational mechanics of the left ventricle in Al amyloidosis. Echocardiography. Oct 2010;27(9):1061-1068.

[93] Migrino RQ, Harmann L, Woods T, Bright M, Truran S, Hari P. Intraventricular dyssynchrony in light chain amyloidosis: a new mechanism of systolic dysfunction assessed by 3-dimensional echocardiography. Cardiovasc Ultrasound. 2008;6:40.

[94] Kim WH, Otsuji Y, Yuasa T, Minagoe S, Seward JB, Tei C. Evaluation of right ventricular dysfunction in patients with cardiac amyloidosis using Tei index. J Am Soc Echocardiogr. Jan 2004;17(1):45-49.

[95] Abdelmoneim SS, Bernier M, Bellavia D, et al. Myocardial contrast echocardiography in biopsy-proven primary cardiac amyloidosis. Eur J Echocardiogr. Mar 2008;9(2): 338-341.

[96] Santarone M, Corrado G, Tagliagambe LM, et al. Atrial thrombosis in cardiac amyloidosis: diagnostic contribution of transesophageal echocardiography. J Am Soc Echocardiogr. Jun 1999;12(6):533-536.

[97] Dubrey S, Pollak A, Skinner M, Falk RH. Atrial thrombi occurring during sinus rhythm in cardiac amyloidosis: evidence for atrial electromechanical dissociation. Br Heart J. Nov 1995;74(5):541-544.

[98] Roberts WC, Waller BF. Cardiac amyloidosis causing cardiac dysfunction: analysis of 54 necropsy patients. Am J Cardiol. Jul 1983;52(1):137-146.

[99] Sloan KP, Bruce CJ, Oh JK, Rihal CS. Complications of echocardiography-guided endomyocardial biopsy. J Am Soc Echocardiogr. Mar 2009;22(3):324 e321-324.

[100] Dubrey SW, Bilazarian S, LaValley M, Reisinger J, Skinner M, Falk RH. Signal-averaged electrocardiography in patients with AL (primary) amyloidosis. Am Heart J. Dec 1997;134(6):994-1001.

[101] Kyle RA. Amyloidosis. Circulation. Feb 15 1995;91(4):1269-1271.

[102] Falk RH, Rubinow A, Cohen AS. Cardiac arrhythmias in systemic amyloidosis: correlation with echocardiographic abnormalities. J Am Coll Cardiol. Jan 1984;3(1): 107-113.

[103] Reyners AK, Hazenberg BP, Reitsma WD, Smit AJ. Heart rate variability as a predictor of mortality in patients with AA and AL amyloidosis. Eur Heart J. Jan 2002;23(2): 157-161.

[104] Kinoshita O, Hongo M, Saikawa Y, et al. Heart rate variability in patients with familial amyloid polyneuropathy. Pacing Clin Electrophysiol. Dec 1997;20(12 Pt 1): 2949-2953.

[105] Takigawa M, Hashimura K, Ishibashi-Ueda H, et al. Annual electrocardiograms consistent with silent progression of cardiac involvement in sporadic familial amyloid polyneuropathy: a case report. Intern Med. 2010;49(2):139-144.

[106] Selvanayagam JB, Leong DP. MR Imaging and Cardiac Amyloidosis Where to Go From Here? JACC Cardiovasc Imaging. Feb 2010;3(2):165-167.

[107] Syed IS, Glockner JF, Feng D, et al. Role of cardiac magnetic resonance imaging in the detection of cardiac amyloidosis. JACC Cardiovasc Imaging. Feb 2010;3(2):155-164.

[108] Maceira AM, Joshi J, Prasad SK, et al. Cardiovascular magnetic resonance in cardiac amyloidosis. Circulation. Jan 18 2005;111(2):186-193.

[109] Vogelsberg H, Mahrholdt H, Deluigi CC, et al. Cardiovascular magnetic resonance in clinically suspected cardiac amyloidosis: noninvasive imaging compared to endomyocardial biopsy. J Am Coll Cardiol. Mar 11 2008;51(10):1022-1030.

[110] Hosch W, Bock M, Libicher M, et al. MR-relaxometry of myocardial tissue: significant elevation of T1 and T2 relaxation times in cardiac amyloidosis. Invest Radiol. Sep 2007;42(9):636-642.

[111] Pellikka PA, Holmes DR, Jr., Edwards WD, Nishimura RA, Tajik AJ, Kyle RA. Endomyocardial biopsy in 30 patients with primary amyloidosis and suspected cardiac involvement. Arch Intern Med. Mar 1988;148(3):662-666.

[112] Mekinian A, Lions C, Leleu X, et al. Prognosis assessment of cardiac involvement in systemic AL amyloidosis by magnetic resonance imaging. Am J Med. Sep 2010;123(9):864-868.

[113] Austin BA, Tang WH, Rodriguez ER, et al. Delayed hyper-enhancement magnetic resonance imaging provides incremental diagnostic and prognostic utility in suspected cardiac amyloidosis. JACC Cardiovasc Imaging. Dec 2009;2(12):1369-1377.

[114] Falk RH, Dubrey SW. Amyloid heart disease. Prog Cardiovasc Dis. Jan-Feb 2010;52(4):347-361.

[115] Zou Z, Zhang HL, Roditi GH, Leiner T, Kucharczyk W, Prince MR. Nephrogenic systemic fibrosis: review of 370 biopsy-confirmed cases. JACC Cardiovasc Imaging. Nov 2011;4(11):1206-1216.

[116] Glaudemans AW, Slart RH, Zeebregts CJ, et al. Nuclear imaging in cardiac amyloidosis. Eur J Nucl Med Mol Imaging. Apr 2009;36(4):702-714.

[117] Perugini E, Guidalotti PL, Salvi F, et al. Noninvasive etiologic diagnosis of cardiac amyloidosis using 99mTc-3,3-diphosphono-1,2-propanodicarboxylic acid scintigraphy. J Am Coll Cardiol. Sep 20 2005;46(6):1076-1084.

[118] Lachmann HJ, Booth DR, Booth SE, et al. Misdiagnosis of hereditary amyloidosis as AL (primary) amyloidosis. N Engl J Med. Jun 6 2002;346(23):1786-1791.

[119] Duston MA, Skinner M, Shirahama T, Cohen AS. Diagnosis of amyloidosis by abdominal fat aspiration. Analysis of four years' experience. Am J Med. Mar 1987;82(3): 412-414.

[120] Libbey CA, Skinner M, Cohen AS. Use of abdominal fat tissue aspirate in the diagnosis of systemic amyloidosis. Arch Intern Med. Aug 1983;143(8):1549-1552.

[121] Westermark P, Stenkvist B. A new method for the diagnosis of systemic amyloidosis. Arch Intern Med. Oct 1973;132(4):522-523.

[122] Nordlinger M, Magnani B, Skinner M, Falk RH. Is elevated plasma B-natriuretic peptide in amyloidosis simply a function of the presence of heart failure? Am J Cardiol. Oct 1 2005;96(7):982-984.

[123] Miller WL, Wright RS, McGregor CG, et al. Troponin levels in patients with amyloid cardiomyopathy undergoing cardiac transplantation. Am J Cardiol. Oct 1 2001;88(7): 813-815.

[124] Takemura G, Takatsu Y, Doyama K, et al. Expression of atrial and brain natriuretic peptides and their genes in hearts of patients with cardiac amyloidosis. J Am Coll Cardiol. Mar 15 1998;31(4):754-765.

[125] Kristen AV, Giannitsis E, Lehrke S, et al. Assessment of disease severity and outcome in patients with systemic light-chain amyloidosis by the high-sensitivity troponin T assay. Blood. Oct 7 2010;116(14):2455-2461.

[126] Dispenzieri A, Gertz MA, Kyle RA, et al. Serum cardiac troponins and N-terminal pro-brain natriuretic peptide: a staging system for primary systemic amyloidosis. J Clin Oncol. Sep 15 2004;22(18):3751-3757.

[127] Dispenzieri A, Gertz MA, Kyle RA, et al. Prognostication of survival using cardiac troponins and N-terminal pro-brain natriuretic peptide in patients with primary systemic amyloidosis undergoing peripheral blood stem cell transplantation. Blood. Sep 15 2004;104(6):1881-1887.

[128] Dispenzieri A, Kyle RA, Gertz MA, et al. Survival in patients with primary systemic amyloidosis and raised serum cardiac troponins. Lancet. May 24 2003;361(9371): 1787-1789.

[129] Palladini G, Lavatelli F, Russo P, et al. Circulating amyloidogenic free light chains and serum N-terminal natriuretic peptide type B decrease simultaneously in association with improvement of survival in AL. Blood. May 15 2006;107(10):3854-3858.

[130] Palladini G, Barassi A, Klersy C, et al. The combination of high-sensitivity cardiac troponin T (hs-cTnT) at presentation and changes in N-terminal natriuretic peptide type B (NT-proBNP) after chemotherapy best predicts survival in AL amyloidosis. Blood. Nov 4 2010;116(18):3426-3430.

[131] Kumar S, Dispenzieri A, Lacy MQ, et al. Serum uric acid: novel prognostic factor in primary systemic amyloidosis. Mayo Clin Proc. Mar 2008;83(3):297-303.

[132] Kumar SK, Gertz MA, Lacy MQ, et al. Recent improvements in survival in primary systemic amyloidosis and the importance of an early mortality risk score. Mayo Clin Proc. Jan 2011;86(1):12-18.

[133] Dispenzieri A, Lacy MQ, Katzmann JA, et al. Absolute values of immunoglobulin free light chains are prognostic in patients with primary systemic amyloidosis undergoing peripheral blood stem cell transplantation. Blood. Apr 15 2006;107(8): 3378-3383.

[134] Cassidy JT. Cardiac amyloidosis. Two cases with digitalis sensitivity. Ann Intern Med. Dec 1961;55:989-994.

[135] Rubinow A, Skinner M, Cohen AS. Digoxin sensitivity in amyloid cardiomyopathy. Circulation. Jun 1981;63(6):1285-1288.

[136] Gertz MA, Falk RH, Skinner M, Cohen AS, Kyle RA. Worsening of congestive heart failure in amyloid heart disease treated by calcium channel-blocking agents. Am J Cardiol. Jun 1 1985;55(13 Pt 1):1645.

[137] Griffiths BE, Hughes P, Dowdle R, Stephens MR. Cardiac amyloidosis with asymmetrical septal hypertrophy and deterioration after nifedipine. Thorax. Sep 1982;37(9):711-712.

[138] Pollak A, Falk RH. Left ventricular systolic dysfunction precipitated by verapamil in cardiac amyloidosis. Chest. Aug 1993;104(2):618-620.

[139] Berk JL, Keane J, Seldin DC, et al. Persistent pleural effusions in primary systemic amyloidosis: etiology and prognosis. Chest. Sep 2003;124(3):969-977.

[140] Modesto KM, Dispenzieri A, Cauduro SA, et al. Left atrial myopathy in cardiac amyloidosis: implications of novel echocardiographic techniques. Eur Heart J. Jan 2005;26(2):173-179.

[141] Dhoble A, Khasnis A, Olomu A, Thakur R. Cardiac amyloidosis treated with an implantable cardioverter defibrillator and subcutaneous array lead system: report of a case and literature review. Clin Cardiol. Aug 2009;32(8):E63-65.

[142] Epstein AE, DiMarco JP, Ellenbogen KA, et al. ACC/AHA/HRS 2008 Guidelines for Device-Based Therapy of Cardiac Rhythm Abnormalities: a report of the American College of Cardiology/American Heart Association Task Force on Practice Guidelines (Writing Committee to Revise the ACC/AHA/NASPE 2002 Guideline Update for Implantation of Cardiac Pacemakers and Antiarrhythmia Devices) developed in collaboration with the American Association for Thoracic Surgery and Society of Thoracic Surgeons. J Am Coll Cardiol. May 27 2008;51(21):e1-62.

[143] Mathew V, Olson LJ, Gertz MA, Hayes DL. Symptomatic conduction system disease in cardiac amyloidosis. Am J Cardiol. Dec 1 1997;80(11):1491-1492.

[144] Strickberger SA, Conti J, Daoud EG, et al. Patient selection for cardiac resynchronization therapy: from the Council on Clinical Cardiology Subcommittee on Electrocardiography and Arrhythmias and the Quality of Care and Outcomes Research Interdisciplinary Working Group, in collaboration with the Heart Rhythm Society. Circulation. Apr 26 2005;111(16):2146-2150.

[145] Siegenthaler MP, Westaby S, Frazier OH, et al. Advanced heart failure: feasibility study of long-term continuous axial flow pump support. Eur Heart J. May 2005;26(10):1031-1038.

[146] De Lorenzi E, Giorgetti S, Grossi S, Merlini G, Caccialanza G, Bellotti V. Pharmaceutical strategies against amyloidosis: old and new drugs in targeting a "protein misfolding disease". Curr Med Chem. Apr 2004;11(8):1065-1084.

[147] Sanchorawala V, Wright DG, Seldin DC, et al. High-dose intravenous melphalan and autologous stem cell transplantation as initial therapy or following two cycles of oral chemotherapy for the treatment of AL amyloidosis: results of a prospective randomized trial. Bone Marrow Transplant. Feb 2004;33(4):381-388.

[148] Gertz MA, Lacy MQ, Dispenzieri A. Therapy for immunoglobulin light chain amyloidosis: the new and the old. Blood Rev. Mar 2004;18(1):17-37.

[149] Palladini G, Perfetti V, Obici L, et al. Association of melphalan and high-dose dexamethasone is effective and well tolerated in patients with AL (primary) amyloidosis who are ineligible for stem cell transplantation. Blood. Apr 15 2004;103(8):2936-2938.

[150] Sanchorawala V, Wright DG, Seldin DC, et al. Low-dose continuous oral melphalan for the treatment of primary systemic (AL) amyloidosis. Br J Haematol. Jun 2002;117(4):886-889.

[151] Seldin DC, Choufani EB, Dember LM, et al. Tolerability and efficacy of thalidomide for the treatment of patients with light chain-associated (AL) amyloidosis. Clin Lymphoma. Mar 2003;3(4):241-246.

[152] Skinner M, Sanchorawala V, Seldin DC, et al. High-dose melphalan and autologous stem-cell transplantation in patients with AL amyloidosis: an 8-year study. Ann Intern Med. Jan 20 2004;140(2):85-93.

[153] Goodman HJ, Gillmore JD, Lachmann HJ, Wechalekar AD, Bradwell AR, Hawkins PN. Outcome of autologous stem cell transplantation for AL amyloidosis in the UK. Br J Haematol. Aug 2006;134(4):417-425.

[154] Lachmann HJ, Gallimore R, Gillmore JD, et al. Outcome in systemic AL amyloidosis in relation to changes in concentration of circulating free immunoglobulin light chains following chemotherapy. Br J Haematol. Jul 2003;122(1):78-84.

[155] Kyle RA, Wagoner RD, Holley KE. Primary systemic amyloidosis: resolution of the nephrotic syndrome with melphalan and prednisone. Arch Intern Med. Aug 1982;142(8):1445-1447.

[156] Zeier M, Perz J, Linke RP, et al. No regression of renal AL amyloid in monoclonal gammopathy after successful autologous blood stem cell transplantation and significant clinical improvement. Nephrol Dial Transplant. Dec 2003;18(12):2644-2647.

[157] Kyle RA, Gertz MA, Greipp PR, et al. A trial of three regimens for primary amyloidosis: colchicine alone, melphalan and prednisone, and melphalan, prednisone, and colchicine. N Engl J Med. Apr 24 1997;336(17):1202-1207.

[158] Moreau P. Autologous stem cell transplantation for AL amyloidosis: a standard therapy? Leukemia. Dec 1999;13(12):1929-1931.

[159] Moreau P, Leblond V, Bourquelot P, et al. Prognostic factors for survival and response after high-dose therapy and autologous stem cell transplantation in systemic AL amyloidosis: a report on 21 patients. Br J Haematol. Jun 1998;101(4):766-769.

[160] Saba N, Sutton D, Ross H, et al. High treatment-related mortality in cardiac amyloid patients undergoing autologous stem cell transplant. Bone Marrow Transplant. Oct 1999;24(8):853-855.

[161] Comenzo RL, Gertz MA. Autologous stem cell transplantation for primary systemic amyloidosis. Blood. Jun 15 2002;99(12):4276-4282.

[162] Cohen AD, Zhou P, Chou J, et al. Risk-adapted autologous stem cell transplantation with adjuvant dexamethasone +/- thalidomide for systemic light-chain amyloidosis: results of a phase II trial. Br J Haematol. Oct 2007;139(2):224-233.

[163] Palladini G, Russo P, Lavatelli F, et al. Treatment of patients with advanced cardiac AL amyloidosis with oral melphalan, dexamethasone, and thalidomide. Ann Hematol. Apr 2009;88(4):347-350.

[164] Terrier B, Jaccard A, Harousseau JL, et al. The clinical spectrum of IgM-related amyloidosis: a French nationwide retrospective study of 72 patients. Medicine (Baltimore). Mar 2008;87(2):99-109.

[165] Lamm W, Willenbacher W, Lang A, et al. Efficacy of the combination of bortezomib and dexamethasone in systemic AL amyloidosis. Ann Hematol. Sep 7 2010.

[166] Kastritis E, Wechalekar AD, Dimopoulos MA, et al. Bortezomib with or without dexamethasone in primary systemic (light chain) amyloidosis. J Clin Oncol. Feb 20 2010;28(6):1031-1037.

[167] Reece DE, Sanchorawala V, Hegenbart U, et al. Weekly and twice-weekly bortezomib in patients with systemic AL amyloidosis: results of a phase 1 dose-escalation study. Blood. Aug 20 2009;114(8):1489-1497.

[168] Kpodonu J, Massad MG, Caines A, Geha AS. Outcome of heart transplantation in patients with amyloid cardiomyopathy. J Heart Lung Transplant. Nov 2005;24(11): 1763-1765.

[169] Dubrey SW, Burke MM, Hawkins PN, Banner NR. Cardiac transplantation for amyloid heart disease: the United Kingdom experience. J Heart Lung Transplant. Oct 2004;23(10):1142-1153.

[170] Gillmore JD, Goodman HJ, Lachmann HJ, et al. Sequential heart and autologous stem cell transplantation for systemic AL amyloidosis. Blood. Feb 1 2006;107(3): 1227-1229.

[171] Maurer MS, Raina A, Hesdorffer C, et al. Cardiac transplantation using extended-donor criteria organs for systemic amyloidosis complicated by heart failure. Transplantation. Mar 15 2007;83(5):539-545.

[172] Dey BR, Chung SS, Spitzer TR, et al. Cardiac transplantation followed by dose-intensive melphalan and autologous stem-cell transplantation for light chain amyloidosis and heart failure. Transplantation. Oct 27 2010;90(8):905-911.

[173] Kristen AV, Sack FU, Schonland SO, et al. Staged heart transplantation and chemotherapy as a treatment option in patients with severe cardiac light-chain amyloidosis. Eur J Heart Fail. Oct 2009;11(10):1014-1020.

[174] Suhr OB, Herlenius G, Friman S, Ericzon BG. Liver transplantation for hereditary transthyretin amyloidosis. Liver Transpl. May 2000;6(3):263-276.

[175] Stangou AJ, Hawkins PN. Liver transplantation in transthyretin-related familial amyloid polyneuropathy. Curr Opin Neurol. Oct 2004;17(5):615-620.

[176] Ruygrok PN, Gane EJ, McCall JL, Chen XZ, Haydock DA, Munn SR. Combined heart and liver transplantation for familial amyloidosis. Intern Med J. Jan-Feb 2001;31(1): 66-67.

[177] Barreiros AP, Post F, Hoppe-Lotichius M, et al. Liver transplantation and combined liver-heart transplantation in patients with familial amyloid polyneuropathy: a single-center experience. Liver Transpl. Mar 2010;16(3):314-323.

[178] Miller SR, Sekijima Y, Kelly JW. Native state stabilization by NSAIDs inhibits transthyretin amyloidogenesis from the most common familial disease variants. Lab Invest. May 2004;84(5):545-552.

[179] Lachmann HJ, Hawkins PN. Novel pharmacological strategies in amyloidosis. Nephron Clin Pract. 2003;94(4):c85-88.

[180] Jones D. Modifying protein misfolding. Nat Rev Drug Discov. Nov 2010;9(11): 825-827.

[181] Gillmore JD, Lovat LB, Persey MR, Pepys MB, Hawkins PN. Amyloid load and clinical outcome in AA amyloidosis in relation to circulating concentration of serum amyloid A protein. Lancet. Jul 7 2001;358(9275):24-29.

[182] Gottenberg JE, Merle-Vincent F, Bentaberry F, et al. Anti-tumor necrosis factor alpha therapy in fifteen patients with AA amyloidosis secondary to inflammatory arthritides: a followup report of tolerability and efficacy. Arthritis Rheum. Jul 2003;48(7): 2019-2024.

[183] Zemer D, Pras M, Sohar E, Modan M, Cabili S, Gafni J. Colchicine in the prevention and treatment of the amyloidosis of familial Mediterranean fever. N Engl J Med. Apr 17 1986;314(16):1001-1005.

[184] Lachmann HJ, Gilbertson JA, Gillmore JD, Hawkins PN, Pepys MB. Unicentric Castleman's disease complicated by systemic AA amyloidosis: a curable disease. QJM. Apr 2002;95(4):211-218.

[185] Dember LM, Hawkins PN, Hazenberg BP, et al. Eprodisate for the treatment of renal disease in AA amyloidosis. N Engl J Med. Jun 7 2007;356(23):2349-2360.

[186] Manenti L, Tansinda P, Vaglio A. Eprodisate in amyloid A amyloidosis: a novel therapeutic approach? Expert Opin Pharmacother. Aug 2008;9(12):2175-2180.

Chapter 4

# Dialysis-Related Amyloidosis: Pathogenesis and Clinical Features in Patients Undergoing Dialysis Treatment

Suguru Yamamoto, Junichiro James Kazama,
Hiroki Maruyama and Ichiei Narita

Additional information is available at the end of the chapter

http://dx.doi.org/10.5772/53390

## 1. Introduction

Amyloidosis is defined as an insoluble protein fibril that is deposited, mainly, in the extracellular spaces of organs and tissues as a result of a sequence of changes in protein folding. Precursor proteins change their conformation that forms amyloid fibrils, then deposited amyloid induce organ damage with disease specific conditions.

To date, there are 27 types of amyloidosis known extracellular fibril proteins in human, and each amyloidosis is characterized amyloid protein precursor, systemic (S) or localized organ (L), and syndrome or involved tissues [1]. In the nomenclature, dialysis-related amyloidosis (DRA) is defined as $\beta_2$-microglobulin-related (A$\beta_2$M) amyloid which precursor protein is $\beta_2$-microglobulin ($\beta_2$-m). It is associated to dialysis, a kidney replacement therapy, and deposits in systemic (S), mainly joint tissues [1].

Long-term dialysis treatment for end-stage kidney disease often induces the A$\beta_2$-m amyloid deposition in mainly osteoarticular tissues that induces various disorders, such as carpal tunnel syndrome (CTS), destructive spondyloarthropathy (DSA), and cystic bone lesions as well as in systemic organs such as heart and gastrointestinal tract when disease advances. Several biomolecules including $\beta_2$-m as well as clinical risk factors are thought to relate with A$\beta_2$M amyloidogenesis (Figure 1). Recent progress of dialysis therapy has improved survival of dialysis patients, however, older age and long-term dialysis treatment may increase the onset and acceleration of DRA. In this article, we described about DRA focused on pathogenesis, clinical manifestations and treatment, and showed DRA is still one of serious complications for patients undergoing long-term dialysis treatment.

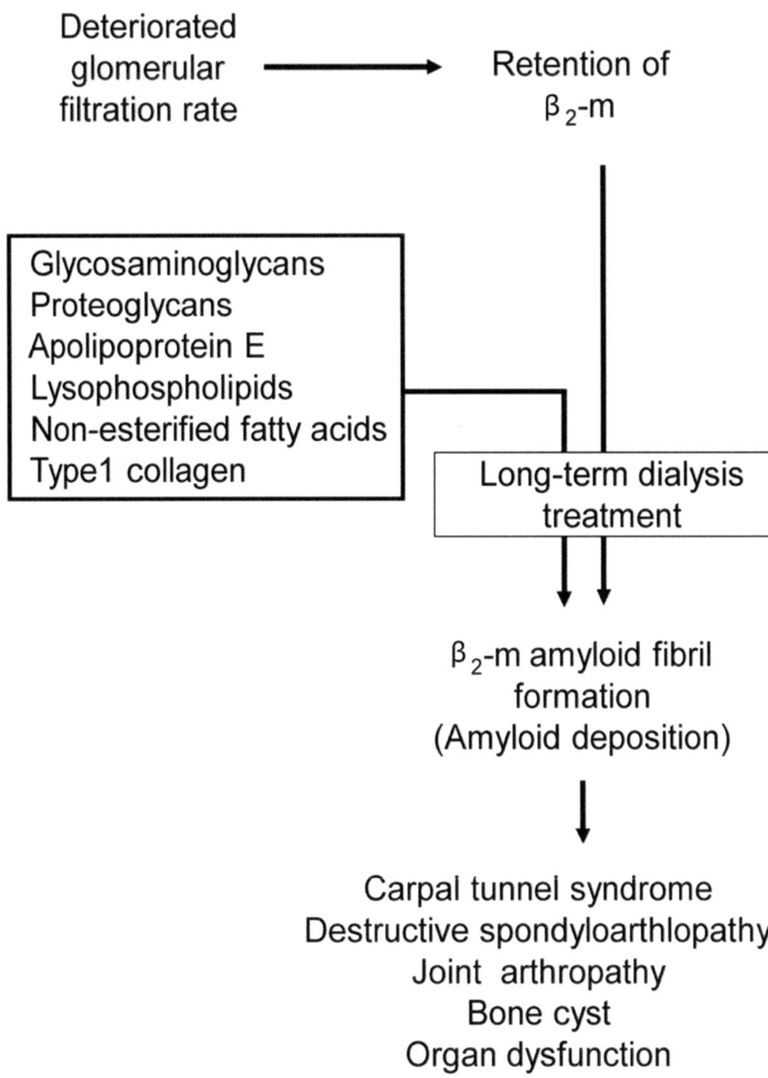


**Figure 1.** Pathogenesis of dialysis-related amyloidosis (DRA). DRA is induced not only accumulation of $\beta_2$-microglobulin but also several biomolecules and clinical risk factors.

## 2. Pathogenesis of dialysis-related amyloidosis

### 2.1. $\beta_2$-microglobulin

$\beta_2$-m is a polypeptide of 99 residues that has a molecular weight of 11.8 kDa. It forms the beta chain of the human leukocyte antigen (HLA) class I molecule and has a well-known β-sandwich structure that involves a 7-strand β-pleated structure stabilized with a single disulphide bond (Cys25-Cys80). $\beta_2$-m changes the conformation under various *in vivo* or *in vitro* conditions, such as acidic pH [2], 2,2,2-trifluoroethanol (TFE) [3], sodium dodecyl sulfate (SDS) [4], lysophospholipids [5], non-esterified fatty acids [6], heating [7] and agitation [8]. Proper dose of those molecules induce conformational intermediate that is required for A$\beta_2$M amyloid fibril formation/extension (see below section).

### 2.2. Retention of conformational intermediate-$\beta_2$-m

$\beta_2$-m is a component of MHC class I molecules, which are present on all nucleated cells. Most $\beta_2$-m is normally eliminated by the kidney via glomerular filtration and subsequent tubular catabolism with Megalin [9]. Thus, severe kidney damage induces the retention of $\beta_2$-m in serum due to impaired excretion from the kidney.

Some clinical studies have attempted to identify the conformational intermediate form of circulating $\beta_2$-m. Capillary electrophoresis reveals that patients undergoing hemodialysis due to end-stage kidney disease, but not healthy control subjects, have the conformational intermediate form of $\beta_2$-m in serum [10]. The level of predialysis serum $\beta_2$-m intermediate was 2.7±1.4 mg/L and native $\beta_2$-m was 29.4±6.8 mg/L in 31 hemodialysis patients. Hemodialysis using a polymethylmethacrylate and online hemodiafiltration with a polysulfone membrane decreased the level of the native form, while any change in the intermediate form was variable [10]. These results suggest that intermediate $\beta_2$-m is increased in hemodialysis patients and is difficult to remove with dialysis treatment. It may suggest that the intermediate form is immobilized in the extracellular space where A$\beta_2$-m amyloid has a marked affinity for joint tissues (cartilage, capsule, and synovium). In addition, immunoaffinity–liquid chromatography–mass spectrometry analysis and immunoassay revealed the generation of lysine-58–cleaved and truncated $\beta_2$-m ($\Delta$K58-$\beta_2$-m), which was found in serum from 20–40% HD patients but not in serum from control subjects [11]. However, this truncated form has not been demonstrated in the tissue containing A$\beta_2$-m amyloid [12]. It is not certain whether the conformational intermediate or the truncated form of $\beta_2$-m has a critical role of onset/progress of DRA, and future studies will be needed to understand the pathogenesis for A$\beta_2$-m amyloid fibrils formation/extension.

### 2.3. A$\beta_2$-m amyloid fibril formation and extension

A nucleation-dependent polymerization model explains the general mechanisms of amyloid fibril formation in vitro, in various types of amyloidosis [13-18]. This model consists of two phases, i.e., nucleation and extension phases. Nucleus formation requires a series of association steps of monomers, which are thermodynamically unfavorable, representing the rate-limiting step in amyloid fibril formation in vitro. Once the nucleus (n-mer) has been formed, further addition of monomers to the nucleus becomes thermodynamically favorable, resulting in rapid extension of amyloid fibrils according to a first-order kinetic model, i.e., via the consecutive association of precursor proteins onto the ends of existing fibrils [14, 17, 18].

In the mechanism of amyloidogenesis from $\beta_2$-m, natively folded proteins, partial unfolding of protein is prerequisite to its assembly into amyloid fibrils [3, 13, 19, 20]. The extension of

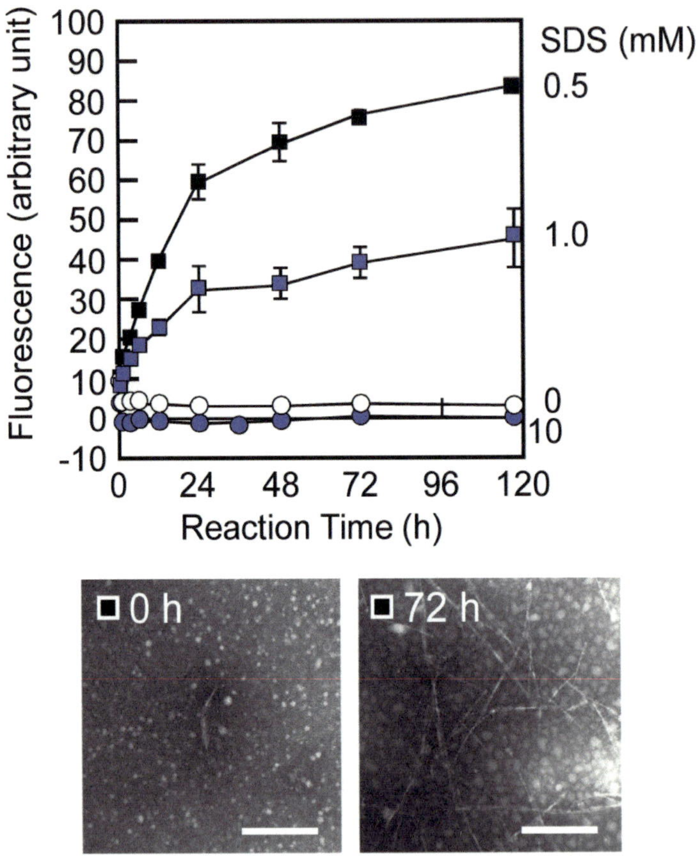


**Figure 2.** $\beta_2$-microglobulin-related ($A\beta_2M$) amyloid fibril extension in vitro. Sub-micellar concentration of sodium dodecyl sulfate (SDS) induces $A\beta_2M$ amyloid fibrils extension at a neutral pH while micellar concentration induces amyloid fibril depolimerization in vitro. The amount of extended fibrils is measured by Thioflavin T (A), and observed by electron microscopy (B). Bar shows 250 nm.

$A\beta_2M$ amyloid fibrils, as well as the formation of the fibrils from $\beta_2$-m are greatly dependent on the pH of the reaction mixture, with the optimum pH around 2.0-3.0 [13, 14]. At pH 2.5, where the extension of $A\beta_2M$ amyloid fibrils is optimum, $\beta_2$-m loses much of the secondary and tertiary structures observed at pH 7.5 [13, 19]. $A\beta_2M$ amyloid fibrils readily depolymerize into monomeric $\beta_2$-m at a neutral pH [19], however, low concentration of TFE [3] and sub-micellar concentration of SDS [4] induced $A\beta_2M$ amyloid fibrils extension with changing conformation of $\beta_2$-m monomer and inhibiting depolymerization of amyloid fibrils at a neutral pH in vitro (Figure 2). While TFE and SDS are organic compounds, several biomolecules could induce $A\beta_2M$ amyloidogenesis in vivo, such as apolipoprotein E, proteoglycans, glicosaminoglycans, type1 collagen, non-esterified fatty acid, and lysophospholipids. [4-6, 21, 22]. For example, some lysophospholipids, especially lysophosphatidic acid (LPA) induces both

http://dx.doi.org/10.5772/53390

amyloid fibril formation and extension at a neutral pH [5]. The mechanism of amyloidogenesis is due to make $\beta_2$-m monomer into partially unfolding the compact structure as well as stabilizing the extended fibrils in vitro. Clinically, plasma LPA concentration is higher in patients undergoing hemodialysis treatment as compare to healthy subjects [5]. It's unclear the local concentration of lysophospholipids in the lesion that A$\beta_2$M amyloid deposits, it may be reasonable to consider the reaction between $\beta_2$-m and lysophospholipids that are increased in chronic kidney disease (CKD) undergoing dialysis treatment. Joint tissues that A$\beta_2$M amyloid deposits at early stage in dialysis patients, contains many kinds of glycosaminoglycans and proteoglycans. Depolymerization of A$\beta_2$M amyloid fibrils at a neutral pH in vitro was inhibited dose-dependently by the presence of some glycosaminoglycans (heparin, dermatan sulfate or heparin sulfate) or proteoglycans (biglycan, decorin or keratan sulfate proteoglycan) [21]. In addition, some glycosaminoglycans, especially heparin, enhanced the A$\beta_2$M amyloid fibril extension induced by low concentration of TFE at a neutral pH [3]. These results suggest that some glycosaminoglycans and proteoglycans stabilize extended A$\beta_2$M amyloid fibrils possibly by binding directly to the surface of the fibrils in vivo. Heparin is widely used for the hemodialysis treatment as an anticoagulant. Although no significant difference in the prevalence of A$\beta_2$M amyloidosis was found between continuous ambulatory peritoneal dialysis patients and hemodialysis patients carefully matched for time on dialysis and age at the onset of dialysis [23], our study may suggest that heparin could exert a subtle effect for the development of A$\beta_2$M amyloidosis under some clinical conditions.

Those molecules are picked up from the results of in vitro amyloid fibril formation, extension, and depolymerization, and further studies will be needed to analyze the histological relationship between those biomolecules and A$\beta_2$M amyloid in the lesion.

### 2.4. Progress of bone disease after deposition of amyloid fibrils

It is not clearly understood the progress of bone disease after deposition of amyloid fibrils. Deposited amyloidosis induces compression that induced CTS and joint arthropathy. Also amyloid deposition induces local osteolysis that induced bone cysts and DSA. The progress through synovial inflammation and subsequent osteoclastogenesis and/or osteoclast activation through three possible pathways: (i) indirect action of inflammatory cytokines through the expression in osteoblasts of receptor activator of nuclear factor-κB ligand/osteoprotegerin ligand (RANKL/OPGL), (ii) direct action of inflammatory cytokines, and (iii) RANKL/OPGL expression in inflammatory cells.

## 3. Clinical manifestations

### 3.1. Serum $\beta_2$-m levels in patients undergoing dialysis treatment

Advanced CKD induces the serum level of $\beta_2$-m to elevate due to the impaired metabolism and excretion in the kidney. The average serum concentration levels of $\beta_2$-m in patients undergoing dialysis is significantly higher compared to those in normal subjects (25–45 vs. 1–2 mg/L) [10, 24-27]. It is clearly understood that the impairment of metabolism in the kidney is the main cause of fluid retention in HD patients; however, it is not clear whether the production of $\beta_2$-m is increased with CKD and/or dialysis treatment. However, a study shows that the amount of $\beta_2$-m on the surface of granulocytes, lymphocytes and monocytes in hemodialysis patients is higher than that in control subjects while mRNA expression of $\beta_2$-m in blood cells is no significant difference between them [28]. This result shows the possibility that increased binding of $\beta_2$-m to blood cells is one of major cause of retention of $\beta_2$-m in dialysis patients. Thus continuous higher serum levels of $\beta_2$-m could induced DRA after long-term dialysis treatment [24, 29].

### 3.2. Risk factors of DRA

Risk factors of DRA are (i) long-term dialysis treatment, (ii) initiation dialysis treatment in young age, (iii) hemodialysis treatment with low purity dialysate, (iv) use of low-flux dialysis membrane [30], while the pathogenesis of DRA with those risk factors is still incompletely understood. Recently it has trend to use high-flux dialysis membrane and high purity dialysate in hemodialysis treatment. However, progress of dialysis treatment as well as treatment for other diseases makes better survival of dialysis patients and older initiation of dialysis treatment. Thus long-term and old age dialysis patients increase, and DRA is still one of serious complications for patients undergoing dialysis treatment.

Serum level of $\beta_2$-m, precursor protein of DRA, increase in dialysis patients and is believed most important for onset and progress of DRA. While cross sectional study shows no relation between onset of DRA and serum level of $\beta_2$-m [24], DRA may be onset after accumulation of $\beta_2$-m with long duration of dialysis treatment [29].

### 3.3. Clinical manifestations

Long-term dialysis treatment for end-stage kidney disease often induces the A$\beta_2$-m amyloid deposition in mainly osteoarticular tissues that induces various disorders, such as CTS, DSA, and cystic bone lesions as well as in rarely systemic organs such as heart [31] and gastrointestinal tract [32] when disease is advanced. CTS is induced by the deposition of A$\beta_2$-m amyloid around synovium in carpal tunnel and the compression of median nerve. DSA is induced by the deposition of A$\beta_2$-m amyloid and the defect of bone in spine. It is radiographically characterized by severe narrowing of the intervertebral disk space and erosions as well as cysts of the adjacent vertebral plates. DSA lesions are mostly detected in the highly mobile areas, such as C5–C7 and L3–L5 [33]. Cystic lesions occur in bones, such as carpal and femur that A$\beta_2$-m amyloid deposition is found around them. Cystic lesions as well as mineral bone disorder associated with CKD increase the risk of bone fracture.

DRA, induce various osteo-articular disorders, is one of serious complications in patients undergoing long-term dialysis treatment even improvement of dialysis treatment such as dialysis membrane and dialysate [34, 35]. For example, we researched over a four year period 359 end-stage kidney disease patients undergoing dialysis treatment were admitted in our center for the treatment of their dialysis-related complications [34]. DSA was a major cause of hospital admission in the patients undergoing dialysis therapy for 20 years or more, and the

http://dx.doi.org/10.5772/53390

rate increased along with the increasing duration of dialysis therapy. The incidence rate of histories of surgeries for osteoarticular disorders, related to DRA was 25.0, 66.0, and 77.8 % in 20-24 years, 25-29 years, and 30 years or more after the initiation of dialysis therapy, respectively (Figure 3). In the patients undergoing dialysis therapy for 30 years or more, the incidence rate of histories of surgeries for CTS, DSA, and joint arthropathy was 72.2%, 50.0%, and 22.2%, respectively that indicated they had analogous histories of surgeries for various osteoarticular disorders (Figure 4). These results indicate that the frequency and severity of osteoarticular disorders which may be caused by DRA accelerated with the increasing duration of dialysis therapy especially for the patients undergoing dialysis therapy for 30 years or more.

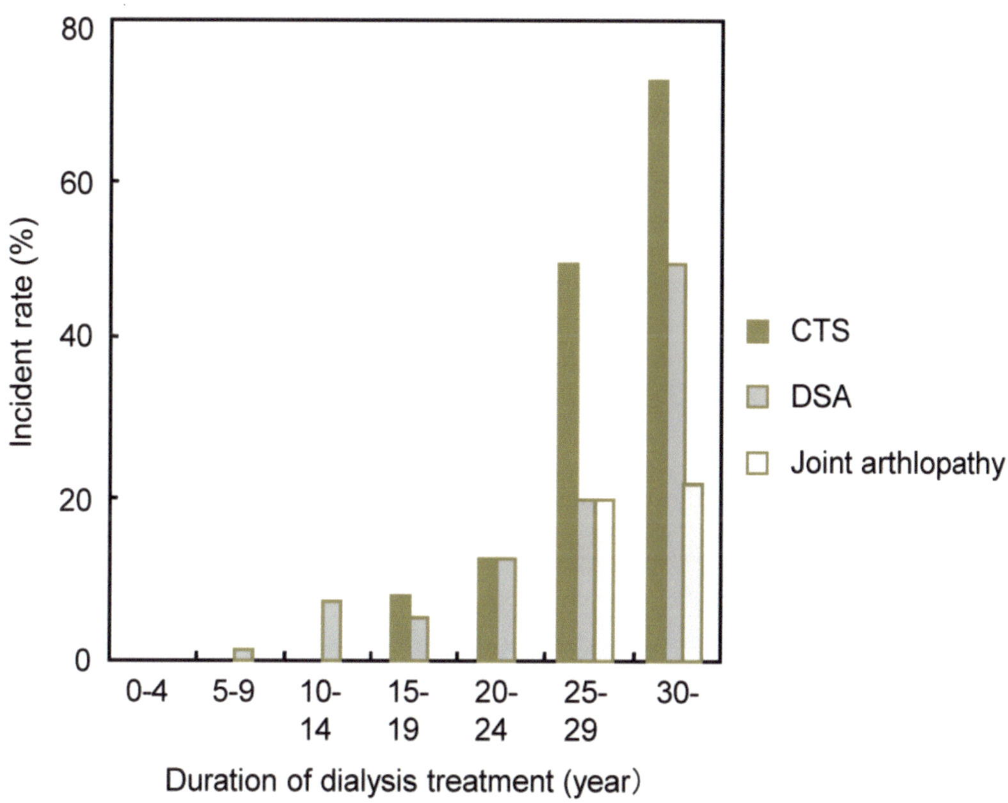


**Figure 3.** The incidence rate of histories of surgeries for osteo-articular disorders, related to dialysis-related amyloidosis (DRA). The rate is 25.0, 66.0, and 77.8 % in 20-24 years, 25-29 years, and 30 years or more after the initiation of dialysis therapy, respectively. In the patients undergoing dialysis therapy for 30 years or more, the rate for carpal tunnel syndrome (CTS), destructive spondyloarthropathy (DSA), and joint arthropathy was 72.2%, 50.0%, and 22.2%, respectively.

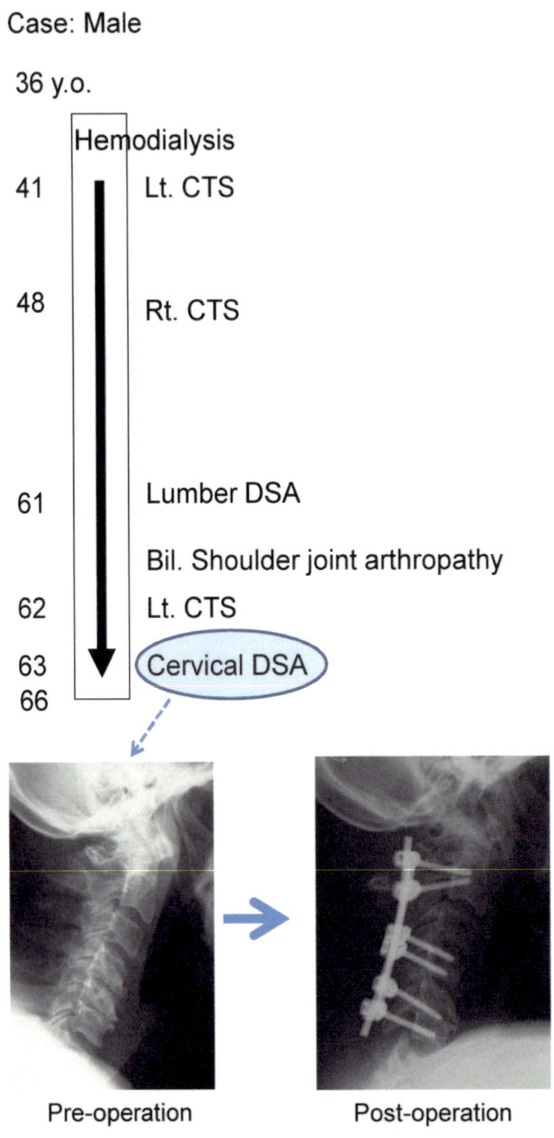


**Figure 4.** A case of long-term dialysis patients complicated with various osteo-articular disorders related to dialysis-related amyloidosis (DRA). A man had end-stage kidney disease due to chronic glomerulo nephritis and received hemodialysis treatment for 30 years. He had various DRA-related osteo-articlular disorders, such as carpal tunnel syndrome (CTS), joint artholopathy, and destructive spondyloartholopahty (DSA) that needed surgical treatment.

Next, we researched 102 patients undergoing dialysis treatment for 30 years or more in our related hospitals, and their complication of osteoarticular disorders. The age at initiation of dialysis therapy was 27.3 ± 7.7 years, and the duration of dialysis therapy was 32.3 ± 1.8 years. The surgery for CTS was done for 80 patients (76%) in 21.6 ± 5.5 years after the initiation of dialysis therapy. All of those patients received the surgeries more than 2 times, furthermore, some of them received more than 4 times for 30 years or more. The surgery for DSA was done for 17 patients (16%) in 27.1 ± 4.7 years after initiation of dialysis treatment. There is dissociation in the incidence of history of surgery for DSA between in our center [34] and in our related hospitals while that for CTS was similar. The main reason may be that our center is a university teaching hospital and severe patients are referred to our hospital. This is a major limitation, however, it should be remembered that one of the main causes for admission was DSA in the patients undergoing long-term dialysis therapy. Our results may suggest that DRA is one of most serious complications in the patients undergoing dialysis therapy for 30 years or more. Further study will be needed about the detail of DRA in the in long-term dialysis patients. In our studies, the main factor associated with osteoarticular disorders which may be caused by DRA was the duration of dialysis therapy despite the younger age at initiation of dialysis therapy [34]. Other risk factors, such as dialyzer and dialysate could not be considered because of the consistent improvements in the technologies from year to year. For example, long-term dialysis patients had used the low-flux dialyzer for several years since initiating therapy, but now use a high-flux dialyzer. Short-term patients however, have used the high-flux dialyzer since the initiation of dialysis therapy.

In summary of our clinical research, the frequency and seriousness of osteoarticular disorders which may be caused by DRA were accelerated with the duration of dialysis therapy, especially in cases treated for 30 years or more.

## 4. Treatment for DRA

Main purpose of treatment for DRA is a) to prevent the deposition of A$\beta_2$-m amyloid fibrils in the lesions, and b) to relieve symptoms induced by A$\beta_2$-m amyloid deposition. Remove $\beta_2$-m with dialysis treatment and suppression of systemic/local inflammation are beneficial to prevent the deposition of A$\beta_2$-m amyloid fibrils. Practically, it should be used biocompatible high-flux dialysis membrane and high purity dialysate in hemodialysis treatment. In addition, hemofiltration, hemodiafiltration, and use of $\beta_2$-m adsorption column have much effect to reduce $\beta_2$-m and to improve symptoms [36]. Non-steroidal anti-inflammatory drugs or low dose of steroid sometimes show relief of symptoms induced by A$\beta_2$-m amyloid deposition while use of steroid for long duration has risk to induce adverse effect, such as infection and osteoporosis. Surgical treatments are needed when A$\beta_2$-m amyloid deposition induces severe osteoarticular symptoms.

### 4.1. Hemodialysis/hemodiafiltration

The use of high-flux dialyzer membrane leads to a reduction in the serum level of $\beta_2$-m as compared to using low-flux dialyzer membrane. In the HEMO Study [26], the predialysis serum $\beta_2$-m level was lower in the high-flux membrane group than in the low-flux membrane group. In another study, switching of dialyzer from conventional to high-flux membrane reduced the predialysis serum $\beta_2$-m level [37]. Clinically, Küchle et al [38]examined the effect of polysulfone high-flux dialysis membrane in hemodialysis treatment, and showed less onset of CTS, arthropathy and bone cysts as well as lower concentration of serum $\beta_2$-m as compare to use of low-flux dialysis membrane. The reason why high-flux membrane produces a lower level of serum $\beta_2$-m is not only that it promotes better clearance, but that it also increases the binding of $\beta_2$-m to blood cells, such as granulocytes, lymphocytes and monocytes [28]. High purity dialysate with low endotoxin reduced serum $\beta_2$-m, pentosidine, C-reactive protein, and interleukin-6 [39] that probably accelerates A$\beta_2$-m amyloid deposition.

Hemodiafiltration has better clearance of middle size molecules than HD and is known to reduce the risk of progression of DRA. A recent multicenter prospective randomized study revealed that on line HDF showed greater efficiency than HD with low-flux membrane in reducing the basal level of $\beta_2$-m [40].

### 4.2. HD with $\beta_2$-m adsorption column

A $\beta_2$-m adsorption column has been developed as a way to directly eliminate serum $\beta_2$-m. This adsorption column system is designed for direct hemoperfusion (Figure 5). Adsorption of $\beta_2$-m by this column is a result both of hydrophobic and molecular size-dependent interactions between the ligand in the column and $\beta_2$-m molecule. The effects of this column show the reduction rate; 60.0-78.9 %, the amount of adsorption; 157-300 mg, serum $\beta_2$-m after treatment; 6.8-13.5 mg/L with single treatment [41-43].

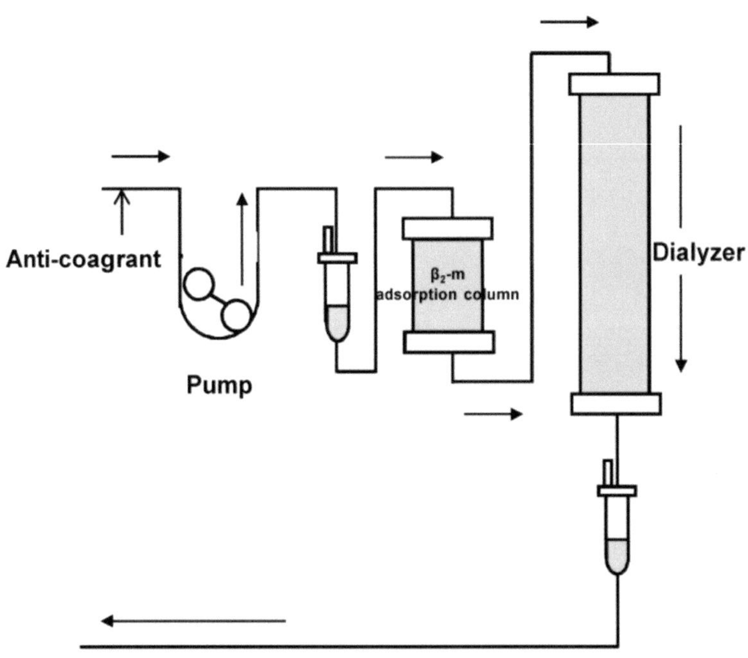


**Figure 5.** A schematic representation of hemodialysis treatment with $\beta_2$-microglobulin ($\beta_2$-m) adsorption column. The $\beta_2$-m adsorption column is placed in series with the dialyzer, with blood flowing through the column first.

According to a prospective multicenter study, a $\beta_2$-m adsorption column that was placed in series with a polysulfone dialyzer increased serum $\beta_2$-m reduction in patients undergoing hemodialysis as compare to hemodialysis treatment without $\beta_2$-m adsorption column [42]. This study also showed improvements of DRA-related symptoms, such as joint pain and activity of daily living, and it may suggest that the column absorbs not only $\beta_2$-m, but also other molecules related to inflammation. Furthermore, a clinical study showed shrink the size of bone cysts when they are checked by X-ray [43].

### 4.3. Other kidney replacement therapies

A significant inverse relationship is observed between residual renal function and serum $\beta_2$-m level [44]. This suggests that peritoneal dialysis may keep lower serum levels of $\beta_2$-m because of better maintenance of intrinsic renal function, but not peritoneal function, than hemodialysis. However the prevalence of histological DRA in peritoneal dialysis patients is not significantly different from that observed in a group of hemodialysis patients matched for age and dialysis duration [23]. End-stage kidney disease patients can do peritoneal dialysis only for 5-10 years, and it is difficult to discuss which treatment shows benefit to prevent DRA. A radical approach for DRA is kidney transplantation that reduces serum $\beta_2$-m, improves symptoms related to DRA and inhibits the progression [45]. The effects of kidney transplantation on DRA probably due to not only recover of kidney function but also effect of immunosuppression therapy.

### 4.4. Medical and surgical treatment

Use of steroid shows beneficial effect for the pain induced by DRA while surgical treatment will be needed for advanced CTS and DSA. However, DSA induces serious neurological symptoms and it is sometimes hard to relief them with surgery. For example, 95 of 865 patients undergoing dialysis treatment had surgeries for DSA, while rate of post-operative complications, such as infection and cardiac events, was much higher than those without DSA [46].

## 5. DRA, a part of chronic kidney disease-mineral and bone disorder

Chronic kidney disease-mineral and bone disorder (CKD-MBD) is a systemic disorder, which consists from abnormal levels of mineral-related bicochemistries, bone abnormalities, and soft tissue calcification [47]. Various types of bone abnormalities are observed in CKD patients, such as high-turnover bone disease and osteomalacia. DRA causes bone abnormalities in patients undergoing dialysis treatment. Bone cyst, joint arthropathy, and DSA are frequency and specifically found in patients especially undergoing long-term hemodialysis therapy [48]. It remains controversial whether DRA and related osteopathy should be included in CKD-MBD. However, DRA is at least closely involved with CKD-MBD, from the view point of preventing osteoarticular complications in dialysis patients (Figure 6).

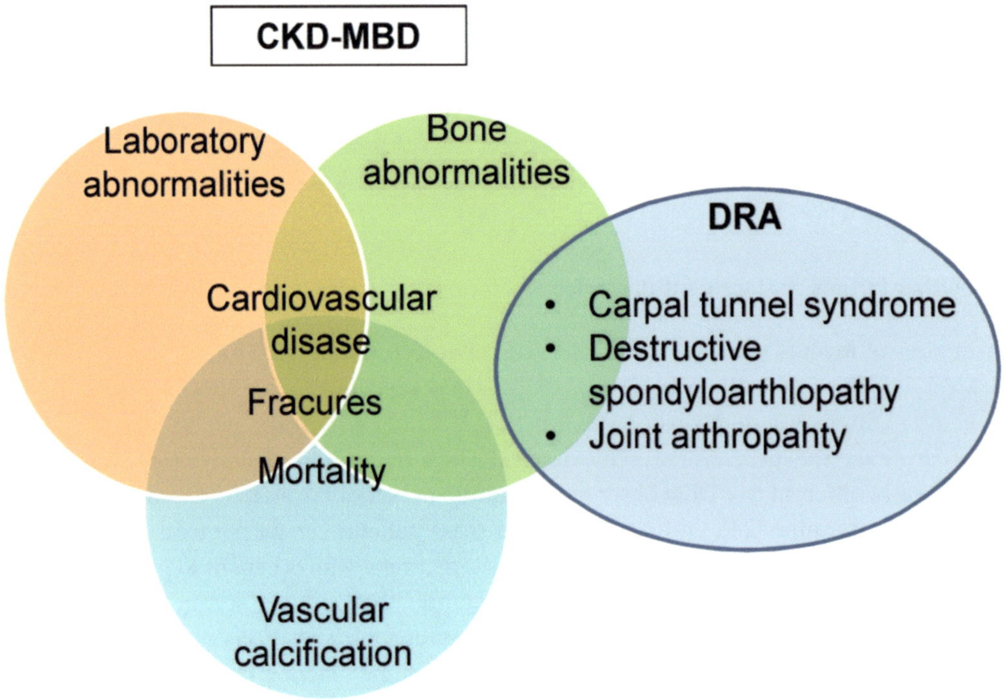


**Figure 6.** Dialysis-related amyloidosis (DRA) in chronic kidney disease-mineral bone disorder (CKD-MBD). CKD-MBD as well as DRA contains various types of bone abnormalities. Furthermore, $\beta_2$-microglobulin/DRA may be involved with cardiovascular disease, bone fracture, and mortality which are clinical outcomes of CKD-MBD. In the view point of bone abnormalities, DRA may be related strongly with CKD-MBD.

CKD- MBD contains various types of bone abnormalities, such as high-turnover bone disease, osteomalacia, and adyanmic bone disease. DRA, such as bone cyst, joint arthropathy and DSA, also causes bone abnormalities and is included in renal osteodystorphy. Recently, some groups reported the relation between serum levels of $\beta_2$-m and atherosclerosis [49] or mortality [26], thus $\beta_2$-m/DRA may be involved with cardiovascular disease, bone fracture, and mortality which are clinical outcomes of CKD-MBD. In the view point of bone abnormalities, DRA related osteopathy may enhance the serious bone disorder, such as bone fractures and DSA, in the presence of other bone abnormalities, such as high-turnover bone disease and osteomalacia. DRA is a serious complication in patients who are receiving long-term dialysis therapy and obviously seems more harmful than other osteodystrophy in terms of maintenance of their ADL and quality of life. Further studies will be needed for this assumption.

## 6. Conclusion

DRA is still one of major and serious complications in end-stage kidney disease patients undergoing long-term dialysis treatment. Several biomolecules that may relate to A$\beta_2$M amyloidogenesis are raised from in vitro studies, and that will be needed to investigate the

http://dx.doi.org/10.5772/53390

involvement in amyloid deposition in vivo. These findings will develop more beneficial prevention and treatment for DRA as well as improvement of dialysis treatment.

## Author details

Suguru Yamamoto, Junichiro James Kazama, Hiroki Maruyama and Ichiei Narita

Department of Clinical Nephroscience, Niigata University Graduate School of Medical and Dental Sciences, Niigata, Japan

Blood Purification Center, Niigata University Medical and Dental Hospital, Niigata, Japan

Division of Clinical Nephrology and Rheumatology, Niigata University Graduate School of Medical and Dental Science, Niigata, Japan

## References

[1] Sipe JD, Benson MD, Buxbaum JN, Ikeda S, Merlini G, Saraiva MJ, et al. Amyloid fibril protein nomenclature: 2010 recommendations from the nomenclature committee of the International Society of Amyloidosis. Amyloid : the international journal of experimental and clinical investigation : the official journal of the International Society of Amyloidosis. 2010;17(3-4):101-4.

[2] Yamaguchi I, Hasegawa K, Naiki H, Mitsu T, Matuo Y, Gejyo F. Extension of A beta2M amyloid fibrils with recombinant human beta2-microglobulin. Amyloid : the international journal of experimental and clinical investigation : the official journal of the International Society of Amyloidosis. 2001;8(1):30-40.

[3] Yamamoto S, Yamaguchi I, Hasegawa K, Tsutsumi S, Goto Y, Gejyo F, et al. Glycosaminoglycans enhance the trifluoroethanol-induced extension of beta 2-microglobulin-related amyloid fibrils at a neutral pH. J Am Soc Nephrol. 2004;15(1):126-33.

[4] Yamamoto S, Hasegawa K, Yamaguchi I, Tsutsumi S, Kardos J, Goto Y, et al. Low concentrations of sodium dodecyl sulfate induce the extension of beta 2-microglobulin-related amyloid fibrils at a neutral pH. Biochemistry. 2004;43(34):11075-82.

[5] Ookoshi T, Hasegawa K, Ohhashi Y, Kimura H, Takahashi N, Yoshida H, et al. Lysophospholipids induce the nucleation and extension of beta2-microglobulin-related amyloid fibrils at a neutral pH. Nephrol Dial Transplant. 2008;23(10):3247-55.

[6] Hasegawa K, Tsutsumi-Yasuhara S, Ookoshi T, Ohhashi Y, Kimura H, Takahashi N, et al. Growth of beta(2)-microglobulin-related amyloid fibrils by non-esterified fatty acids at a neutral pH. Biochem J. 2008;416(2):307-15.

[7] Sasahara K, Naiki H, Goto Y. Exothermic effects observed upon heating of beta2-microglobulin monomers in the presence of amyloid seeds. Biochemistry. 2006;45(29): 8760-9.

[8] Sasahara K, Yagi H, Sakai M, Naiki H, Goto Y. Amyloid nucleation triggered by agitation of beta2-microglobulin under acidic and neutral pH conditions. Biochemistry. 2008;47(8):2650-60.

[9] Orlando RA, Rader K, Authier F, Yamazaki H, Posner BI, Bergeron JJ, et al. Megalin is an endocytic receptor for insulin. J Am Soc Nephrol. 1998;9(10):1759-66.

[10] Uji Y, Motomiya Y, Ando Y. A circulating beta 2-microglobulin intermediate in hemodialysis patients. Nephron Clin Pract. 2009;111(3):c173-81.

[11] Corlin DB, Johnsen CK, Nissen MH, Heegaard NH. A beta2-microglobulin cleavage variant fibrillates at near-physiological pH. Biochem Biophys Res Commun. 2009;381(2):187-91.

[12] Giorgetti S, Stoppini M, Tennent GA, Relini A, Marchese L, Raimondi S, et al. Lysine 58-cleaved beta2-microglobulin is not detectable by 2D electrophoresis in ex vivo amyloid fibrils of two patients affected by dialysis-related amyloidosis. Protein Sci. 2007;16(2):343-9.

[13] Kad NM, Thomson NH, Smith DP, Smith DA, Radford SE. Beta(2)-microglobulin and its deamidated variant, N17D form amyloid fibrils with a range of morphologies in vitro. J Mol Biol. 2001;313(3):559-71.

[14] Naiki H, Hashimoto N, Suzuki S, Kimura H, Nakakuki K, Gejyo F. Establishment of a kinetic model of dialysis-related amyloid fibril extension in vitro. Amyloid : the international journal of experimental and clinical investigation : the official journal of the International Society of Amyloidosis. 1997;4:223-32.

[15] Naiki H, Gejyo F, Nakakuki K. Concentration-dependent inhibitory effects of apolipoprotein E on Alzheimer's beta-amyloid fibril formation in vitro. Biochemistry. 1997;36(20):6243-50.

[16] Jarrett JT, Lansbury PT, Jr. Seeding "one-dimensional crystallization" of amyloid: a pathogenic mechanism in Alzheimer's disease and scrapie? Cell. 1993;73(6):1055-8.

[17] Naiki H, Higuchi K, Nakakuki K, Takeda T. Kinetic analysis of amyloid fibril polymerization in vitro. Lab Invest. 1991;65(1):104-10.

[18] Naiki H, Nakakuki K. First-order kinetic model of Alzheimer's beta-amyloid fibril extension in vitro. Lab Invest. 1996;74(2):374-83.

[19] Yamaguchi I, Hasegawa K, Takahashi N, Gejyo F, Naiki H. Apolipoprotein E inhibits the depolymerization of beta 2-microglobulin-related amyloid fibrils at a neutral pH. Biochemistry. 2001;40(29):8499-507.

[20] Kelly JW. Alternative conformations of amyloidogenic proteins govern their behavior. Current opinion in structural biology. 1996;6(1):11-7.

[21] Yamaguchi I, Suda H, Tsuzuike N, Seto K, Seki M, Yamaguchi Y, et al. Glycosaminoglycan and proteoglycan inhibit the depolymerization of beta2-microglobulin amyloid fibrils in vitro. Kidney Int. 2003;64(3):1080-8.

[22] Relini A, De Stefano S, Torrassa S, Cavalleri O, Rolandi R, Gliozzi A, et al. Heparin strongly enhances the formation of beta2-microglobulin amyloid fibrils in the presence of type I collagen. J Biol Chem. 2008;283(8):4912-20.

[23] Jadoul M, Garbar C, Vanholder R, Sennesael J, Michel C, Robert A, et al. Prevalence of histological beta2-microglobulin amyloidosis in CAPD patients compared with hemodialysis patients. Kidney Int. 1998;54(3):956-9.

[24] Gejyo F, Homma N, Suzuki Y, Arakawa M. Serum levels of beta 2-microglobulin as a new form of amyloid protein in patients undergoing long-term hemodialysis. N Engl J Med. 1986;314(9):585-6.

[25] Ikee R, Honda K, Oka M, Maesato K, Mano T, Moriya H, et al. Association of heart valve calcification with malnutrition-inflammation complex syndrome, beta-microglobulin, and carotid intima media thickness in patients on hemodialysis. Ther Apher Dial. 2008;12(6):464-8.

[26] Cheung AK, Rocco MV, Yan G, Leypoldt JK, Levin NW, Greene T, et al. Serum beta-2 microglobulin levels predict mortality in dialysis patients: results of the HEMO study. Journal of the American Society of Nephrology : JASN. 2006;17(2):546-55.

[27] Okuno S, Ishimura E, Kohno K, Fujino-Katoh Y, Maeno Y, Yamakawa T, et al. Serum beta2-microglobulin level is a significant predictor of mortality in maintenance haemodialysis patients. Nephrol Dial Transplant. 2009;24(2):571-7.

[28] Traut M, Haufe CC, Eismann U, Deppisch RM, Stein G, Wolf G. Increased binding of beta-2-microglobulin to blood cells in dialysis patients treated with high-flux dialyzers compared with low-flux membranes contributed to reduced beta-2-microglobulin concentrations. Results of a cross-over study. Blood purification. 2007;25(5-6):432-40.

[29] Dember LM, Jaber BL. Dialysis-related amyloidosis: late finding or hidden epidemic? Seminars in dialysis. 2006;19(2):105-9.

[30] Davison AM. beta 2-microglobulin and amyloidosis: who is at risk? Nephrol Dial Transplant. 1995;10 Suppl 10:48-51.

[31] Takayama F, Miyazaki S, Morita T, Hirasawa Y, Niwa T. Dialysis-related amyloidosis of the heart in long-term hemodialysis patients. Kidney international Supplement. 2001;78:S172-6.

[32] Araki H, Muramoto H, Oda K, Koni I, Mabuchi H, Mizukami Y, et al. Severe gastrointestinal complications of dialysis-related amyloidosis in two patients on long-term hemodialysis. American journal of nephrology. 1996;16(2):149-53.

[33] Maruyama H, Gejyo F, Arakawa M. Clinical studies of destructive spondyloarthropathy in long-term hemodialysis patients. Nephron. 1992;61(1):37-44.

[34] Yamamoto S, Kazama JJ, Maruyama H, Nishi S, Narita I, Gejyo F. Patients undergoing dialysis therapy for 30 years or more survive with serious osteoarticular disorders. Clin Nephrol. 2008;70(6):496-502.

[35] Otsubo S, Kimata N, Okutsu I, Oshikawa K, Ueda S, Sugimoto H, et al. Characteristics of dialysis-related amyloidosis in patients on haemodialysis therapy for more than 30 years. Nephrol Dial Transplant. 2009;24(5):1593-8.

[36] Nakai S, Iseki K, Tabei K, Kubo K, Masakane I, Fushimi K, et al. Outcomes of hemodiafiltration based on Japanese dialysis patient registry. Am J Kidney Dis. 2001;38(4 Suppl 1):S212-6.

[37] Koda Y, Nishi S, Miyazaki S, Haginoshita S, Sakurabayashi T, Suzuki M, et al. Switch from conventional to high-flux membrane reduces the risk of carpal tunnel syndrome and mortality of hemodialysis patients. Kidney Int. 1997;52(4):1096-101.

[38] Kuchle C, Fricke H, Held E, Schiffl H. High-flux hemodialysis postpones clinical manifestation of dialysis-related amyloidosis. Am J Nephrol. 1996;16(6):484-8.

[39] Furuya R, Kumagai H, Takahashi M, Sano K, Hishida A. Ultrapure dialysate reduces plasma levels of beta2-microglobulin and pentosidine in hemodialysis patients. Blood Purif. 2005;23(4):311-6.

[40] Pedrini LA, De Cristofaro V, Comelli M, Casino FG, Prencipe M, Baroni A, et al. Long-term effects of high-efficiency on-line haemodiafiltration on uraemic toxicity. A multicentre prospective randomized study. Nephrol Dial Transplant.26(8):2617-24.

[41] Gejyo F, Homma N, Hasegawa S, Arakawa M. A new therapeutic approach to dialysis amyloidosis: intensive removal of beta 2-microglobulin with adsorbent column. Artif Organs. 1993;17(4):240-3.

[42] Gejyo F, Kawaguchi Y, Hara S, Nakazawa R, Azuma N, Ogawa H, et al. Arresting dialysis-related amyloidosis: a prospective multicenter controlled trial of direct hemoperfusion with a beta2-microglobulin adsorption column. Artif Organs. 2004;28(4):371-80.

[43] Homma N, Gejyo F, Hasegawa S, Teramura T, Ei I, Maruyama H, et al. Effects of a new adsorbent column for removing beta-2-microglobulin from circulating blood of dialysis patients. Contrib Nephrol. 1995;112:164-71.

[44] Yamamoto S, Kasai A, Shimada H. High peritoneal clearance of small molecules did not provide low serum beta2-microglobulin concentrations in peritoneal dialysis patients. Perit Dial Int. 2003;23 Suppl 2:S34-6.

[45] Mourad G, Argiles A. Renal transplantation relieves the symptoms but does not reverse beta 2-microglobulin amyloidosis. J Am Soc Nephrol. 1996;7(5):798-804.

[46] Chikuda H, Yasunaga H, Horiguchi H, Takeshita K, Kawaguchi H, Matsuda S, et al. Mortality and morbidity in dialysis-dependent patients undergoing spinal surgery: analysis of a national administrative database in Japan. The Journal of bone and joint surgery American volume. 2012;94(5):433-8.

[47] Moe S, Drueke T, Cunningham J, Goodman W, Martin K, Olgaard K, et al. Definition, evaluation, and classification of renal osteodystrophy: a position statement from Kidney Disease: Improving Global Outcomes (KDIGO). Kidney Int. 2006;69(11): 1945-53.

[48] Koch KM. Dialysis-related amyloidosis. Kidney Int. 1992;41(5):1416-29.

[49] Zumrutdal A, Sezer S, Demircan S, Seydaoglu G, Ozdemir FN, Haberal M. Cardiac troponin I and beta 2 microglobulin as risk factors for early-onset atherosclerosis in patients on haemodialysis. Nephrology (Carlton). 2005;10(5):453-8.

# Chapter 5

# Ocular Presentations of Amyloidosis

Hesam Hashemian, Mahmoud Jabbarvand, Mehdi Khodaparast,
Elias Khalilipour and Hamid Riazi Esfehani

Additional information is available at the end of the chapter

http://dx.doi.org/10.5772/53910

## 1. Introduction

Amyloidosis is a term used for some clinical disorders that result from deposition of insoluble amyloid fibrils in extra- and intracellular spaces leading to many tissue dysfunctions and disrupt tissue architectures in human body. These set of disorders with similar pathophysiology, and involvement of metabolic pathways result in protein deposition in different tissue.[1-3]

Amyloid deposits in various groups of amyloidosis have these common findings:

1. Homogeneous granular, filamentous eosinophilia in hematoxylin and eosin staining.
2. Metachromasia in crystal violet staining.
3. Ultraviolet fluorescence in Thioflavin-T staining
4. Orange-red staining with Congo red, which exhibits two additional properties – Birefringence (ability to rotate polarized light by 90°) and Dichroism (red to green color change under polarized light).

These amyloid proteins can be classified into:

a. Immunoglobulin light chains (AL) in primary systemic amyloidosis.

b. Amyloid A protein (AA) in secondary amyloidosis.

c. Transthyretine in familial amyloidosis.

d. A protein known as Amyloid P component (AP ). These conditions may be primary or secondary, localized or systemic, and familial or nonfamilial. Primary systemic amyloidosis includes so many clinical disorders like heart failure, gastrointestinal tract involvement, neuropathies, and other disorders. Secondary systemic amyloidosis results from chronic inflammatory diseases such as tuberculosis or syphilis. [4-8]

Various ocular structures may be involved in any subgroup of systemic amyloidosis, as well as in localized amyloidosis limited to the eye. We will discuss in detail in this chapter about ocular manifestations of amyloidosis. Table-1 summarizes ocular involvements of different subgroups of amyloidosis.

| Structure | Involvement | Amyloidosis Classification | Comment |
|---|---|---|---|
| Eyelids ,Orbit & Adnexa | Waxy eyelid papules with purpura, | Primary Systemic | |
| | Proptosis, diplopia, Ptosis, accommodative paresis | Primary localized, primary systemic | |
| | Keratoconjunctivitis sicca, upper lid mass | Primary localized, primary systemic, secondary systemic | |
| Conjunctiva | Tumefactive or diffuse yellow infiltrative masses | Primary localized, secondary localized, primary systemic | |
| Cornea | Polymorphic Amyloid Degeneration | Primary localized | Secondary to climatic Effects |
| | Primary Gelatinous Drop-Like Dystrophy | Primary localized | Autosomal-Dominant Inheritance |
| | Lattice Stromal Dystrophy (Type I, III) | Primary localized | Autosomal-Dominant Inheritance |
| | Lattice Stromal Dystrophy (Type II = Meretoja Syndrome ) | Primary systemic | Autosomal-Dominant Inheritance with Systemic Symptoms |
| Anterior Chamber | Particulate glaucoma | Heredofamilial (neuropathic) | |
| | Scalloped pupils, amyloid particles pupillary margin | Heredofamilial (neuropathic), primary systemic | |
| Retina and Vitrous | Fundus abnormalities, decreased vision | Heredofamilial, I and II (neuropathic) | |

**Table 1.** Amyloidosis presentations in different ocular tissue

## 1.1. Periorbital and orbital amyloidosis

Ophthalmic presentations of Amyloidosis are not a common entity. Amyloidosis can affect any ocular and periocular structures with multifarious clinical presentations so reaching to correct diagnosis is often an arduous task. Periocular and orbital amyloidosis is generally a slowly progressive disease, but it potentially can lead to devastating ocular complications.

The most common signs and symptoms include: visible or palpable periocular mass or tissue infiltration and ptosis. Other less common signs are; pain or periocular discomfort, recurrent periocular subcutaneous haemorrhages, keratoconjunctivitis sicca, ocular motility disturbances, pupillary abnormalities, proptosis and globe displacement. Proptosis may result from a localized orbital mass or from diffuse amyloid infiltration. Mild pain or painless status in clinical presentations of ocular amyloidosis can differentiate this disease from idiopathic inflammatory pseudotumor.[9-11]

In this section different involvements of periorbital tissues by amyloidosis will be discussed in detail.

## 2. Eyelid involvement

Dermal and ocular amyloidosis can affect eyelid skin either as a part of primary systemic amyloidosis or secondary to dermal conditions like basal cell carcinoma, Bowen's disease and seborrhoeic keratosis.

Nodular or diffuse deposits of amyloid in eyelids are either unilateral or bilateral. Eyelids can be either isolated site of involvement or get involved beside the other sites (e.g. scalp, head and neck or axillae).

Eyelid skin is the preferred site of amyloid deposits both in primary and secondary (reactive) amyloidosis; so unlike other periocular amyloidoses, eyelid skin involvement indicates systemic workup for presence of systemic disease and even some ophthalmologists believe that cutaneous involvement of the eyelid is a sign of primary systemic amyloidosis unless otherwise proved; on the other hand periocular involvements that spares eyelid skin is probably localized.

Amyloid protein deposits in the eyelid skin vessel walls and secondarily increase their fragility, making them very susceptible to hemorrhage after minor trauma (or even spontaneously), so waxy eyelid papules with hemorrhagic appearance can be diagnostic clue of systemic amyloidosis.

Dermatologic conditions like basal cell carcinoma, Bowen's disease, and seborrheic keratosis can lead to secondary localized forms of amyloid deposits in the eyelids although this condition is a histopathologically incidental finding.

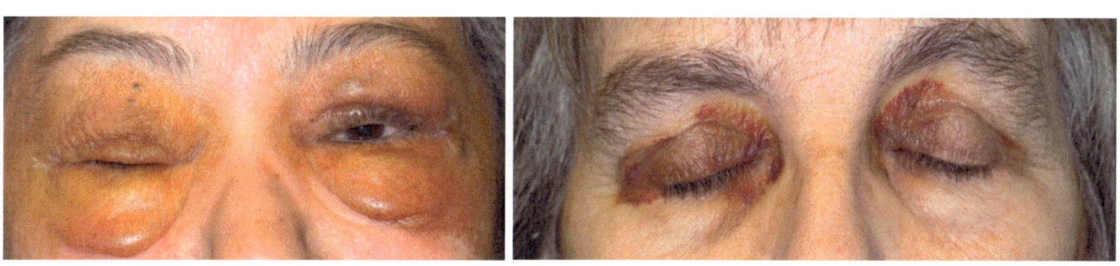

(a) (b)

**Figure 1.** Waxy eyelid papules (A ) with hemorrhagic appearance (B ) in systemic amyloidosis Sophie R Silverstein MB BChir MA; Primary, systemic amyloidosis and the dermatologist: Where classic skin lesions may provide the clue for early diagnosis; Dermatology Online Journal 11 (1): 5

Primary localized cutaneous amyloidosis of eyelid is not a common condition and can be overlooked easily. In this condition we can see Amyloid light chains (AL) deposits in the tissue. As this condition is usually associated with B-cell or Plasma cell proliferation so plasma cell dyscrasia must be excluded.[9,11,12-16]

## 3. Orbital involvement

Orbital involvement is more common in primary compared to secondary amyloidosis and is rare in hereditary/familial or senile amyloidosis. Localized amyloidosis is a rare condition usually affecting head and neck region and only 4% of them involve orbital region. Although some sight threatening complications like secondary glaucoma and optic neuropathy have been reported, orbital localized amyloidosis is usually considered a benign condition with a slowly progressive nature.

Two types of localized orbital amyloidosis have been described. One type presents with progressive proptosis and limitation of ocular movements and is associated with bilateral nodular infiltration of extraorbital muscles and nearby adnexal tissues. Second form is rare cases of Amyloidoma that occurs usually in anterior orbital region next to lacrimal glands. These Amyloidomas have yellow waxy appearances with fragile consistency that shows calcification in orbital CT-scan. [10, 17-22]

Ptosis and Ophthalmoplegia are two common clinical presentations of periocular involvement that can occur coincidentally or respectively (ophthalmoplegia may follow the ptosis by weeks or months). These two manifestations are due to infiltration and secondary necrosis of extraocular muscles, including levator and Muller's Muscles.

Although Extra-Ocular muscle involvements can present with proptosis, ocular motility restrictions or diplopia, in some cases no prominent signs suggestive of this involvement can be found and Orbital imaging is necessary to make the accurate diagnosis.[9-11,23]

Lacrimal gland involvement is not common in amyloidosis and most commonly presents with hard and mobile Superior-temporal orbital mass, rarely fixated to periocular bones. Other manifestations include proptosis, ocular motility disorders, keratoconjunctivitis Sicca and mild pain.

Amyloid deposits in systemic Amyloidosis involve lacrimal glands bilaterally, whereas primary localized amyloidosis usually affects them unilaterally. Lacrimal Gland involvement can mimic disorders like vascular malformations, dacryoadenitis, or lacrimal gland neoplasms.

Computed tomography and MRI although not diagnostic but are important in localizing the involved orbital structures. Lacrimal gland involvement on orbital CT scan usually presents as a homogenous mass, with a slightly higher density than brain with involvement of nearby extra-ocular muscles, although sometimes lobulated gland with areas of calcification and orbital wall erosion can be seen.

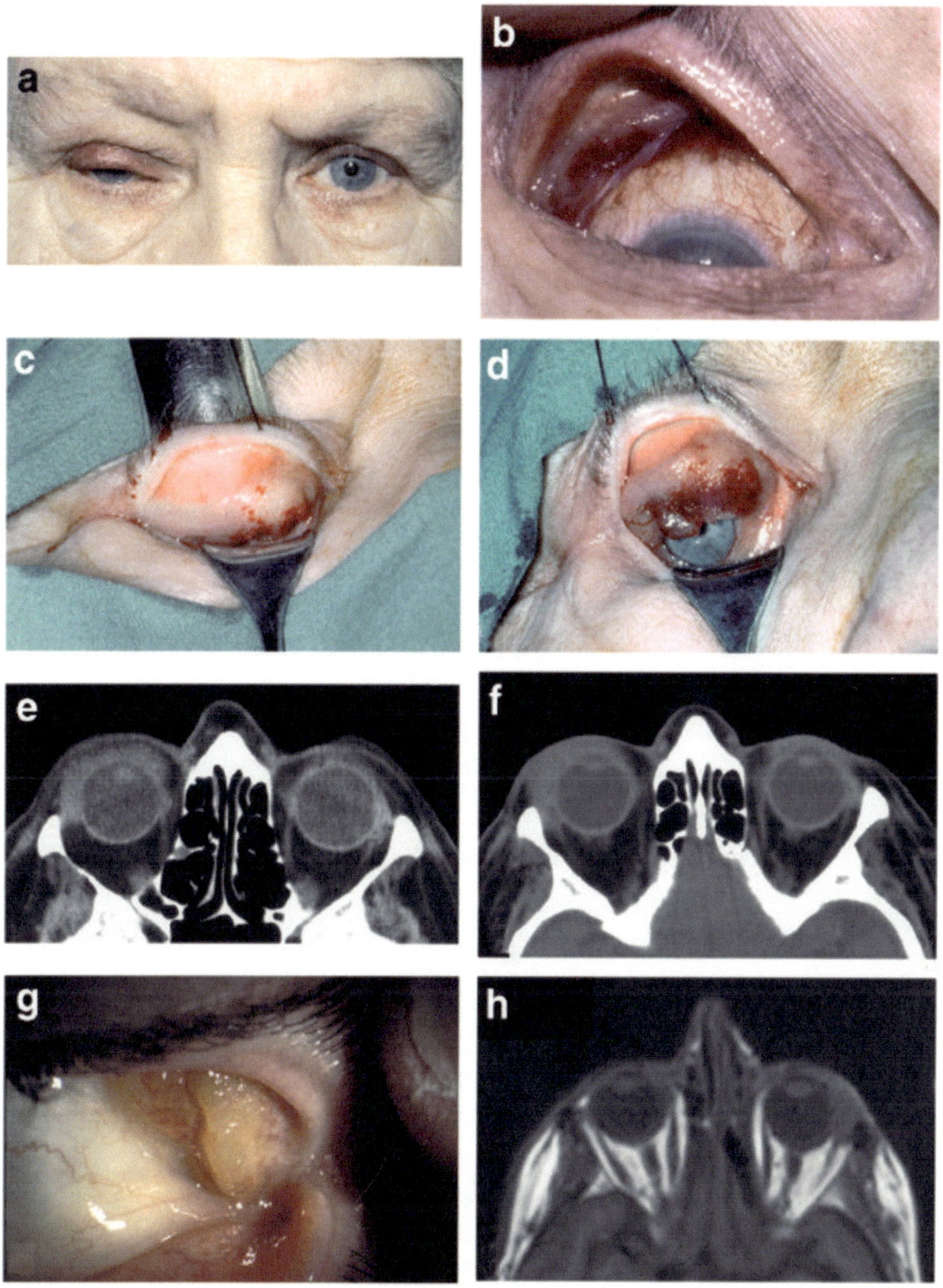


**Figure 2.** Patient-1. (a) Right-sided ptosis. (b) Orbital mass prolapsing through the right upper fornix. (c) and (d) Intra-operative photographs at the time of biopsy. (e) First CT orbits showing the right-sided orbital mass. (f) Repeat CT 9 years later showing the mass to be unchanged. Patient-2. (g). Translucent, yellow, and nodular orbital mass prolapsing through the left upper fornix. (h) MRI of orbits showing the mass in the left orbit. S Dinakaran, A D Singh and I G Rennie: Orbital amyloidosis presenting as ptosis; Eye (2005) 19, 110–112. doi:10.1038/sj.eye.6701411

Although both CT and MRI can be useful in detecting the involvement of periocular tissue in amyloidosis, CT scan is generally more informative than MRI because of the higher sensitivity in detecting specific bone changes and calcifications.

The mass effect can cause globe displacement. Extraocular muscle enlargement, soft tissue infiltration/mass, and calcifications are also characteristic findings on imaging and are seen almost always in orbital involvement.

Other signs of extra-ocular muscle involvement include highly irregular nodular enlargement of muscles with extension to nearby fat tissue with a reticular pattern, fusiform enlargement of muscles with islands of calcification. Extraocular muscle tendons usually are spared. and muscle involvement may be either unilateral or bilateral. [ 9,11,22-26]

## 4. Optic nerve involvement

Although orbital amyloidosis rarely involves optic nerve primarily, orbital or muscular amyloid masses especially those located at the orbital apex can involve optic nerve secondarily and can lead to vision loss. Moreover compressive optic neuropathy secondary to dural infiltration is another cause of optic nerve involvement. As a rule, the neuropathic amyloidosis spares the optic nerve.[9-11]

## 5. Conjunctival involvement

A primary localized form of Amyloidosis is Amyloid plaque deposition in substantia propria of the conjunctiva that usually occurs in healthy young and middle-aged persons with no sex predilection.

The conjunctiva can either be the only site of involvement or involve as well as other structures like the orbicularis occuli or levator muscles. Nodular or diffuse amyloid deposits in these structures can clinically present with Salmon patch nodules and blephariptosis. Conjunctival amyloidosis usually involves the fornixes (superior fornix more than inferior) and tarsal conjunctiva. Amyloid deposits may be unilateral or bilateral and have firm or rubbery and waxy appearance.

Conjunctival deposits are usually painless, but may cause epiphora or significant local swelling and irritation. Recurrent subconjunctival haemorrhages is another presenting symptom of conjunctival amyloidosis that can be missed easily and is usually due to increased fragility of orbital vasculature secondary to amyloid deposits.

Although initial systemic evaluation for primary systemic amyloidosis in patients with conjunctival deposits is usually negative, progression of a local primary-amyloidosis to a systemic disease has been reported and should be kept in mind when following a presumed localized amyloid patient. Although disorders like trachoma, recurrent bacterial conjunctivitis, or immune conjunctival involvements like GVHD can lead to secondary conjunctival Amyloidosis, this is not a common phenomenon.

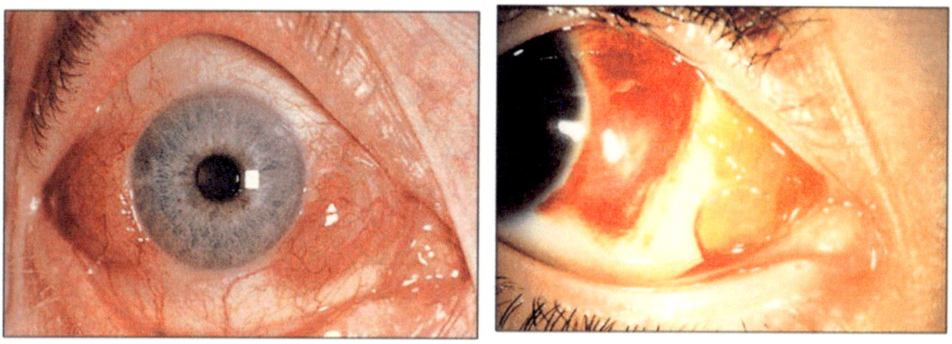

(a) (b)

**Figure 3.** A. Tumefactive conjunctival amyloidosis.B. Nodular amyloid infiltration of the conjunctiva with spontaneous hemorrhage. Albert & Jakobiec's Principles & Practice of Ophthalmology- 3rd Ed,2008,Vol 3,chapter 331,Page 4524,4525

In review of literatures some reports can be seen about conjunctival amyloid deposits after recent strabismus surgery and conjunctival involvement secondary to reactive systemic amyloidosis in rheumatoid arthritis.[9-11, 27-33]

## 6. Management of periocular and ocular amyloidosis

For diagnosis of periorbital and orbital amyloidosis usually tissue biopsy is required and Congo red staining shows characteristic red-green dichroism in unidirectional polarized light.

The first step in management of periocular amyloidosis is determining the type of disease and coincidental systemic involvement. Some treatment modalities like Surgical debulking, radiotherapy and observation have been descried for localized amyloidosis but surgical debulking remained mainstay of treatments in patients with symptomatic diseases including ocular motility disturbances, compressive optic neuropathy, and unacceptable cosmetic appearance.

In patients with medical contraindications for surgery or with extensive infiltrative disease, radiotherapy either with or without surgical debulking may be useful.

Observation is a choice of treatment in asymptomatic or mildly symptomatic patients with localized amyloidosis.

Because complete surgical excision of periocular masses is not possible in most patients, and some case reports showed significant progression after surgical debulking, often symptom revealing treatments for restoration of visual functions and prevention of ocular complications is the goal of treatment.

For Extensive conjunctival infiltration close follow-up is the best option because surgical removal and other modalities are not effective for these lesions.[9-11]

## 7. Anterior chamber involvement

Anterior chamber involvement is usually accompanied by vitroretinal involvement in hereditary systemic amyloidosis. Clinical manifestations in this form of involvement include white flocculent debris in aqueous, anterior lens capsule and on the iris surface and scalloped pupil borders that indicate amyloid deposition in iris stroma or disruption of parasympathetic innervation of the iris sphincter.

Hallmark of ocular amyloidosis presenting in anterior chamber is amyloid glaucoma that is very similar to pseudoexfoliation syndrome and only microscopic studies can differentiate these entities. A close relationship between the onset of glaucoma and pupillary abnormalities has been described in this condition. This is a unilateral asymmetric condition with multiple mechanisms involved in its pathophysiology. Increased episcleral venous pressure secondary to perivascular amyloid deposition and increased resistance to aqueous outflow are two probable mechanisms of increased intra-ocular pressure (IOP) in this situation. Familial amyloid polyneuropathy (FAP) is often complicated with glaucoma and vitreous opacity.

As previously mentioned amyloid deposition on the pupil border is a strong predictor of glaucoma. It is proposed that fringed pupil may be secondary to high amount of amyloid deposit on the pupil border and these deposits may involve trabecular meshwork, reduce aqueous outflow and secondarily increase intra-ocular pressure (IOP).

Medical management with aqueous suppressants is treatment of choice to decrease IOP but vitrectomy may have some benefits in aphakic eyes. [34-40]

## 8. Iris involvement

As in amyloid glaucoma, iris stromal deposits originated from blood vessels in amyloidosis is associated with vitreoretinal diseases and usually occur in familial amyloid polyneuropathy (FAP ).

Scalloped border pupils have been found to be the classic sign of iris involvement in amyloidosis, although not a pathognomonic sign.

Secondary localized Amyloidosis has been reported after conditions like recurrent or chronic uveitis and rare disease like ocular leprosy.

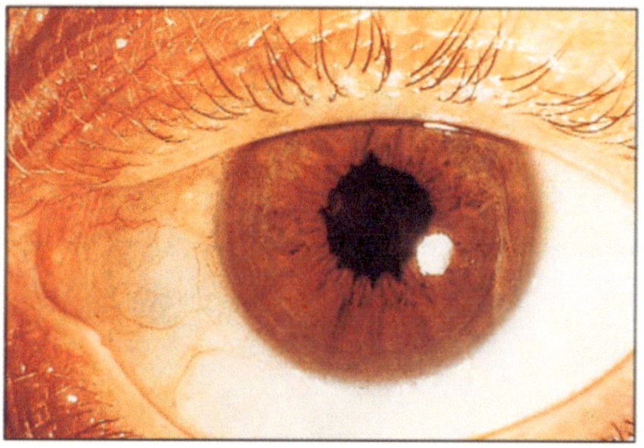

**Figure 4.** Scalloped pupil seen in heredofamilial neuropathic amyloidoses. From Lessell S, Wolf PA, Benson MD, Cohen AS: Scalloped pupils in familial amyloidosis. Reprinted from the New England Journal of Medicine, 1975; 293:914–915.

Histopathological review of eyes from patients with rheumatoid arthritis has showed amyloid deposition in iris and posterior uvea. More than the iris, the choroid may also be infiltrated with amyloid in patients with primary systemic amyloidosis.

There are some reports of pupillary abnormality such as pupillary deformity, decrease in pupillary reaction to light, and amyloid deposition in the pupillary border. [34-35,41,42]

## 9. Vitreoretinal involvement

Vitreous Amyloidosis as a rare condition usually presents in Familial Amyloid Polyneuropathy (FAP) but isolated vitreous deposits in the absence of a family history (primary nonfamilial amyloidosis of the vitreous) are extremely rare. FAP usually results from mutations in transthyretin (TTR) gene and is the most common form of hereditary amyloidosis. Although TTR (also known as prealbumin) is usually produced in the liver, retinal pigment epithelium and choroid plexus of brain can synthesize this protein too. TTR transfers thyroxine and retinol binding proteins in plasma.

Vitreous opacities, manifested as bilateral (but highly asymmetric) cobweb-like or sheet-like veils or string of pearls white opacities are the most common presentations of this condition, and density of this opacities determines severity of visual symptoms. These symptoms include glare, floater, blurred vision and acute decrease in vision secondary to dislocation of these opacities to the visual axis. These vitreous opacities usually spread from cortical vitreous to the center and are often the only sign of ocular involvement but can be in association with other signs like Iris deposits, choroidal infiltration and amyloid glaucoma. Unfortunately this condition can be misdiagnosed easily with uveitis, vitritis, intra-ocular lymphoma, and vasculitis. In FAP, vitreous opacity incidence is variable between 5.4% and 35%. Vitreous involvement in FAP may be accompanied by other organs involvement so systemic workup is necessary.

Retinal vessels usually appear normal in vitreous involvement, although sometimes these opacities may involve perivascular regions and appear as focal plaques, tortuosity, beading or vascular sheathing. Retinal vasoocclussive accidents that appear as cotton-wool spots and neovascularizations have been reported too.

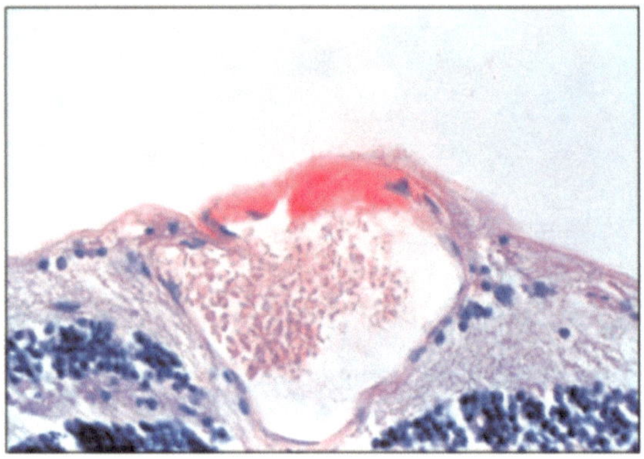

**Figure 5.** Congo red preparation of amyloid infiltration of outer retinal vessel wall. From Schwartz MF, Green WR, Michels RG, et al: An unusual case of ocular involvement in primary systemic nonfamilial amyloidosis. Ophthalmology 1982; 89:394–401.

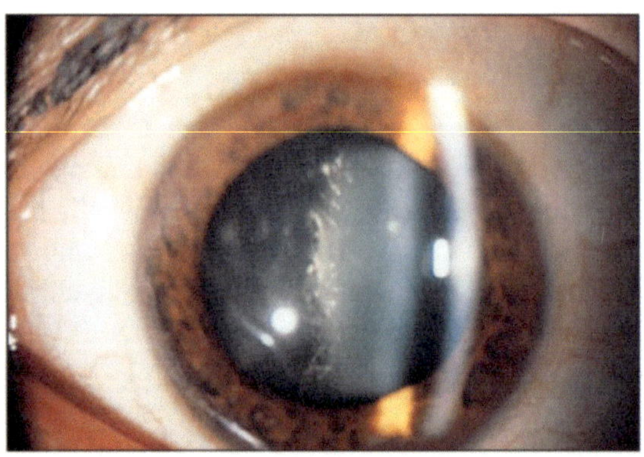

**Figure 6.** Typical lens footplates seen in advanced vitreous amyloidosis (deposits aligning themselves on posterior lens capsule). From Doft BH, Machemer R, Skinner M, et al: Pars plana vitrectomy for vitreous amyloidosis. Ophthalmology 1987; 94:607–611.

Retinal hemorrhages with dot and linear shapes may be seen. In angiography, retinal vascular involvement present with blockage from vasocclusive abnormalities and focal or diffuse leakage that is more prominent in posterior pole than retinal periphery. Another clinical presentation of vitreous amyloidosis is central vitreous opacities that make footplate-like opacities on the posterior lens capsule.

http://dx.doi.org/10.5772/53910

In OCT (optical coherence tomography) veil like vitreous opacities shows needle-shaped deposits on the retinal surface that extend to the vitreous cavity and immunohistochemistry studies demonstrate amyloid-light chain deposits.

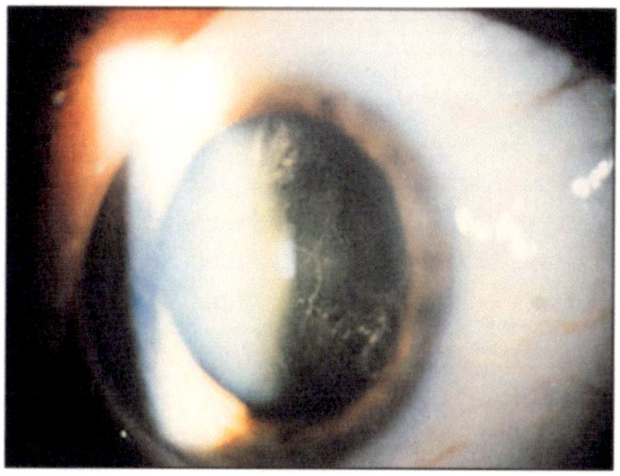

**Figure 7.** Magnified view of vitreous opacification. From Schwartz MF, Green WR, Michels RG, et al: An unusual case of ocular involvement in primary systemic nonfamilial amyloidosis. Ophthalmology 1982;89:394–401.

Treatment modalities for vitreous amyloidosis is limited to vitrectomy and leads to significant visual improvement, but unfortunately opacities can reoccur in one-fourth of patients over months. Incomplete vitrectomy proposed as the reason of this amyloid reaccumulation. Tight adhesion of these opacities to the perivascular regions potentially can lead to formation of retinal breaks during surgery.

Glaucoma as an independent condition in vitreous amyloidosis or concurrently developed complication, can be managed with filtering surgery at the time of vitrectomy or at any time postoperatively.[43-55]

## 10. Amyloidosis of the cornea

The Cornea as an important transparent structure of human visual system can be affected in Systemic and localized amyloidosis, either as a primary site of Amyloid deposition or secondarily.

*Primary localized corneal amyloidosis* consists of two localized inherited corneal involvements, gelatinous droplike dystrophy and lattice corneal dystrophy types I and III. In these dystrophies the amyloidosis is localized to the cornea without systemic manifestations.

*Primary systemic amyloidosis* is known as lattice corneal dystrophy type II (LCD II), (also known as familial amyloidotic polyneuropathy type IV, or Meretoja syndrome.)

*Secondary localized corneal amyloidosis* has been observed in a variety of corneal and ocular diseases such as trichiasis, trachoma, leprosies, sarcoidosis, interstitial keratitis, phlyctenular keratitis, uveitis, chronic post-traumatic inflammation, glaucoma, and keratoconus.

*Secondary systemic amyloidosis* does not affect the cornea.[56-59]

## 11. Gelatinous drop-like corneal dystrophy

Gelatinous drop-like corneal dystrophy (GDCD),( also known as : Lattice corneal dystrophy type III, Familial subepithelial corneal amyloidosis, primary familial amyloidosis of the cornea) is a rare corneal dystrophy,first described by Nakaizumi in 1914 and mainly affects Asian descent but can occurs in diverse ethnic groups throughout the US, Europe and the Asia.[14,15]

Inheritance pattern of this dystrophy is Autosomal Dominant and its gene ( TACSTD2 gene ) located on 1p32. Although More than 25 mutations in TACSTD2 gene encoding *Tumor-associated calcium signal transducer 2* have been described,some patients with this corneal dystrophy doesn't have this mutation suggesting genetic heterogenicity and probability involvement of other genes in this autosomal recessive disease.

This dystrophy presents in young adulthood (within the 1st and 2nd decades ) and tends to be slowly progressive.

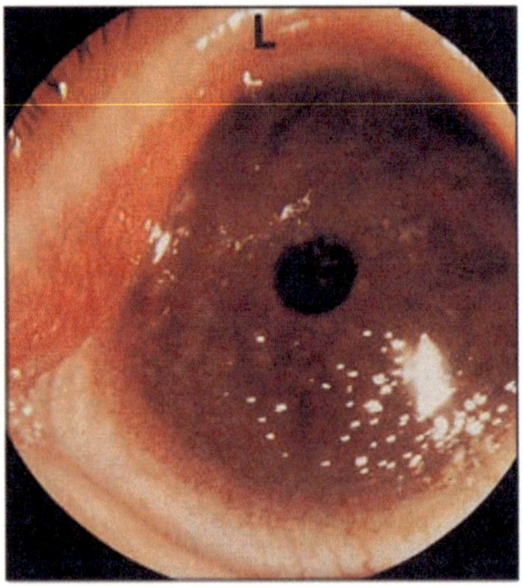


**Figure 8.** Primary, gelatinous droplike dystrophy of the cornea. From Ohnishi Y, Shinoda Y, Ishibashi T, Taniguchi Y: The origin of amyloid in gelatinous drop-like corneal dystrophy. Curr Eye Res 1982–1983; 2:225–231.

Cornea of this patients on slit-lamp biomicroscopy shows gelatinous white deposits of amyloid in the subepithelial and Bowman Layer, gives multilobulated mulberry-like appearance to the cornea. These deposits spread laterally and deeply within the stroma with time and can make larger nodular lesions leading to photophobia, vision loss and foreign body sensation. These lesions marked on with fluorescein staining and sometimes superficial vascularization appears on the cornea. Sever vision loss is secondary to coalescence of this deposits on the cornea surface. Some cases of cataract have been reported in young patients with this dystrophy. Fusiform appearance of deposits in corneal stroma of some patients resembles Lattice Corneal Dystrophy (LCD) and some ophthalmologists categorize Gelatinous Drop-like dystrophy as LCD type III. In this disease, the amyloid contains lactoferrin, but the disease is not linked to the lactoferrin gene.

Treatment is with repeated superficial keratectomy because of early recurrences on corneal grafts. In GDCD, the response to both lamellar and penetrating keratoplasty as well as to a superficial keratectomy is unsatisfactory as amyloid deposition recurs in the graft within about 5 years. Soft contact lenses are effective in managing the abnormal epithelial permeability to decrease recurrences.[56-69]

## 12. Lattice Corneal Dystrophy (LCD)

Lattice corneal dystrophy is the second form of inherited localized amyloidosis and is the most common form of corneal stromal dystrophies. This dystrophy typically is a bilateral disease with an autosomal dominant inheritance which presents at the first and second decade of life with symptoms like recurrent corneal erosion and decreased vision.

The term of Lattice for this dystrophy has been originated for the network of thin and delicate interdigitating branching opacities of the cornea in two separate common types of this stromal dystrophy. Lattice Corneal Dystrophy type 1 (LCD I ) and its variants are due to a specific mutation in the TGFBI gene and patients with this form of corneal dystrophy have no systemic manifestations, but in LCD type II systemic manifestations are inevitable part of corneal disease and this form resulting from a mutation in Gelsolin (GSN) gene.

Five subtypes of LCD have been identified,we will discuss in this section about Lattice corneal dystrophy type I, II,III. Other sub-types of this dystrophy are very rare disorders. [56,70,75]

### 12.1. Lattice dystrophy type ( I )

This type of LCD is the most common form and also known as Biber-Haab-Dimmer corneal dystrophy. LCD1 usually presents its manifestations at the end of the first decade of life, but occasionally it begins in middle life and rarely in infancy and typically is a bilateral disease although occasional unilateral involvement may occur. Corneal sensation is often decreased and the network of interdigitating corneal filamentous opacities has some similarity to nerves, although these lesions are not apparent in all affected members of families with LCD1. Although LCD 1 is seen most often in the western world but some cases have been reported from Bulgaria, Spain and China.

| Characteristics | Lattice Corneal Dystrophy | | | Gelatinous drop-like corneal dystrophy |
|---|---|---|---|---|
| | *Type I* | *Type II* | *Type III* | |
| **Usual age at onset** | <10 years | >20 years | >40 years | <20 years |
| **Visual acuity** | Markedly impaired by age 40–60 years | Usually good until after age 65 years | Impaired after 60 years | Markedly impaired by age 10–30 years |
| **Systemic amyloidosis** | No | Yes | No | No |
| **Mode of inheritance** | Autosomal dominant | Autosomal dominant | Autosomal recessive | Autosomal recessive |
| **Facies** | Normal | Masklike facial expression, blepharochalasis, floppy ears, protruding lips | Normal | Normal |
| **Nervous system** | Normal | Cranial and peripheral nerve palsies | Normal | Normal |
| **Skin** | Normal | Dry, itchy, and lax with amyloid deposits | Normal | Normal |
| **Cornea** | Delicate interdigitating network of filaments; no lines present at early stage; lines difficult to see at late stage | Thick and radially oriented lines | Thick lines | Multiple prominent subepithelial nodules |
| **Episodic corneal erosion** | Yes | Yes | No | No |

From Hida K, Tsubota Kigasawa K, et al: Clinical features of a newly recognized type of lattice dystrophy. Am J Ophthalmol 1987; 104:241–248, 1987.

**Table 2.** Comparison of Inherited Varieties of Corneal Amyloidosis.

At the time of presentation in the first or second decade of life Rod-like fine glassy opacities in the anterior stroma appear and over time this opacities become denser and combine together and make a network of linear branching and interdigitating opacities. These opacities usually are denser anteriorly and centrally but peripheral cornea is usually spared and classical branching lattice figures may not be present in all cases. The lines are relatively fine, as opposed to the more ropy opacities seen in lattice dystrophy Type III.

LCD I in light microscopy reveals Amyloid deposits in anterior stroma and subepithelial region that may lead to poor adhesion between corneal epithelium and stroma and secondary recurrent corneal erosion. Other pathologic features of this dystrophy in light microscopy include epithelial atrophy and disruption, degeneration of basal epithelial cells, and focal thinning or absence of Bowman layer increasing progressively with age and presence of an eosinophilic layer between the epithelial basement membrane and Bowman layer. Stromal deposition of the amyloid substance can lead to distortion of the corneal lamellar architecture. Amyloid deposition in this dystrophy shows typical Amyloid histopathologic features including metachromasia with crystal violet; ultraviolet fluorescence (yellow-green) with Thioflavin T; and orange-red staining with Congo red and stain with periodic acid-Schiff, and Masson's trichrome, exhibits dichroism and birefringence previously mentioned in this chapter.

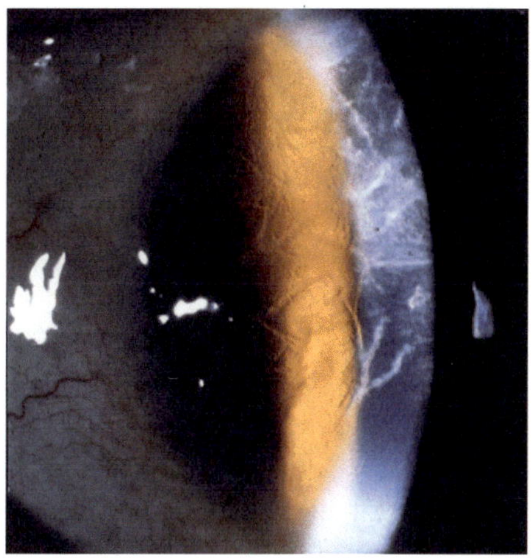

**Figure 9.** Lattice corneal dystrophy type I. Klintworth Orphanet Journal of Rare Diseases 2009 4:7 doi: 10.1186/1750-1172-4-7

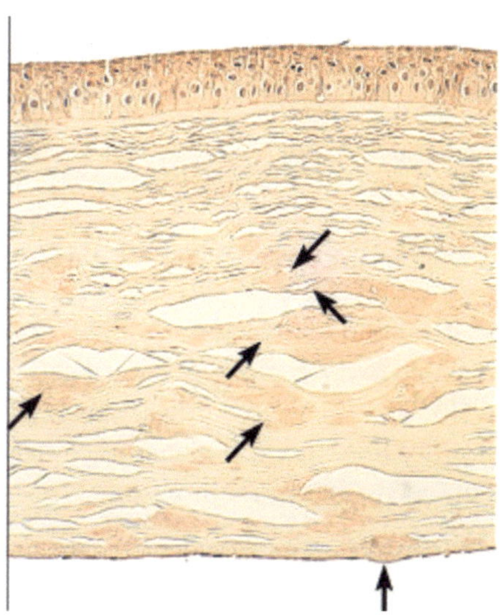

**Figure 10.** Lattice dystrophy Type 1.HistopathologyusingCongoredstain showstheamyloidaccumulationsthroughout-thestromaarrows Yanoff & Duker: Textbook of Ophthalmology, 3rd ed. )

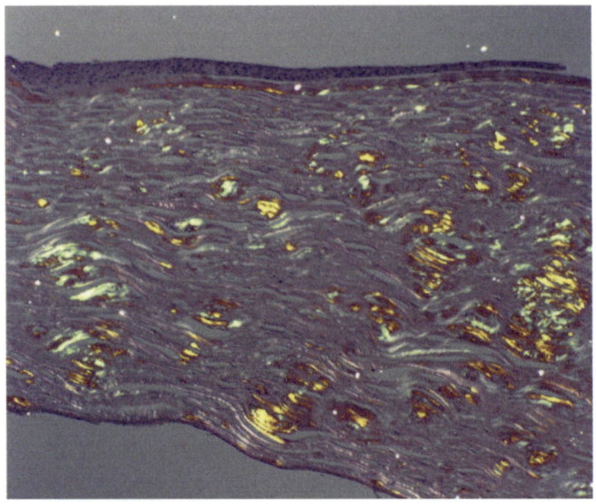

**Figure 11.** Lattice corneal dystrophy type I variant. Deposits of amyloid throughout the corneal stroma due to a p. Ala546Asp mutation in the TFGFBI gene in a patient with a variant of LCD type 1. Eifrig DE Jr, Afshari NA, Buchanan HW IV, Bowling BL, Klintworth GK: Polymorphic corneal amyloidosis: a disorder due to a novel mutation in the TGFBI (BIGH3) gene. Ophthalmology 2004, 111:1108-1114

Diagnosis of LCD I is based on clinical findings. As mentioned before; this dystrophy has an autosomal dominant inheritance and is due to mutation in the TGFBI gene resulting in isolated amyloid deposition in the cornea without any systemic manifestation.

Recurrent corneal erosions as a common complication of this dystrophy can be manage with options like therapeutic contact lenses, superficial keratectomy or phototherapeutic keratectomy. Despite the fact that this dystrophy may recur in the corneal grafts, severe cases of lattice dystrophy with decreased vision can be treated with lamellar keratoplasty (DALK) or Penetrating Keratoplasty (PK).[56,70-79]

### 12.2. lattice dystrophy type II

(Familial amyloid polyneuropathy Type IV (Finnish type), also known as Meretoja's syndrome)

This dystrophy as a part of systemic disease involves corneal stroma bilaterally and is similar to LCD I, histopathologically and clinically but fine glass-like lines are randomly scattered, radially oriented, less numerous, and more delicate, than those in LCD I. Stromal lattice lines in this dystrophy reach to the peripheral cornea and limbus and central cornea is almost spared in contrast to LCD I. Although corneal sensitivity and nerve density is reduced in this type of LCD, Lattice lines are not related to corneal nerves. Patients with this disease are at increased risk of Open-Angle Glaucoma.

This dystrophy is secondary to the GSN (Gelsolin) gene mutation located on chromosome 9. Gelsolin is an actin severing protein and the abnormal Gelsolin molecule leads to deposition of highly amyloidogenic protein throughout the body. Amyloid deposits in this systemic disease can be seen in the conjunctiva, sclera, and ciliary body, along the choriocapillaris, in the ciliary nerves and vessels, and in the optic nerve. Extraocularly, amyloid is detected in arterial walls, peripheral nerves, and glomeruli. The amyloid in this condition is related to Gelsolin and does not stain for type AA or AP.

LCD II present usually after second decade of life but patients that are homozygous for mutated GSN gene may reveal symptoms earlier. Recurrent corneal erosions are not a common complication in LCD II and vision loss does not significantly occur before sixth decade of life. The pathology is similar to lattice dystrophy Type I. Light microscopy shows amyloid in the lattice lines as a discontinuous band under Bowman layer and within the sclera.

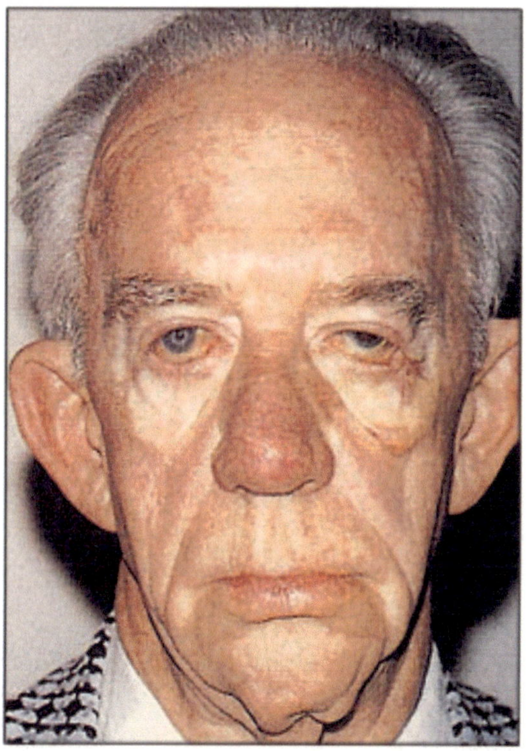

**Figure 12.** Mask like facies of patient with familial amyloid polyneuropathy type IV (Meretoja, Finnish type). From Purcell JJ Jr,Rodrigues M, Chishti MI,et al: Lattice cornealndystrophy associated with familial systemic amyloidosis.Ophthalmology 1983;90:1512–1517.)

Treatment modalities are similar to LCD type I, but exposure keratopathy secondary to facial neuropathy in some patients may need additional considerations. [56,80-87]

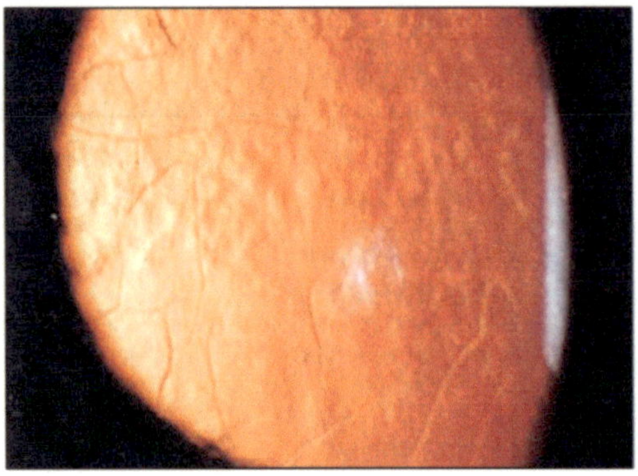

**Figure 13.** Corneal deposits of Meretoja's syndrome (lattice type II, familial amyloidotic polyneuropathy type IV). Note the location along the course of corneal nerves. From Purcell JJ, Jr, Rodrigues M, Chishti MI, et al: Lattice corneal dystrophy associated with familial systemic amyloidosis. Ophthalmology 1983;90:1512–1517.

### 12.3. Lattice dystrophy type III & IV

Lattice dystrophy Type III is an autosomal recessive disease that presents often after forth decade of life (later that LCD type I). Lattice lines in this dystrophy are thicker than type I and corneal erosions rarely occur. Amyloid usually deposits in the superficial stroma and beneath the Bowman's layer and also can be found in mid-stroma.

LCD IIIA has been described with autosomal dominant inheritance and corneal changes similar to LCD type III; but in this subtype recurrent corneal erosions are more prevalent. This disorder is due to a defect in the keratoepithelin gene, demonstrated at various codons.

LCD IV is a late-onset corneal dystrophy that has been reported in Japanese population and is secondary to mutation in TGFBI gene. In this subtype of LCD amyloid deposition is in deeper stromal layers of cornea.[88-91]

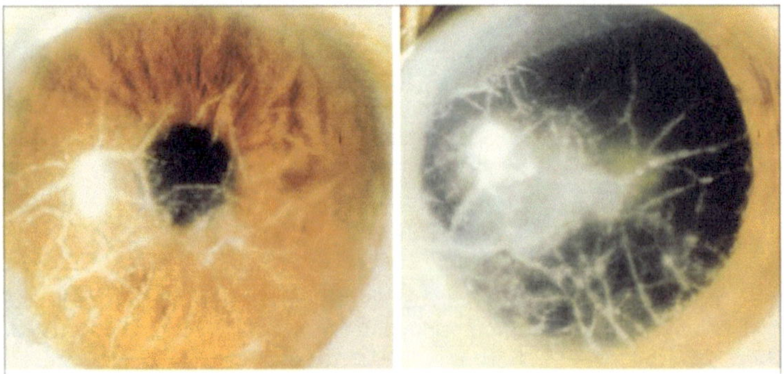

**Figure 14.** Thick ropy lattice lines in patient with LCD III. From Hida T, Tsubota K, Kigasawa T, et al: Clinical features of a newly recognized type of lattice corneal dystrophy. Am J Ophthalmol 1987; 104:241-248.

## 13. Polymorphic amyloid degeneration

This is a specific type of corneal amyloid degeneration that generally occurs after fifth decade of life. This condition is usually bilateral and incidental finding in elderly without much affect on vision. In slit-lamp biomicroscopy deposits with punctate glass-like appearance can be seen in central corneal stroma with extension to descemet's membrane. Sometimes these deposits resemble lattice dystrophy although usually these deposits are less denser than LCD. Histopathologically there is a similarity between polymorphic degeneration and LCD. The reason of this degeneration has not been clearly described and no treatment is usually required for this patients.

Climatic proteoglycan stromal keratopathy is another condition similar to spheroidal degeneration of cornea first time described in Saudi Arabia. Patients with this condition have bilateral oval, central horizontal haziness in anterior stroma that may accompany with refractile stromal lines but does not usually affect vision. In histopathologic review of these patients proteoglycan and amyloid deposits have been found.[92,93]

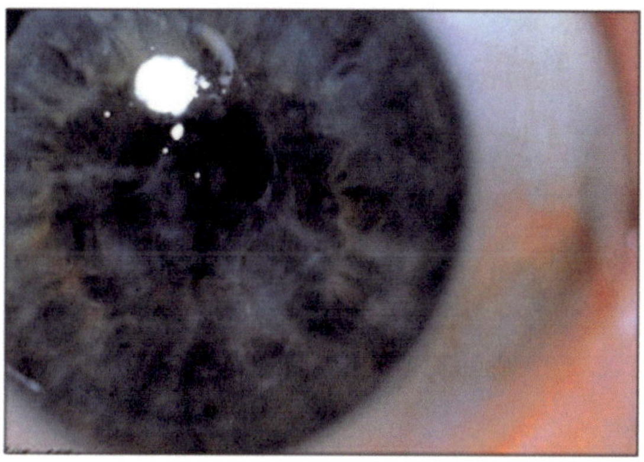

**Figure 15.** Polymorphic amyloid degeneration of the cornea. From Ohnishi Y, Shinoda Y, Ishibashi T, Taniguchi Y: The origin of amyloid in gelatinous drop-like dystrophy. Curr Eye Res 1982–1983; 2:225–231.

## 14. Secondary localized amyloidosis

Wide variety of chronic ocular disorders can lead to corneal amyloid deposition including; keratoconus, trachoma, phlyctenulosis, leprosy, bullous keratopathy (of any etiology), prolonged contact lens wear, trichiasis, uveitis, and severe retinopathy of prematurity with glaucoma.

Amyloid Deposits secondary to these conditions are usually subepithelial and appear as cream-colored nodules very similar to Gelatinous-drop like corneal dystrophy. Corneal vascularization in relation to primary disorder can be seen. Genetic work up must be done to rule out systemic inherited amyloidosis.

Keratoconjunctivitis sicca may be associated with amyloidosis with several mechanisms. The first mechanism is lacrimal gland infiltration in primary localized amyloidosis, with secondary hyposecretion of tears. The second mechanism is orbital nerve infiltration with associated autonomic neuropathy. Reactive (secondary) systemic amyloidosis has been reported with Sjögren syndrome, a condition frequently heralded by dry eyes. Finally, a systemic immunocyte dyscrasia, with or without systemic amyloidosis may result in neoplastic infiltration of the lacrimal gland and associated dry eye.[94-96]

## Author details

Hesam Hashemian, Mahmoud Jabbarvand, Mehdi Khodaparast, Elias Khalilipour and Hamid Riazi Esfehani

Farabi Eye Hospital, Tehran University of Medical Sciences, Iran

## References

[1] Pepys, MB ; Pathogenesis, diagnosis and treatment of systemic amyloidosis. Philos. Trans. R. Soc. Lond., B, Biol. Sci. 2001, 356, 1406:203-10.

[2] Glenner GG: Amyloid deposits and amyloidosis. The beta-fibrilloses (first of two parts). N Engl J Med 1980; 302:1283-1292.

[3] Picken MM. Amyloidosis-where are we now and where are we heading?. Arch Pathol Lab Med. Apr 2010;134(4):545-51

[4] Rosenzweig M, Landau H. Light chain (AL) amyloidosis: update on diagnosis and management. J Hematol Oncol. Nov 18 2011;4:47.

[5] Westermark P, Benson MD, Buxbaum JN, Cohen AS, Frangione B, Ikeda S, et al. A primer of amyloid nomenclature. Amyloid. Sep 2007;14(3):179-83.

[6] Buxbaum JN. The systemic amyloidoses. Curr Opin Rheumatol. Jan 2004;16(1):67-75.

[7] Breathnach SM. Amyloid and amyloidosis. J Am Acad Dermatol. 1988;18(1 Pt 1):1-16.

[8] Campos EC, Melato M, Manconi R, Antonutto G. Pathology of ocular tissues in amyloidosis. Ophthalmologica. 1980;181(1):31-40

[9] I Leibovitch, D Selva, RA Goldberg, TJ Sullivan, P Saeed, G Davis, JD McCann, A McNab, J Rootman : Periocular and orbital amyloidosis: clinical characteristics, management, and outcome : Ophthalmology, 2006, Sep,, 113(9): 1657-64.

[10] I E Murdoch, T J Sullivan, I Moseley, P N Hawkins, M B Pepys, S Y Tan, A Garner, and J E Wright; Primary localised amyloidosis of the orbit; Br J Ophthalmol. 1996 December; 80(12): 1083–1086.

[11] Taban M, Piva A, See RF, Sadun AA, Quiros PA. Review: orbital amyloidosis. Ophthal Plast Reconstr Surg. 2004;20(2):162-165.

[12] Lamkin JC, Jakobiec FA. Amyloidosis and the eye. In: Aiello LM, Albert DM, Dallow RL et al, editors. Principles and Practice of Ophthalmology. WB Saunders; 1994. p. 2963-70.

[13] Brownstein MH, Elliott R, Helwig EB. Ophthalmic aspects of amyloidosis. Am J Ophthalmol 1970; 69: 423-30.

[14] Lemke BN, Woog JJ, Stasior OG, Dortbach RK. Amyloidosis of the orbit and adnexa. In: Hornblass A, ed. Oculoplastic, Orbital and Reconstructive Surgery: Orbit and Lacrimal System. Baltimore: Williams & Wilkins; 1990. p. 907-14

[15] Slagle GA, Lupton GP: Postproctoscopic periorbital purpura. Primary systemic amyloidosis. Arch Dermatol 1986; 122:464–468.

[16] Rubinow A, Cohen AS. Skin involvement in generalized amyloidosis. A study of clinically involved and uninvolved skin in 50 patients with primary and secondary amyloidosis. Ann Intern Med. 1978;88(6):781-785.

[17] Knowles DM, II, Jakobiec FA, Rosen M, Howard G: Amyloidosis of the orbit and adnexae. Surv Ophthalmol 1975;19:367–384.

[18] Levine MR, Buckman G: Primary localized orbital amyloidosis. Ann Ophthalmol 1986;18:165–167.

[19] Erie JC, Garrity JA, Norman ME: Orbital amyloidosis involving the extraocular muscles. Arch Ophthalmol 1989;107:1428–1429.

[20] Holstrom GE, Nyman KG: Primary orbital amyloidosis localised to an extraocular muscle. Br J Ophthalmol 1987; 71:32–33.

[21] Katz B, Leja S, Melles RB, et al: Amyloid ophthalmoplegia. Ophthalmoparesis secondary to primary systemic amyloidosis. J Clin Neuroophthalmol 1989;9:39–42.

[22] Dithmar S, Linke RP, Kolling G, Volcker HE, Helmke B: Ptosis from localized A-lambda amyloid deposits in the levator palpebrae muscle. Ophthalmology 2004; 111:1043–1047.

[23] Cohen MM, Lessell S: Amyloid tumor of the orbit. Neuroradiology 1979; 18:157–159.

[24] Motta AO, Han JS, Levine M, Benton JE: Primary amyloid tumor of the lacrimal gland: CT findings. J Comput AssistTomogr 1983; 7:1079–1080.

[25] Cooper JH, Rootman J, Ramsey MS: Extramedullary plasmacytoma (amyloidtumor) of the caruncle. Can J Ophthalmol 1989; 24:166–168.

[26] Hamidi Asl K, Liepnieks JJ, Nunery WR, et al. Kappa III immunoglobulin light chain origin of localized orbital amyloidosis. Amyloid2004;11:179–83.

[27] Hakan D, Shields CL, Eagle RC, Shields JA. Conjunctival Amyloidosis: Report of six cases and review of the literature. Surv Ophthalmol 2006;51:419-33.

[28] Mesa-Gutiérrez JC, Huguet TM, Garcia NB, Ginebreda JA. Primary localized conjunctival amyloidosis: A case report with ten-year follow-up. Clinical Ophthalmology 2:685-7.

[29] B Eshraghi, H Hashemian, A Sadeghi, F Asadi Amoli;Primary Localized Conjunctival Amyloidosis Presenting with Unilateral Ptosis ; Journal of Ophthalmic & Vision Research 22,1-2

[30] Shields JA, Eagle RC, Shields CL, Green M, Singh AD. Systemic amyloidosis presenting as a mass of the conjunctival semilunar fold. Am J Ophthalmol 2000;130:523-525.

[31] Duke JR, Paton D. Primary familial amyloidosis: Ocular manifestations with histopathological observations. Tr Am Ophthalmol 1965;63:146-67.

[32] Leibovitch I, et al. Periocular and orbital amyloidosis. Ophthalmology 2006:113:1657-64.

[33] Lee HM, et al. Primary localized conjunctival amyloidosis presenting with recurrent subconjunctival hemorrhage. Am J Ophthalmol 2000;129:244-5.

[34] Schwartz MF, Green WR, Michels RG, et al: An unusual case of ocular involvement in primary systemic nonfamilial amyloidosis. Ophthalmology 1982; 89:394–401.

[35] Ando E, Ando Y, Okamura R, Uchino M, Ando M, Negi A. Ocular manifestations of familial amyloidotic polyneuropathy type I: long-term follow up. Br J Ophthalmol. 1997;81295- 298.

[36] Ciulla TA, Tolentino F, Morrow JF, Dryja TP. Vitreous amyloidosis in familial amyloidotic polyneuropathy: report of a case with the Val30Met transthyretin mutation. Surv Ophthalmol. 1995;40197- 206

[37] Nelson GA, Edward DP, Wilensky JT. Ocular amyloidosis and secondary glaucoma. Ophthalmology. 1999;1061363- 1366

[38] Silva-Araujo AC, Tavares MA, Cotta JS, Castro-Correia JF. Aqueous outflow system in familial amyloidotic polyneuropathy, Portuguese type. Graefes Arch Clin Exp Ophthalmol. 1993;231131- 135

[39] Kimura A, Ando E, Fukushima M, Koga T, Hirata A, Arimura K, Ando Y, Negi A, Tanihara H. Secondary glaucoma in patients with familial amyloidotic polyneuropathy. Arch Ophthalmol. 2003 Mar;121(3):351-6

[40] Streeten BW, Bookman L, Ritch R, et al: Pseudoexfoliative fibrillopathy in the conjunctiva. A relation to elastic fibers and elastosis. Ophthalmology 1987;94:1439–1449

[41] Futa R, Inada K, Nakashima H, et al: Familial amyloidotic polyneuropathy: ocular manifestations with clinicopathological observation. Jpn J Ophthalmol 1984; 28:289–298.

[42] Char DH, Crawford JB, Howes E, Carolan JA. Amyloid Mass of the Ciliary Body. Arch Ophthalmol. 2006 Jun;124(6):908-10.

[43] Qiao CY, Lu L, Wei WB. A case of vitreous amyloidosis complicated with glaucoma. Yanke. 2004;13(4):199–200.

[44] Ma HJ, Tang SB, Li T, Hu J. Long-term follow-up for vitreous amyloidosis. Zhongguo Shiyong Yanke Zazhi. 2010;28(12):1374–1375.

[45] Chen L, Lu L, Zhang P, Li Y, Lin J. Transthyretin Arg-83 mutation in vitreous amyloidosis. Yanke Xuebao. 2008;24(1):65–67.

[46] Zambarakji HJ, Charteris DG, Ayliffe W, Luthert PJ, Schon F, Hawkins PN. Vitreous amyloidosis in alanine 71 transthyretin mutation. Br J Ophthalmol. 2005;89(6):773–774.

[47] Dunlop AA, Graham SL: Familial amyloidotic polyneuropathy presenting with rubeotic glaucoma. Clin Experiment Ophthalmol 2002; 30:300–302.

[48] Wang X, Li JY, Li F, Liu WL, Xie P, Hao XY. The effect of vitrectomy for vitreous amyloidosis in a family. Yanke Yanjiu. 2010;28(10):931–932.

[49] Doft BH, Machemer R, Skinner M, et al: Pars plana vitrectomy for vitreous amyloidosis. Ophthalmology 1987; 94:607–611.

[50] Fan DS. Vitrectomy for 3 cases of vitreous amyloidosis. Yanke Xingjinzhan. 2007;27(5):398–399.

[51] Doft BH, Machemer R, Skinner M, et al: Pars plana vitrectomy for vitreous amyloidosis. Ophthalmology 1987; 94:607–611.

[52] Koga T, Ando E, Hirata A, Fukushima M, Kimura A, Ando Y, Negi A, Tanihara H. Vitreous Opacities and Outcome of Vitreous Surgery in Patients With Familial Amyloidotic Polyneuropathy. Am J Ophthalmol. 2003;135(2):188–193.

[53] Schweitzer K, Ehmann D, Garcia R, Alport E. Oculoleptomeningeal amyloidosis in 3 individuals with the transthyretin variant Tyr69His. Can J Ophthalmol. 2009;44(3): 317–319.

[54] Komatsuzaki Y, Tanaka M, Sakuma T, Kiyokawa M, Takebayashi H. Retinal vessel changes in a patient with primary systemic nonfamilial amyloidosis. Ophthalmic Surg Lasers Imaging. 2003 Jul-Aug;34(4):321-3.

[55] Hattori T, Shimada H, Yuzawa M, Kinukawa N, Fukuda T, Yasuda N. Needle-shaped deposits on retinal surface in a case of ocular amyloidosis. Eur J Ophthalmol. 2008 May-Jun;18(3):473-5

[56] Klintworth GK : Corneal Dystrophies. Orphanet J Rare Dis. 2009 Feb 23;4:7.

[57] Jay H. Krachmer. Disorders of Amino Acid, Nucleic Acid, and Protein Metabolism. Cornea, 3rd edn.Vol.1.Mosby Company:2011, pp

[58] Lin PY, Kao SC, Hsueh KF, Chen WY, Lee SM, Lee FL, Shiuh WM. Localized amyloidosis of the cornea secondary to trichiasis: clinical course and pathogenesis. Cornea. 2003; 22:491-4.

[59] Starck T, et al: Clinical and histopathologic studies of two families with lattice corneal dystrophy and familial systemic amyloidosis (Meretoja syndrome). Ophthalmology 1991; 98:1197-1206.

[60] Nakaizumi, K. : A rare case of corneal dystrophy. Acta. Soc. Ophthal. Jpn. 18: 949-950, 1914

[61] Fujiki K, Nakayasu K, Kanai A. Corneal dystrophies in Japan. J Hum Genet. 2001; 46:431-5

[62] Tsujikawa M, Kurahashi H, Tanaka T, Nishida K, Shimomura Y, Tano Y, Nakamura Y. Identification of the gene responsible for gelatinous drop-like corneal dystrophy. Nat Genet. 1999; 21:420-3.

[63] Bei Zhang, Yu-Feng Yao. Gelatinous drop-like corneal dystrophy with a novel mutation of TACSTD2 manifested in combination with spheroidal degeneration in a Chinese patient. Molecular Vision 2010; 16:1570-1575

[64] Li S., Edward D.P., Ratnakar K.S., et al: Clinicohistopathological findings of gelatinous droplike corneal dystrophy among Asians. Cornea 1996; 15:355-362.

[65] Ide T, Nishida K, Maeda N, Tsujikawa M, Yamamoto S, Watanabe H, Tano Y. A spectrum of clinical manifestations of gelatinous drop-like corneal dystrophy in Japan. Am J Ophthalmol. 2004; 137:1081-4.

[66] Kinoshita S, Nishida K, Dota A, et al. Epithelial barrier function and ultrastructure of gelatinous drop -like corneal dystrophy. Cornea. 2000;19(4):551 – 555

[67] Weber FL, Babel J: Gelatinous drop-like dystrophy. A form of primary corneal amyloidosis. Arch Ophthalmol 1980, 98:144-148.

[68] Klintworth GK, Sommer JR, Obrian G, Han L, Ahmed MN, Qumsiyeh MB, Lin PY, Basti S, Reddy MK, Kanai A, Hotta Y, Sugar J, Kumaramanickavel G, Munier F, Schorderet DF, El ML, Iwata F, Kaiser-Kupfer M, Nagata M, Nakayasu K, Hejtmancik JF, Teng CT: Familial subepithelial corneal amyloidosis (gelatinous drop-like corneal dystrophy): exclusion of linkage to lactoferrin gene.Mol Vis 1998, 4:31.

[69] Ren Z, Lin P-Y, Klintworth GK, Munier FL, Shorderet DF, el Matri L, Kaiser-Kupfer M, Hejtmancik JF: Mutations of the M1S1 gene on chromosome 1P in autosomal recessive gelatinous drop-like corneal dystrophy. [abstract].Proc Internat Soc Eye Res 2000, 71:S108P.

[70] Sturrock GD: Lattice corneal dystrophy: a source of confusion. Br J Ophthalmol 1983; 67:629.

[71] Dubord PJ, Krachmer JH: Diagnosis of early lattice corneal dystrophy. Arch Ophthalmol 1982; 100:788.

[72] Durand L, Resal R, Burillon C: Focus on an anatomoclinical entity: Biber-Haab-Dimmer lattice dystrophy. J Fr Ophtalmol 1985; 8:729.

[73] Zechner EM, Croxatto JO, Malbran ES: Superficial involvement in lattice corneal dystrophy. Ophthalmologica 1986; 193:193.

[74] Folberg R., Stone E.M., Sheffield V.C., Mathers W.D.: The relationship between granular, lattice type I and Avellino corneal dystrophies. A histopathologic study. Arch Ophthalmol 1994; 112:1080-1085.

[75] Lisch W, Seitz B : The Clinical Landmarks of Corneal Dystrophies. Dev Ophthalmol. 2011;48:9-23. Epub 2011 Apr 26.

[76] Kivela T, Tarkkanen A, McLean I, et al: Immunohistochemical analysis of lattice corneal dystrophy type I and II. Br J Ophthalmol 1993; 77:799.

[77] Aldave AJ, Gutmark JG, Yellore VS, Affeldt JA, Meallet MA, Udar N, Rao NA, Small KW, Klintworth GK. Lattice corneal dystrophy associated with the Ala546Asp and Pro551Gln missense changes in the TGFBI gene. Am J Ophthalmol. 2004 Nov;138(5): 772-81.

[78] Marcon AS, Cohen E], Rapuano C], Laibson PRo Recurrence of corneal stromal dystrophies after penetrating keratoplasty. Cornea. 2003;22( I): 19- 21.

[79] Pihlamaa T, Suominen S, Kiuru-Enari S. Familial amyloidotic polyneuropathy type IV - gelsolin amyloidosis. Amyloid. 2012 Apr 18. [Epub ahead of print].

[80] Meretoja J. Genetic aspects of familial amyloidosis with corneal lattice dystrophy and cranial neuropathy. Clin Genet. 1973;4(3):173-185.

[81] Rosenberg ME, Tervo TM, Gallar J, Acosta MC, Müller LJ, Moilanen JA, Tarkkanen AH, Vesaluoma MH. Corneal morphology and sensitivity in lattice dystrophy type II(familial amyloidosis, Finnish type). Invest Ophthalmol Vis Sci. 2001 Mar;42(3): 634-41.

[82] Kivela T, Tarkkanen A, McLean I, et al: Immunohistochemical analysis of lattice corneal dystrophy type I and II. Br J Ophthalmol 1993; 77:799.

[83] Levy E, Haltia M, Fernandez-Madrid I, et al: Mutation in gelsolin gene in Finnish hereditary amyloidosis. J Exp Med 1990; 172:1865.

[84] de la Chapelle A, et al: Familial amyloidosis, Finnish type: G654-a mutation of the gelsolin gene in Finnish families and an unrelated American family. Genomics 1992; 13:898-901.

[85] Steiner RD, et al: Asp187Asn mutation of gelsolin in an American kindred with familial amyloidosis, Finnish type (FAP IV). Hum Genet 1995; 95:327-330.

[86] Maury CPJ, Nurmiaho-Lassila E-L: Creation of amyloid fibrils from mutant Asnl87 gelsolin peptides. Biochem Biophys Res Commun 1992; 183:227-231.

[87] Hida T., Proia A.D., Kigasawa K., et al: Histopathologic and immunological features of lattice corneal dystrophy Type III. Am J Ophthalmol 1987; 104:249-254.

[88] Stock E.L., Feder R.S., O'Grady R.B., et al: Lattice corneal dystrophy type III A: Clinical and histopathologic correlations. Arch Ophthalmol 1991; 109:354-358.

[89] Kawasaki S., Nishida K., Quantock A.J., et al: Amyloid and Pro 501 Thr-mutated Big-h3 gene product colocalize in lattice corneal dystrophy type IIIA. Am J Ophthalmol 1999; 127:456-458.

[90] Fukuoka H, Kawasaki S, Yamasaki K, Matsuda A, Fukumoto A, Murakami A, Kinoshita S. Lattice corneal dystrophy type IV (p.Leu527Arg) is caused by a founder mutation of the TGFBI gene in a single Japanese ancestor. Invest Ophthalmol Vis Sci. 2010 Sep;51(9):4523-30. Epub 2010 Mar 31.

[91] Mannis M.J., Krachmer J.H., Rodriguez M.M., et al: Polymorphic amyloid degeneration of the cornea. Arch Ophthalmol 1981; 99:1217-1223.

[92] Waring G.O., Malaty A., Grossniklaus H., et al: Climatic proteoglycan stromal keratopathy, a new

[93] Lin PY, Kao SC, Hsueh KF, Chen WY, Lee SM, Lee FL, Shiuh WM ; Localized amyloidosis of the cornea secondary to trichiasis: clinical course and pathogenesis; Cornea. 2003 Jul;22(5):491-4.

[94] Hayasaka S, Setogawa T, Ohmura M; Secondary localized amyloidosis of the cornea caused by trichiasis; Ophthalmologica. 1987;194(2-3):77-81.

[95] Dutt S, Elner VM, Soong HK, Meyer RF, Sugar A ; Secondary localized amyloidosis in interstitial keratitis. Clinicopathologic findings ; Ophthalmology. 1992 May;99(5): 817-23.

Section 2

# The Mechanism of the Disease

Chapter 6

# Transthyretin-Related Amyloidoses: A Structural and Thermodynamic Approach

Estefania Azevedo, Priscila F. Silva,
Fernando Palhano, Carolina A. Braga and
Debora Foguel

Additional information is available at the end of the chapter

http://dx.doi.org/10.5772/53148

## 1. Introduction

The amyloidoses comprise a spectrum of diseases caused by the systemic or localised deposition of characteristic fibrillar material, termed amyloid fibrils [1]. These deposits can be found in various organs and tissues throughout the body [1]. Each amyloidosis is classified according to the chemical nature of the protein that forms the initial amyloid fibril deposit (Table 1). Amyloid fibrils are ubiquitous structures that are rich in cross β-sheets and typically have a fibrillar morphology, which can vary in length and diameter [1]. Amyloid fibrils are detected *in vitro* and *in vivo* using specific-binding molecules, namely Congo Red [1], thiophene derivatives [2] and Thioflavin-S and T [1]. The most common amyloidoses are Alzheimer's and Parkinson's disease and type 2 diabetes, in which amyloid fibrils are found deposited in the central nervous system and in beta cells from the pancreas, respectively [1]. This chapter will cover the transthyretin (TTR)-related amyloidoses, a group of diseases that roughly affects approximately 8,000-10,000 people worldwide [3]. These amyloidoses are caused by the aggregation of TTR, an amyloidogenic protein that can give rise to amyloid fibrils [4].

Transthyretin (TTR) was first discovered in the cerebrospinal fluid (CSF) in 1942 [5, 6] and then sequenced in 1984 [7], receiving the name prealbumin because of its electrophoretic migration pattern compared to albumin. Afterwards, aiming to better describe its functionality, its name was changed to transthyretin- the transporter of thyroxine (T4) and retinol [5]. TTR transports retinol through binding to retinol-binding protein (RBP) and T4 due to the formation of a hydrophobic channel, which exists only when TTR is tetrameric (Figure 1). Although its function may vary, TTR is highly conserved from humans to bacteria [8]. TTR is a 55 kDa homotetrameric protein predominantly synthesised by the liver and choroid plexus, which is located in the brain. Although TTR is known primarily as a transporter, emerging evidence has demonstrated that TTR can also act as a protease [9] and a neuroprotective molecule [10].

| Amyloidoses | Amyloidogenic Protein | Tissues Affected |
|---|---|---|
| Alzheimer's Disease | Amyloid-β | Brain |
| Parkinson's Disease | α-synuclein | Brain |
| Primary Systemic Amyloidosis | Immunoglobulin heavy or light chain | Mesenchymal tissue, tongue, heart, skin, gastrointestinal tract |
| Dialysis-related β2-microglobulin Amyloidosis | β2-microglobulin | Kidney |
| Senile Systemic Amyloidosis | Wild-type TTR | Heart |
| Familial Amyloid Cardiomyopathy | Mutated TTR | Heart |
| Familial Amyloid Polyneuropathy | Mutated TTR | Peripheral nervous system |
| Central Nervous System-associated Amyloidosis Or Oculoleptomeningeal Amyloidosis | Mutated TTR | Brain, Meninges |
| Hereditary Fibrinogen Alpha-chain Renal Amyloidoses | Fibrinogen alpha-chain | Kidney |
| Apolipoprotein A Amyloidosis | Apolipoprotein A-I, A-II and A-III | Kidney, liver, heart |
| Hereditary Cistatin C Amyloid Angiopathy | Cistatin C | Brain |
| Gelsolin Amyloidosis | Gelsolin | Peripheral nervous system Heart |
| Familial Renal Amyloidosis Or Lysozyme Amyloidosis | Lysozyme | Kidney |
| Cerebral Amyloid Angiopathy British-type | Abri | Brain |
| Cerebral Amyloid Angiopathy Danish-type | Adan | Brain |
| Spongiform Encephalopathy | Cellular prion protein (Scrapie form) | Brain |
| Medullary Thyroid Carcinoma | Calcitonin | Thyroid |
| Type 2 Diabetes | Islet amyloid polypeptide (amylin) | Pancreas |
| Atrial Amyloidosis | Atrial natriuretic peptide | Heart |
| Age-related Pituitary Amyloidosis | Prolactin | Pituitary |
| Insulinomes | Insulin | Pancreas or insulinome–associated tissue |
| Aortic Medial Amyloidosis | Lactadherin | Heart |
| Hereditary Lattice Corneal Dytrophy | keratoepithelin | Cornea |
| Familial Supepithelial Corneal Amyloidosis | Lactoferrin | Cornea |
| Ameloblast-associated Odontogenic Tumour | Odontogenic protein | Mouth |
| Senile Seminal Amyloidosis | Semenogelin | Seminal Gland |
| Tauopathies associated with ageing or secondary to Alzheimer's Disease | Tau | Brain |
| Huntington's Disease | Hungtintin | Brain |
| Familial Encephalopathy | Neuroserpin | Brain |

**Table 1.** Amyloidogenic proteins and tissues affected in human amyloidoses. Adapted from Hamilton and Benson, 2001.

The crystallographic structure of human TTR, which was solved in 1971 [11], revealed that each TTR monomer is composed of 127 amino acid residues, forming 8 β-strands named from A-H, which are arranged in a β-sandwich of two four-stranded β-sheets and one small $\alpha$-helix found between β-strands E and F [11, 12]. TTR monomers interact via hydrogen bonds between the antiparallel, adjacent β-strands H-H′ and F-F′ to form a dimeric species. The two dimers (A-B and C-D) predominantly form the tetramer through hydrophobic contacts between the residues of the A-B and G-H loops. The tetramer forms a central hydrophobic pocket (T4 channel) with two binding sites for hormones [11, 12]. Each TTR monomer contains one cysteine residue at position 10 and two tryptophan residues at positions 41 and 79, which can be used as a tool for monitoring TTR unfolding [13]. Many groups have studied the structure of TTR and its aggregation process to understand the triggering factors that favour TTR aggregation, which occurs in a non-nucleated manner that is known as a downhill polymerisation reaction because tetramer dissociation into monomers is the rate-liming step of the aggregation reaction [14]. Based on this model, many studies have focused on developing effective and selective TTR ligands that can prevent TTR dissociation and aggregation [15].

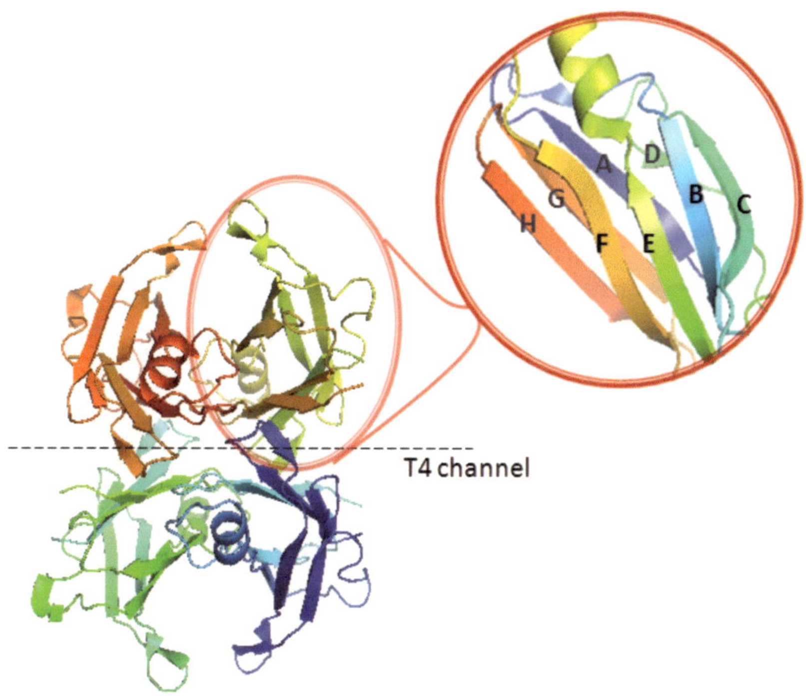


**Figure 1.** X-ray structure of Transthyretin. TTR is a homotetrameric protein composed of four monomers of 127 amino acids. Structurally, in its native state, TTR contains eight stands (A-H) and a small α-helix. The contacts between the dimers form two hydrophobic pockets where T4 binds (T4 channel). As shown in red, each monomer contains one small α-helix and eight β-strands (CBEF and DAGH). Adapted from a model; PDB code 1DVQ.

Thus, in the present review, we aim to appraise the literature related to TTR aggregation and focus on the contribution of the thermodynamics and structural aspects related to tetramer dissociation and monomer unfolding, which appears to be the basis for TTR amyloid formation.

## 2. TTR-related amyloidoses

The TTR gene, which is located on chromosome 18 at position 12.1 [16], presents many polymorphisms, except for one deletion, leading to over 80 amino acid substitutions in the TTR polypeptide sequence [16]. Many TTR variants, such as V30M and L55P, are associated with familial amyloidotic polyneuropathy (FAP), a lethal autosomal dominant disorder in which mutant forms of TTR aggregate to form amyloid fibrils that deposit in tissues, especially the peripheral nervous system (PNS). These amyloid deposits are predominantly composed of intact or fragmented TTR in the form of fibrillar species that progressively accumulate [16, 17]. The initial symptom is typically a sensory peripheral neuropathy in the lower limbs, with pain and severely affected temperature sensation and later followed by motor impairments [17]. Most patients with FAP have early and severe impairment of the autonomic nervous system, commonly manifested by dyshidrosis, sexual impotence, alternating diarrhoea and constipation, orthostatic hypotension, and urinary incontinence [17-19]. The disease onset typically depends on the mutation and the ethnic background of each patient and begins at approximately the third or fourth decade of life, although there are many cases in which the disease onset occurs later in life [17-19]. Not all TTR variant gene carriers develop FAP, indicating that other factors must be involved in the development of clinical symptoms [19].

Not only are most TTR mutants prone to aggregation, wild-type TTR (wt-TTR) possesses an inherent, although low, potential to undergo aggregation and form amyloid fibrils (predominantly in the heart). Hence, it is estimated that approximately 25% of the world population over 80 years old presents some cardiac amyloid deposits composed of wt-TTR [20]. This form of TTR amyloidosis is known as senile systemic amyloidosis (SSA). SSA patients typically present with congestive heart failure and arrhythmia [20, 21]. Recently, it was demonstrated that wt-TTR can aggregate in many tendons and ligaments in aged individuals [22]. Interestingly, among all patients who exhibit SSA symptoms, the male gender predominates, suggesting that gender is a significant disease modifier [20, 22].

Some mutations of TTR, such as V122I, have also been associated with cardiac amyloidosis and are frequently found among African descendants, even though the age of onset varies significantly among patients [23]. This form of TTR-related amyloidosis is termed familial amyloid cardiomyopathy (FAC). FAC symptoms comprise an increase in ventricular wall thickness and an increase in parietal stiffness, which leads to a precipitous increase in ventricular pressure [23, 24].

Although rare, another form of TTR amyloidosis has been described as predominantly affecting the central nervous system and is, therefore, known as central nervous system amyloidosis (CNSA) or oculoleptomeningeal amyloidosis (OA) [25]. Approximately 13 different mutations, such as D18G and A25T, have been associated with the development of CNSA in humans [25, 26]. This form of amyloidosis is believed to occur due to the high instability of TTR mutants, leading to protein degradation by the endoplasmic reticulum-associated degradation (ERAD) pathway in hepatocytes and preferential secretion by the choroid plexus epithelium [27]. This preferential secretion by the choroid plexus is believed to be caused by a higher concentration of T4, which when bound to TTR stabilises the tetramer and favours its secretion by choroid plexus cells [27]. The age of onset is approximately the fourth to fifth decade of life, and amyloid accumulation typically occurs in brain vessels and leptomeninges, predominantly leading to subarachnoideal bleeding [25]. Some affected individuals may also develop hydrocephalus with increased CSF pressure and relatively high CSF protein levels [25]. Leptomeningeal involvement can extend down to the spinal cord, leading to symptoms related to spinal cord or spinal nerve compression [25]. Most patients have little, if any, systemic amyloid deposition. In addition to CNS deposits, TTR amyloid fibrils can also accumulate in the eye vitreous humour, leading to blindness [25].

## 3. Therapies for TTR-related amyloidoses: When and where to inhibit aggregation?

The treatment for TTR-related amyloidoses varies according to the symptoms presented by the patient (cardiac, autonomic or central). Currently, FAP is the only form of TTR-related amyloidoses that has a treatment, which is orthotopic liver transplantation (OLT) [28]. Although a treatment exists, some patients have displayed disease progression after OLT, which has been shown to be due to continued amyloid formation from wt-TTR and is especially true in patients with active FAC symptoms [28, 29]. In addition, after OLT, some patients develop CNSA symptoms [30, 31] due to the production of mutant TTR by the choroid plexus. Another problem related to OLT therapy is that this procedure is also known as "domino liver transplantation", in which the liver of the FAP patient is transplanted into a non-FAP patient. However, the non-FAP liver receptors develop FAP symptoms in less than 5 years and not later in life as expected [32]. These phenomena suggest that OLT therapy is possible but that it is not a fully effective and safe procedure. In addition, for FAC or SSA patients, heart transplantations have only been performed successfully worldwide in a few patients presenting cardiac amyloidosis [33]. In summary, these clinical data emphasise the importance of developing new therapies for TTR-related amyloidosis.

## 4. TTR-stabilisers: A new and powerful approach to stop TTR aggregation

TTR can bind a variety of molecules, from small hydrophobic compounds to large glycosaminoglycans, with great flexibility [15]. As mentioned before, TTR is composed of four identical monomeric subunits that assemble around a central channel; therefore, the tetramer possesses a molecular symmetry with two hormone-binding sites per tetramer (T4 channel). Under physiological conditions, only one of the hormone-binding sites of the T4 channel is occupied by T4 [34]. However, hormone binding is governed by a phenomenon termed negative cooperativity, in which the binding of T4 to the second binding site reduces the hormone-binding affinity of the first hormone-binding site [15, 34]. The fact that TTR is not the only T4 transporter in the human body [34] and that unbound T4 concentrations in blood are very low (less than 0.1 μM, 34) agree with the fact that most TTR *in vivo* does not have T4 bound to its two binding sites. This information has made it possible to design a novel therapy using small molecules that bind to the T4 channel with high affinity and reduce TTR aggregation.

Miroy et al. have shown that the binding of T4 itself stabilises the TTR tetramer and consequently inhibits amyloid formation [35]. Since then, many pharmacological agents and natural products, such as plant flavonoids, nonsteroidal anti-inflammatory drugs (NSAIDs), and inotropic bipyridines, have been tested, and these agents have been demonstrated to be strong competitors for T4 binding to TTR and even possess higher binding affinities than T4 [15, 36, 37]. Interestingly, many of these small molecules share structural similarities with T4, typically presenting one or more aromatic rings. X-ray crystallographic studies have demonstrated that these compounds bind to the TTR hydrophobic channel, similarly to T4, due to the hydrophobic properties of the compounds [15, 36]. As observed for T4 and even RBP, as mentioned above, the binding of NSAIDs to TTR is typically negatively cooperative. However, depending on the ligand, this cooperativity may change. The currently tested NSAIDS include diclofenac, diflunisal and flufenamic acid [15, 36-39]. Interestingly, the first two compounds are currently approved by the Food and Drug Administration (FDA) for the treatment of other pathological conditions. Structural data for TTR complexed with flufenamic acid and diflunisal demonstrate that these compounds mediate hydrophobic and hydrogen bond interactions between the subunits, which stabilise tetrameric TTR [36, 38, 39]. The detailed comparisons of several structures of apo TTR (native TTR) and TTR complexes with small molecules provide insights into the mechanism of ligand-induced conformational changes on ligand binding [40, 41]. Although promising, the chronic use of NSAIDS has been correlated with dyspepsia symptoms, small intestine bleeding and ulcers [42].

Natural polyphenols (curcumin and epigallocatechin gallate) and flavonoids (quercetin and chrisin) have also been successful in inhibiting wt- and V30M TTR aggregation under acidic conditions [43, 44]. Genistein, an isoflavone compound, is also able to inhibit TTR fibril formation by stabilising the native tetramer [45]. Interestingly, both flavonoids and genistein interact with Lys15, Ser117 and Thr119, enhancing tetramer stability [44, 45] and implicating these amino acids in preventing TTR aggregation. In addition, a TTR point mutation (Thr119Met) has been demonstrated to be highly stable to denaturising agents [46], corroborating the idea that the amino acids around the hormone-binding sites aide in tetramer stabilisation.

http://dx.doi.org/10.5772/53148

Recently, a new TTR-stabilising drug, Tafamidis, was approved for use in Europe. This class of compounds functions by preventing the formation of amyloid fibrils, retaining the native tetrameric state of TTR [15, 47, 48]. This mode of action is possible because the most accepted theory regarding amyloid fibril formation is that TTR tetramers need to dissociate to a partially folded monomer, which then rapidly self-assembles to give rise to soluble oligomer intermediates before reaching the amyloid state [12].

There are many studies introducing the use of TTR-stabilising drugs or antisense oligonucleotides (ASO) as new, more effective therapies against TTR amyloidosis. There is currently an on-going trial to test the efficacy of using ASO specifically to target TTR in FAP patients and its safety in healthy subjects [ISIS pharmaceuticals, ISI-$TTR_{rx}$, 49]. The rationale behind ASO therapy and other small interfering RNA (siRNA) therapies [49-51] is that these oligonucleotides interfere with TTR production in the liver and choroid plexus, inhibiting its production and, therefore, its deposition as amyloid fibrils [49, 50, 52]. Data have shown that RNA interference techniques have been successful; however, this technique may still be unsuccessful for dealing with old, existing amyloid deposits.

As mentioned above, the use of various compounds as TTR-stabilisers relies on the hypothesis that TTR needs to dissociate to form fibrils (Figure 2). Although there is evidence supporting this hypothesis, our group has shown that a cycle of compression-decompression using high hydrostatic pressure (HHP) is able to produce an altered wt-TTR species (T4*) that remains tetrameric and that undergoes aggregation under mild acidic conditions (pH 5-5.6), where untreated wt-TTR remains soluble [53] (Figure 2).

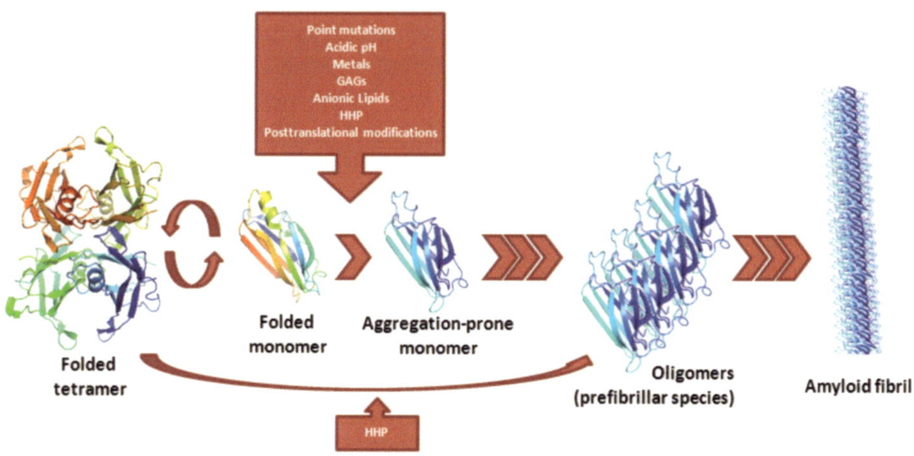


**Figure 2. Transthyretin (TTR) amyloid cascade**. TTR maintains a tetramer to monomer dissociation rate, normally forming folded monomers. These monomers can partially unfold due to point mutations, acidic conditions, metals, glycosaminoglycans (GAGs), anionic lipids, high hydrostatic pressure (HHP) and posttranslational modifications. This unfolded monomer is prone to aggregation, forming prefibrillar species such as oligomers and, consequently, mature amyloid fibrils. In addition, the alternatively folded tetramers formed during a compression-decompression cycle of HHP can aggregate either directly or after dissociating into monomers.

An alternative way to approach this problem is to design drugs that disrupt existing amyloid fibrils. To this end, another class of molecules known as tetracyclines, such as doxycycline, is able to interfere with TTR fibrillogenesis *in vitro* [54], disrupting TTR fibrils. Interestingly, these molecules do not act as inhibitors of TTR fibril formation; however, these molecules disrupt fibrils [54]. The *in vivo* use of doxycycline in a murine FAP model exhibits beneficial effects [54], suggesting that this alternative approach may be as effective as the use of TTR stabilisers. However, it is unclear whether the products of fibril breakdown are toxic. The anthracycline compound described by Palha et al., which is known as 4'-deoxi-4'-iododoxorubicina (IDOX) and which has been used in the treatment of patients diagnosed with monoclonal immunoglobulin light chain (AL) amyloidosis [55], is able to efficiently disrupt TTR amyloid fibrils into amorphous aggregates [56]. Although IDOX displayed promising effects, it was later demonstrated that IDOX is cardiotoxic and is not indicated for use for that reason [57]. However, this new class of compounds has provided a new way of understanding TTR pathogenesis and helped to design new and clinically safer fibril-disrupting drugs.

## 5. Why TTR aggregates?

Although restricted to a single amino acid substitution, TTR mutations may significantly alter the kinetics of TTR aggregation [27]. In trying to understand which features of TTR mutants are responsible for its altered amyloidogenicity, a large amount of crystallographic data has been collected by different groups worldwide. Unfortunately, the conclusion reached was that there was no significant deviation in TTR structure. The only exception to this conclusion was that there were significant deviations for the positions at which the amino acid substitutions took place [58]. However, these single deviations were not significant enough to account for the variability in TTR mutation aggressiveness. Although TTR mutations do not significantly alter the tetrameric structure compared to wt-TTR [58], a single amino acid substitution is enough to alter the thermodynamic stability and rate of dissociation of the tetramer [27]. Many *in vitro* studies using chaotropic agents such as urea or guanidine chloride and HHP have revealed that thermodynamic stability and the rate of tetramer dissociation links certain TTR mutations to variant amyloidogenicity. In one study, Sekijima et al. conducted a global energetic analysis of 23 disease-associated TTR mutants, observing that the rate of tetramer dissociation and the thermodynamic stability in increasing concentrations of urea predicted the aggressiveness of the mutants [27]. Our group has collected supporting data concerning the latter hypothesis that the amyloidogenic mutants A25T and L55P, which exhibit an aggressive phenotype, have lower thermodynamic stabilities than wt-TTR [59, 60]. In addition, we have demonstrated that other amyloidogenic mutants with exacerbated profiles of aggregation and with high tetramer dissociation rates, when HHP is applied, are typically associated with the development of clinically severe FAP [60]. These studies have been corroborated by Hammarstrom et al. [46], who observed that one particular TTR mutation, T119M, which is clinically associated with a phenomenon known as trans-suppression, dissociated at a 40-fold slower rate than wt-TTR. These dissociation rates allow this mutant to be significantly more stable than any of the other described mutants and highly resistant to high urea concentrations for long periods of time [27, 46]. Indeed, this mutation clinically induces trans-suppression, a phenomenon where a patient bearing the V30M mutation, an amyloidogenic variant associated with FAP, along with the T119M mutation does not develop amyloid deposits and, therefore, has no FAP symptoms [46]. In fact, it was later demonstrated that the TTR tetramers that circulated in this patient's bloodstream were hybrids composed of T119M and V30M monomers [46]. These hybrid tetramers gained the characteristic stability of T119M, which overcame the characteristic instability of V30M, and these properties allowed the hybrid tetramers to remain intact and prevent the formation of amyloid fibrils [46].

In addition, the X-ray crystallographic data for the V30M variant, which is also involved in FAP, revealed a perturbation of the β-sheets, which led to a distortion of the T4-binding channel that weakens the hormone interactions [61]. The X-ray structure of another highly amyloidogenic mutant, known as L55P, revealed a disruption of the hydrogen bonds between strands D and A, which produces different interface contacts and, in contrast to what has been mentioned previously, results in eight monomers that have different packing arrangements than that described for wt-TTR [62]. In addition, the highly amyloidogenic, yet engineered, triple mutant G53S/E54D/L55S reveals a new conformation with a novel β-slip conformation, which results in the shift of three residues in strand D and places Leu58 at the position occupied by Leu55. This new conformation impacts the binding interactions with retinol-binding protein [63]. Together, these data lead us to believe that mutations that influence the unfolding of monomers create species that are prone to aggregation. The contribution of the inserted amino acid does not alter the overall structure of the protein but may be capable of interfering with the aggressiveness of the disease, of impacting tetramer stability and dissociation rates and of directing the aggregate to specific tissues such as the peripheral nerves, heart, and meninges.

Although these structural alterations may predict TTR amyloidogenicity, some studies have also shown that because of the presence of cysteine residues (4 per tetramer), TTR is more prone to be posttranslationally modified, such as by S-thiolation and S-sulphonation [64, 65], which have been shown to affect TTR amyloidogenicity. In addition, only 5-15% of circulating TTR is free of posttranslational modifications [66]. One study has also shown that the interaction of TTR with anionic lipids and cholesterol might accelerate the aggregation process [67].

TTR aggregation, especially *in vivo*, does not occur without additional proteins. In fact, in addition to the factors mentioned above, there are many other factors involved in TTR aggregation. The TTR amyloid fibrils from FAP patient deposits and nearly all amyloid fibrils *in vivo* are found to be co-aggregated with many other molecules such as serum amyloid P (SAP), heparan sulphate, and metalloproteinases, which makes it even more difficult to analyse which one of these molecules actually contributes to TTR aggregation and clearance *in vivo* and *in vitro* [1, 68-70]. Among the various molecules that co-aggregate with TTR, glycosaminoglycans (GAGs) are able to accelerate the aggregation of TTR in vitro, and this phenomenon is dependent on the degree of GAG sulphation [69]. Because the GAG composition and concentrations vary among different tissues, this fact might partly explain the specificity of these aggregates for certain tissues [69]. Murakami et al. has described the effect of augmented levels of SAP in the deposition of TTR fibrils in the tissue of TTR transgenic mice [70]. Although SAP was found to be associated with TTR deposits, their findings suggest that SAP does not affect the severity or onset of TTR deposition into the gastrointestinal tract of mice [70]. Our group has recently shown that the TTR fibrils formed from a CNSA-related mutant, A25T, are able to sequester a diversity of molecules from human CSF during aggregation [59]. Many of these molecules are associated with inflammation and coagulation, suggesting that *in vivo* these pathways may also contribute to TTR-related amyloidosis. Indeed, in many of the amyloidotic tissues from FAP patients, an upregulation of inflammation-associated molecules such as inducible nitric oxide synthase (iNOS), IL-1β and TNF-$\alpha$ [68] has been found. Interestingly, a report by Saito et al. showed that nitric oxide (NO) has an important role in TTR amyloid formation because of the S-nitrosylation of cysteine 10 of TTR monomers [71].

TTR aggregation can also be triggered by mild acidification (pH 5.0–4.0) [73], cold storage [74] and the presence of metals such as $Zn^{2+}$ [72, 75]. Using X-ray crystallography, Palaninathan et al. observed that acidic conditions increase the probability that the EF helix–loop of the B monomer of TTR changes its conformation, leading to destabilisation of the TTR tetramer and favouring TTR aggregation [73]. In addition, upon further acidification (< pH 3.9), TTR monomers can adopt a different conformation that may not be in the classic folding pathway of TTR but is able to aggregate without reaching the amyloid fibril [73]. Olofsson et al. have shown that prior to aggregation, the first step in TTR destabilisation occurs in the C-D β-strands, which dislocate when exposed to acidic conditions [76]. More data have shown that not only are the C-D β-strands more susceptible to destabilisation but also the entire β-sheet sandwich CBEF actually dislocates upon acidification [77], suggesting that this region of TTR may be responsible, in part, for the first structural changes preceding TTR dissociation. Recently, Bateman et al. demonstrated that wt-TTR fibril cores were predominantly composed of the C-terminal region and described a different pathway of aggregation that may not require loosening of the above-mentioned TTR regions [78]. Interestingly, the majority of amyloidogenic mutations, which are associated with FAP, FAC or OA, are found within the β-strands of the CBEF β-sheet sandwich [77]. Other groups also believe that acidic conditions may make an important contribution to TTR aggregation both *in vitro* and *in vivo*, in which the amyloid process may take place inside endosomes and lysosomes [79, 80].

Previous data have shown that high concentrations of metals, such as $Zn^{2+}$ and $Cu^{2+}$, can induce TTR amyloid formation *in vitro* [81]. Additionally, chelating agents, such as EDTA or EGTA, are able to disrupt amyloid fibrils, suggesting that metals affect the stability of TTR fibrils [81]. Interestingly, $Zn^{2+}$ was also found in ex vivo ocular amyloid deposits from FAP patients, indicating the possible role of metals in the pathogenesis of FAP [82]. Our group has shown that increasing concentrations of $Zn^{2+}$ are able to perturb, predominantly under acidic conditions, the loop EF helix loop, a region involved in RBP binding [75]. This region has recently been implicated in this phenomenon by two other groups, as the X-ray structures of wt-TTR and two variants, I84A and I84S, demonstrated a structural perturbation in the EF helix loop under acidic conditions [83].

http://dx.doi.org/10.5772/53148

## 6. Conclusion

Although many studies have attempted to infer the conditions that affect TTR stability and amyloidogenicity, why the disease penetrance, pathology and clinical course are so different between mutations is still not completely understood. Herein, we present some of the data obtained by different groups that provides evidence on TTR stability and amyloidogenicity. Many groups have collected data on TTR stability by studying the structure of TTR and designing TTR-binding compounds. However, as further questions have been raised about TTR stability, more evidence has demonstrated that most of the answers with regard to TTR stability lie within its thermodynamic properties and rate of tetramer dissociation.

## Acknowledgements

We would like to thank the funding agencies: Conselho Nacional de Desenvolvimento Científico e Tecnológico (CNPq), Coordenação de Aperfeiçoamento de Pessoal de Nível Superior (CAPES) and Fundação de Amparo a Pesquisa Carlos Chagas Filho do Estado do Rio de Janeiro (FAPERJ).

## Author details

Estefania Azevedo[1], Priscila F. Silva[1], Fernando Palhano[1,2], Carolina A. Braga[1,3] and Debora Foguel[1]

1 Instituto de Bioquimica Medica, Universidade Federal do Rio de Janeiro, Rio de Janeiro, Brazil

2 The Scripps Research Institute, La Jolla, California, USA

3 Polo de Xerem, Universidade Federal do Rio de Janeiro, Duque de Caxias, Brazil

## References

[1] Chiti F, Dobson CM. Protein misfolding, functional amyloid, and human disease. Annual Review of Biochemistry 2006; 75, 333-366.

[2] Aslund A, Sigurdson CJ, Klingstedt T, Grathwohl S, Bolmont T, Dickstein DL, Glimsdal E, Prokop S, Lindgren M, Konradsson P, Holtzman DM, Hof PR, Heppner FL, Gandy S, Jucker M, Aguzzi A, Hammarström P, Nilsson KP. Novel pentameric thio-

phene derivatives for *in vitro* and *in vivo* optical imaging of a plethora of protein aggregates in cerebral amyloidoses. ACS Chem Biol. 2009; 4(8):673-84.

[3] Benson MD, Kincaid JC.The molecular biology and clinical features of amyloid neuropathy. Muscle Nerve. 2007; 36(4):411-23.

[4] Serpell LC, Sunde M, Fraser PE, Luther PK, Morris EP, Sangren O, Lundgren E, Blake CC. Examination of the structure of the transthyretin amyloid fibril by image reconstruction from electron micrographs. Journal of Molecular Biology. 1995; 254(2): 113-8.

[5] Hamilton JA, Benson MD. Transthyretin: a review from a structural perspective.Cellular and Molecular Life Sciences. 2001; 58(10):1491-521.

[6] Kabat EA, Moore DH, Landow H. An electrophoretic study of the protein components in cerebrospinal fluid and their relationship to the serum proteins. Journal of Clinical Investigation. 1942; 21(5):571-7

[7] Mita S, Maeda S, Shimada K, Araki S. Cloning and sequence analysis of cDNA for human prealbumin. Biochemica et Biophysica Research Communications. 1984; 124(2):558-64.

[8] Cendron L, Ramazzina I, Percudani R, Rasore C, Zanotti G, Berni R.Probing the evolution of hydroxyisourate hydrolase into transthyretin through active-site redesign. Journal of Molecular Biology. 2011; 409(4):504-12.

[9] Liz MA, Faro CJ, Saraiva MJ, Sousa MM. Transthyretin, a new cryptic protease. Journal of Biological Chemistry. 2004; 279(20):21431-8.

[10] Said G. Familial amyloid polyneuropathy: mechanisms leading to nerve degeneration. Amyloid. 2003; 1:7-12.

[11] Blake CC, Swan ID, Rerat C, Berthou J, Laurent A, Rerat B. An x-ray study of the subunit structure of prealbumin. Journal of Molecular Biology. 1971; 61(1):217-24

[12] Foss TR, Wiseman RL, Kelly JW. The pathway by which the tetrameric protein transthyretin dissociates. Biochemistry. 2005; 44(47):15525-33.

[13] Silva JL, Cordeiro Y, Foguel D. Protein folding and aggregation: two sides of the same coin in the condensation of proteins revealed by pressure studies. Biochimica et Biophysica Acta. 2006; 1764(3):443-51.

[14] Hurshman AR, White JT, Powers ET, Kelly JW. Transthyretin aggregation under partially denaturing conditions is a downhill polymerization. Biochemistry. 2004;43(23): 7365-81.

[15] Johnson SM, Connelly S, Fearns C, Powers ET, Kelly JW..The transthyretin amyloidoses: from delineating the molecular mechanism of aggregation linked to pathology to a regulatory-agency-approved drug. Journal of Molecular Biology. 2012;421(2-3): 185-203.

[16] Saraiva MJ. Transthyretin mutations in health and disease. Human Mutations. 1995;5(3):191-6.

[17] Ando Y, Suhr OB.Autonomic dysfunction in familial amyloidotic polyneuropathy (FAP). Amyloid. 1998; 5(4):288-300.

[18] Alves IL, Altland K, Almeida MR, Winter P, Saraiva MJ. Screening and biochemical characterization of transthyretin variants in the Portuguese population. Human Mutations. 1997;9(3):226-33.

[19] Tanaka M, Hirai S, Matsubara E, Okamoto K, Morimatsu M, Nakazato M. Familial amyloidotic polyneuropathy without familial occurrence: carrier detection by the radioimmunoassay of variant transthyretin. Journal of Neurology, Neurosurgery and Psychiatry. 1988; 51(4):576-8.

[20] Westermark P, Sletten K, Johansson B, Cornwell GG 3rd. Fibril in senile systemic amyloidosis is derived from normal transthyretin. Proccedings in National Academy of Sciences of United States of America. 1990; 87(7):2843-5.

[21] Sekijima Y, Kelly JW, Ikeda S. Pathogenesis of and therapeutic strategies to ameliorate the transthyretin amyloidoses. Current Pharmaceuthical Design. 2008;14(30): 3219-30.

[22] Sueyoshi T, Ueda M, Jono H, Irie H, Sei A, Ide J, Ando Y, Mizuta H.Wild-type transthyretin-derived amyloidosis in various ligaments and tendons. Human Pathology. 2011;42(9):1259-64.

[23] Rapezzi C, Quarta CC, Riva L, Longhi S, Gallelli I, Lorenzini M, Ciliberti P, Biagini E, Salvi F, Branzi A.Transthyretin-related amyloidoses and the heart: a clinical overview. Nature Review Cardiology. 2010;7(7):398-408.

[24] Dungu JN, Anderson LJ, Whelan CJ, Hawkins PN.Cardiac transthyretin amyloidosis. Heart. 2012 Aug 11.

[25] Benson MD. Leptomeningeal amyloid and variant transthyretins. American Journal of Pathology. 1996;148(2):351-4.

[26] Liepnieks JJ, Dickson DW, Benson MD. A new transthyretin mutation associated with leptomeningeal amyloidosis. Amyloid. 2011; 18 Suppl 1:155-7.

[27] Sekijima Y, Wiseman RL, Matteson J, Hammarström P, Miller SR, Sawkar AR, Balch WE, Kelly JW.The biological and chemical basis for tissue-selective amyloid disease. Cell. 2005;121(1):73-85

[28] Hund E, Linke RP, Willig F, Grau A.Transthyretin-associated neuropathic amyloidosis. Pathogenesis and treatment.Neurology. 2001;56(4):431-5.

[29] Liepnieks JJ, Benson MD.Progression of cardiac amyloid deposition in hereditary transthyretin amyloidosis patients after liver transplantation. Amyloid. 2007;14(4): 277-82.

[30] Liepnieks JJ, Zhang LQ, Benson MD. Progression of transthyretin amyloid neuropathy after liver transplantation. Neurology. 2010; 75(4):324-7.

[31] Munar-Qués M, Salva-Ladaria L, Mulet-Perera P, Solé M, López-Andreu FR, Saraiva MJ.Vitreous amyloidosis after liver transplantation in patients with familial amyloid polyneuropathy: ocular synthesis of mutant transthyretin.Amyloid. 2000;7(4):266-9.

[32] Takei Y, Gono T, Yazaki M, Ikeda S, Ikegami T, Hashikura Y, Miyagawa S, Hoshii Y. Transthyretin-derived amyloid deposition on the gastric mucosa in domino recipients of familial amyloid polyneuropathy liver. Liver Transplantation 2007; 13, 215–18.

[33] Ammirati E, Marziliano N, Vittori C, Pedrotti P, Bramerio MA, Motta V, Orsini F, Veronese S, Merlini PA, Martinelli L, Frigerio M.The first Caucasian patient with p.Val122Ile mutated-transthyretin cardiac amyloidosis treated with isolated heart transplantation.Amyloid. 2012;19(2):113-7.

[34] Bartalena, L. & Robbins, J. (1993). Thyroid hormone transport proteins. Clin. Lab. Med. 13, 583–598.

[35] Miroy GJ, Lai Z, Lashuel HA, Peterson SA, Strang C, Kelly JW.Inhibiting transthyretin amyloid fibril formation via protein stabilization. Procedings of the National Academy of Sciences of the United States of America. 1996;93(26):15051-6

[36] Cody V.Mechanisms of molecular recognition: crystal structure analysis of human and rat transthyretin inhibitor complexes. Clinical Chemistry and Laboratory Medicine. 2002;40(12):1237-43.

[37] Trivella DB, Sairre MI, Foguel D, Lima LM, Polikarpov I.The binding of synthetic triiodo l-thyronine analogs to human transthyretin: molecular basis of cooperative and non-cooperative ligand recognition. Journal of Structural Biology. 2011;173(2): 323-32

[38] Adamski-Werner SL Palaninathan SK, Sacchettini,JC, Kelly J W. Diflunisal analogues stabilize the native state of transthyretin. Potent inhibition of amyloidogenesis. Journal of Medical Chemistry.2004; 47,355–374.

[39] Baures PW, Oza VB, Peterson SA, Kelly JW. Synthesis and evaluation of inhibitors of transthyretin amyloid formation based on the non-steroidal anti-inflammatory drug, flufenamic acid. Bioorganic and Medical Chemistry.1999; 7, 1339–1347.

[40] Almeida MR, Gales L, Damas AM, Cardoso I, Saraiva MJ.Small transthyretin (TTR) ligands as possible therapeutic agents in TTR amyloidoses. Current Drug Targets: CNS and Neurological Disorders. 2005; 4(5):587-96

[41] Neumann P, Cody V, Wojtczak A.Structural basis of negative cooperativity in transthyretin. Acta Biochimica Polonica. 2001; 48(4):867-75.

[42] Graham DY, Opekun AR, Willingham FF, Qureshi WA.Visible small-intestinal mucosal injury in chronic NSAID users. Clinical Gastroenterology and Hepatology. 2005; 3(1):55-9.

[43] Ferreira N, Saraiva MJ, Almeida MR. Natural polyphenols inhibit different steps of the process of transthyretin (TTR) amyloid fibril formation. FEBS Letters. 2011; 585(15):2424-30.

[44] Trivella DB, Dos Reis CV, Lima LM, Foguel D, Polikarpov I.Flavonoid interactions with human transthyretin: Combined structural and thermodynamic analysis. Journal of Structural Biology. 2012; in press.

[45] Trivella DB, Bleicher L, Palmieri Lde C, Wiggers HJ, Montanari CA, Kelly JW, Lima LM, Foguel D, Polikarpov I. Conformational differences between the wild type and V30M mutant transthyretin modulate its binding to genistein: implications to tetramer stability and ligand-binding. Journal of Structural Biology. 2010; 170(3):522-31.

[46] Hammarström P, Schneider F, Kelly JW. Trans-suppression of misfolding in an amyloid disease. Science. 2001; 293(5539):2459-62.

[47] Bulawa CE, Connelly S, Devit M, Wang L, Weigel C, Fleming JA, Packman J, Powers ET, Wiseman RL, Foss TR, Wilson IA, Kelly JW, Labaudinière R. Tafamidis, a potent and selective transthyretin kinetic stabilizer that inhibits the amyloid cascade. Proccedings of the National Academy of Sciences of the Unites States of America. 2012;109(24):9629-34.

[48] Coelho T, Maia LF, Martins da Silva A, Waddington Cruz M, Planté-Bordeneuve V, Lozeron P, Suhr OB, Campistol JM, Conceição IM, Schmidt HH, Trigo P, Kelly JW, Labaudinière R, Chan J, Packman J, Wilson A, Grogan DR.Tafamidis for transthyretin familial amyloid polyneuropathy: A randomized, controlled trial. Neurology. 2012

[49] Benson MD, Pandey S, Witchell D, Jazayeri A, Siwkowski A, Monia B, Kluve-Beckerman B. Antisense oligonucleotide therapy for TTR amyloidosis.Amyloid. 2011; 18; 1-55.

[50] Ackermann EJ, Guo S, Booten S, Alvarado L, Benson M, Hughes S, Monia BP.Clinical development of an antisense therapy for the treatment of transthyretin-associated polyneuropathy. Amyloid. 2012; 1:43-4.

[51] Hayashi Y, Mori Y, Higashi T, Motoyama K, Jono H, Sah DW, Ando Y, Arima H. Systemic delivery of transthyretin siRNA mediated by lactosylated dendrimer/$\alpha$-cyclodextrin conjugates into hepatocyte for familial amyloidotic polyneuropathy therapy.Amyloid. 2012; 1:47-9.

[52] Benson MD, Smith RA, Hung G, Kluve-Beckerman B, Showalter AD, Sloop KW, Monia BP.Suppression of choroid plexus transthyretin levels by antisense oligonucleotide treatment. Amyloid. 2010;17(2):43-9.

[53] Ferrão-Gonzales AD, Souto SO, Silva JL, Foguel D.The preaggregated state of an amyloidogenic protein: hydrostatic pressure converts native transthyretin into the amyloidogenic state. Proccedings of the National Academy of Sciences of the United States of America. 2000;97(12):6445-50.

[54] Cardoso I, Saraiva MJ.Doxycycline disrupts transthyretin amyloid: evidence from studies in a FAP transgenic mice model. FASEB Journal. 2006; 20(2):234-9.

[55] Gertz MA, Lacy MQ, Dispenzieri A, Cheson BD, Barlogie B, Kyle RA, Palladini G, Geyer SM, Merlini G. A multicenter phase II trial of 4'-iodo-4'deoxydoxorubicin (IDOX) in primary amyloidosis (AL). Amyloid. 2002; 9(1):24-30.

[56] Merlini G, Ascari E, Amboldi N, Bellotti V, Arbustini E, Perfetti V, Ferrari M, Zorzoli I, Marinone MG, Garini P, et al. Interaction of the anthracycline 4'-iodo-4'-deoxydoxorubicin with amyloid fibrils: inhibition of amyloidogenesis. Proccedings of the National Academy of Sciences of the United States of America. 1995; 92(7):2959-63.4-9.

[57] Danesi R, Bernardini N, Agen C, Costa M, Macchiarini P, Della Torre P, Del Tacca M.Cardiotoxicity and cytotoxicity of the anthracycline analog 4'-deoxy-4'-iodo-doxorubicin.Toxicology. 1991;70(2):243-53.

[58] Hörnberg A, Eneqvist T, Olofsson A, Lundgren E, Sauer-Eriksson AE.A comparative analysis of 23 structures of the amyloidogenic protein transthyretin. Journal of Molecular Biology. 2000;302(3):649-69.

[59] Azevedo EP, Pereira HM, Garratt RC, Kelly JW, Foguel D, Palhano FL. Dissecting the structure, thermodynamic stability, and aggregation properties of the A25T transthyretin (A25T-TTR) variant involved in leptomeningeal amyloidosis: identifying protein partners that co-aggregate during A25T-TTR fibrillogenesis in cerebrospinal fluid. Biochemistry. 2011; 50(51):11070-83.

[60] Ferrão-Gonzales AD, Palmieri L, Valory M, Silva JL, Lashuel H, Kelly JW, Foguel D.Hydration and packing are crucial to amyloidogenesis as revealed by pressure studies on transthyretin variants that either protect or worsen amyloid disease. Journal of Molecular Biology. 2003;328(4):963-74.

[61] Hamilton JA, Steinrauf LK, Braden BC, Liepnieks J, Benson MD, Holmgren G, Sandgren O, Steen L. The x-ray crystal structure refinements of normal human transthyretin and the amyloidogenic Val-30-->Met variant to 1.7-A resolution. Journal of Biological Chemistry. 1993; 268(4):2416-24.

[62] Sebastião MP, Saraiva MJ, Damas AM. The crystal structure of amyloidogenic Leu55 --> Pro transthyretin variant reveals a possible pathway for transthyretin polymerization into amyloid fibrils.Journal of Biological Chemistry. 1998; 273(38):24715-22.

[63] Karlsson A, Sauer-Eriksson AE. Heating of proteins as a means of improving crystallization: a successful case study on a highly amyloidogenic triple mutant of human

transthyretin. Acta Crystallographica Section F: Structural Biology and Crystallization Communications. 2007; 63(Pt 8):695-700.

[64] Nakanishi T, Yoshioka M, Moriuchi K, Yamamoto D, Tsuji M, Takubo T. S-sulfonation of transthyretin is an important trigger step in the formation of transthyretin-related amyloid fibril. Biochimica et Biophysica Acta. 2010 ;1804(7):1449-56

[65] Lim A, Prokaeva T, McComb ME, Connors LH, Skinner M, Costello CE.Identification of S-sulfonation and S-thiolation of a novel transthyretin Phe33Cys variant from a patient diagnosed with familial transthyretin amyloidosis. Protein Science. 2003; 12(8):1775-85.

[66] Hagen GA, Elliott WJ. Transport of thyroid hormones in serum and cerebrospinal fluid.The Journal of Clinical Endocrinology and Metabolism. 1973; 37(3):415-22.

[67] Hou X, Mechler A, Martin LL, Aguilar MI, Small DH. Cholesterol and anionic phospholipids increase the binding of amyloidogenic transthyretin to lipid membranes. Biochimica et Biophysica Acta. 2008; 1778(1):198-205.

[68] Cardoso I, Brito M, Saraiva MJ.Extracellular matrix markers for disease progression and follow-up of therapies in familial amyloid polyneuropathy V30M TTR-related. Disease Markers. 2008; 25(1):37

[69] Bourgault S, Solomon JP, Reixach N, Kelly JW.Sulfated glycosaminoglycans accelerate transthyretin amyloidogenesis by quaternary structural conversion.Biochemistry. 2011; 15;50(6):1001-15.

[70] Murakami T, Yi S, Maeda S, Tashiro F, Yamamura K, Takahashi K, Shimada K, Araki S.Effect of serum amyloid P component level on transthyretin-derived amyloid deposition in a transgenic mouse model of familial amyloidotic polyneuropathy. American Journal of Pathology. 1992; 141(2):451-6.

[71] Saito S, Ando Y, Nakamura M, Ueda M, Kim J, Ishima Y, Akaike T, Otagiri M.Effect of nitric oxide in amyloid fibril formation on transthyretin-related amyloidosis. Biochemistry. 2005; 44(33):11122-9.

[72] Bonifácio MJ, Sakaki Y, Saraiva MJ. 'In vitro' amyloid fibril formation from transthyretin: the influence of ions and the amyloidogenicity of TTR variants. Biochimica et Biophysica Acta. 1996; 1316(1):35-42

[73] Palaninathan SK, Mohamedmohaideen NN, Snee WC, Kelly JW, Sacchettini JC.Structural insight into pH-induced conformational changes within the native human transthyretin tetramer. Journal of Molecular Biology. 2008; 382(5):1157-67.

[74] Sörgjerd K, Klingstedt T, Lindgren M, Kågedal K, Hammarström P.Prefibrillar transthyretin oligomers and cold stored native tetrameric transthyretin are cytotoxic in cell culture. Biochemical and Biophysical Research Communications. 2008; 377(4): 1072-8

[75] Palmieri Lde C, Lima LM, Freire JB, Bleicher L, Polikarpov I, Almeida FC, Foguel D. Novel Zn2+-binding sites in human transthyretin: implications for amyloidogenesis and retinol-binding protein recognition. Journal of Biological Chemistry. 2010; 285(41):31731-41

[76] Olofsson A, Ippel JH, Wijmenga SS, Lundgren E, Ohman A.Probing solvent accessibility of transthyretin amyloid by solution NMR spectroscopy. Journal of Biological Chemistry. 2004; 279(7):5699-707.

[77] Liu K, Cho HS, Lashuel HA, Kelly JW, Wemmer DE.A glimpse of a possible amyloidogenic intermediate of transthyretin. Nature Structural Biology. 2000 ;7(9):754-7.

[78] Bateman DA, Tycko R, Wickner RB. Experimentally derived structural constraints for amyloid fibrils of wild-type transthyretin. Biophysical Journal. 2011; 101(10):2485-92.

[79] Chang MH, Hua CT, Isaac EL, Litjens T, Hodge G, Karageorgos LE, Meikle PJ.Transthyretin interacts with the lysosome-associated membrane protein (LAMP-1) in circulation. Biochem J. 2004; 382(Pt 2):481-9.

[80] Purkey HE, Dorrell MI, Kelly JW. Evaluating the binding selectivity of transthyretin amyloid fibril inhibitors in blood plasma. Proccedings of the National Academy of Sciences of United States of America. 2001; 98(10):5566-71.

[81] Wilkinson-White LE, Easterbrook-Smith SB. Characterization of the binding of Cu(II) and Zn(II) to transthyretin: effects on amyloid formation. Biochemistry. 2007; 46(31): 9123-32.

[82] Susuki S, Ando Y, Sato T, Nishiyama M, Miyata M, Suico MA, Shuto T, Kai H.Multielemental analysis of serum and amyloid fibrils in familial amyloid polyneuropathy patients. Amyloid. 2008; 15(2):108-16.

[83] Pasquato N, Berni R, Folli C, Alfieri B, Cendron L, Zanotti G. Acidic pH-induced conformational changes in amyloidogenic mutant transthyretin. Journal of Molecular Biology. 2007; 366(3):711-9

Chapter 7

# Anti-Cytokine Therapy for AA Amyloidosis

Keisuke Hagihara, Syota Kagawa, Yuki Kishida and Junsuke Arimitsu

Additional information is available at the end of the chapter

http://dx.doi.org/10.5772/53315

## 1. Introduction

Amyloid A (AA) amyloidosis is a serious complication of chronic inflammatory diseases, including rheumatoid arthritis (RA), juvenile idiopathic arthritis (JIA), inflammatory bowel disease (IBD), familial Mediterranean fever (FMF), and others [1]. Several reports suggest a prevalence of about 3 to 6% in rheumatoid arthritis patients [2-5], about 11 to 13% in FMF patients [6,7], and about 1 to 3% in IBD patients [8]. Serum amyloid A (SAA) is well known as a precursor of amyloid A proteins in AA amyloidosis. Insoluble amyloid fibril deposition is derived from the extracellular aggregation of proteolytic fragments of SAA. Human SAA family proteins are apolipoproteins of high-density lipoprotein molecules. Acute phase SAA consists of SAA1 and SAA2, which are mainly produced by proinflammatory cytokines in the liver such as interleukin-1 (IL-1), tumor necrosis factor-$\alpha$ (TNF-$\alpha$), and interleukin-6 (IL-6), and dramatically increase, by a magnitude of up to 1000 times during inflammation [9, 10]. Long-term overproduction of the SAA protein is a key component of the resultant pathogenic cascade [1]. The physiological roles of the various SAA isotypes remain unclear, but analysis of AA amyloid deposits has shown that SAA1 is the main amyloidogenic factor [11] and SAA1 genotypes are involved in the development of AA amyloidosis [12, 13]. In fact, it is reported that serum levels of SAA are associated with relative risk of death in AA amyloidosis patients. Relatively favorable outcomes are reported in patients with SAA concentrations remaining in the low-normal range (<4 mg per liter) [14, 15]. In Figure 1, the suppression of SAA levels by anti-cytokine therapy that may lead to clinical amelioration of symptoms, prevention of progressive organ deterioration, or recovery from damage caused by amyloid A deposits in the pathogenic cascade of AA amyloidosis is schematically represented. Anti-cytokine therapies have been used for rheumatoid arthritis (RA) and other chronic inflammatory diseases, and, as noted, their efficacy has been established in several clinical trials [16], although the best choice of biologic for AA amyloidosis remains controversial.

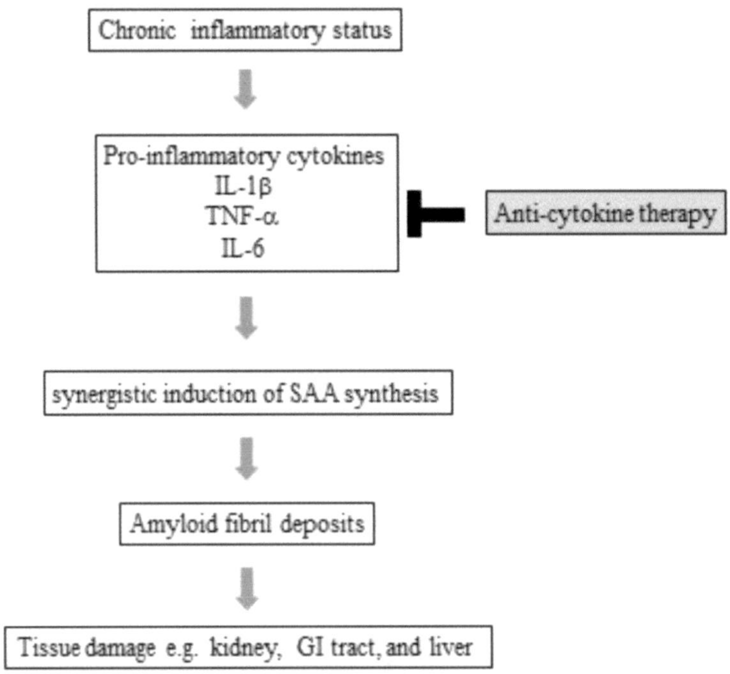


**Figure 1.** Anti-cytokine therapy for the pathogenesis of AA amyloidosis

In this chapter, we outline the clinical effect of anti-cytokine therapy for AA amyloidosis. We summarize animal models of AA amyloidosis association with pro-inflammatory cytokines, and finally, we show results elucidating the cytokine-driven induction mechanism of SAA. The formation of a transcriptional complex with signal transducer and activator of transcription 3 (STAT3) and nuclear factor κB (NF-κB) p65 play a critical role in the synergistic induction of SAA by IL-1, TNF-$\alpha$, and IL-6. These results provide a rationale for IL-6 blocking therapy as a highly reasonable candidate to normalize the serum levels of SAA in the treatment of AA amyloidosis.

## 2. Clinical effect of anti-cytokine therapy for AA amyloidosis

In The European League Against Rheumatism (EULAR) recommendations 2010 for the management of RA, the efficacy and safety of biologics were reviewed in patients with RA. We summarize the biologics against TNF-$\alpha$, IL-1, and IL-6 in Table 1. Five anti-TNF drugs are available, but golimumab and certolizumab have not been reported in the treatment of AA amyloidosis, and we found only 1 report of treatment with adalimumab in a patient with AA amyloidosis complicating JIA [17].

| Anti-TNF drugs | Characteristic | Dosage |
|---|---|---|
| Infliximab (IFX) | Chimeric (mouse/human)mAb IgG1 | div. once 8 weekly 3-10mg/kg |
| Adalimumab (ADA) | Human mAb, IgG1 | s.c. once biweekly 40-80mg/body |
| Etanercept (ETN) | Fusion protein of TNF receptor 2 and IgG1 Fc component | s.c. once weekly 25-50mg/body |
| Golimumab (GLM) | Human mAb, IgG1 | s.c. once monthly 50-100mg/body |
| Certolizumab (CZP) | Humanized Fab' fragment conjugated to a polyethylene glycol | s.c. once monthly 400 mg /body |
| IL-1 receptor antagonist | | |
| Anakinra (ANA) | non-glycosylated version of human IL-1RA | s.c. once or twice daily 100mg/body |
| Anti-IL-6 receptor antibody | | |
| Tocilizumab (TCZ) | Humanized mAb, IgG1 | div. once 4 weekly 8mg/kg |

**Table 1.** Examples of biologics for inflammatory cytokines

### 2.1. Anti-TNF therapy for AA amyloidosis

Several studies have reported that the efficacy of various anti-TNF drugs in the treatment of patients with AA amyloidosis, and infliximab (IFX) and etanercept (ETN) have been used in many of them (Table 2). In 2002, Elkayam et al. first reported successful treatment of an AA amyloidosis patient with IFX. A 67-year-old woman with RA developed moderately active disease and significant proteinuria. AA amyloidosis was diagnosed by a renal biopsy. After 14 weeks with IFX the patient's SAA decreased from the pre-therapy level of 29 mg/L to 4.5 mg/L. In addition, clinical remission of the nephrotic syndrome was observed as along with stabilization of amyloid deposits confirmed by $^{123}$I-labeled SAP scintigraphy after 1 year [18]. In 2003, Verschueren et al. reported that a 26-year-old man with JIA and IBD associated with spondyloarthropathy (HLA B27+) developed significant proteinuria. AA amyloidosis was diagnosed by a renal biopsy. IFX improved the proteinuria after 9 months, but amyloid deposits in renal specimens remained almost the same in the mesangium and in the subendothelial and subepithelial spaces after IFX therapy [19]. Ortiz-Santamaria et al. reported the clinical effect of IFX on 6 patients with AA amyloidosis (5 patients with related RA and 1 with ankylosing spondylitis (AS)). Three patients were withdrawn from the therapy in the first 2 months, 2 because they required hemodialysis and 1 because of an anaphylactic reaction. Serum creatinine levels and proteinuria stabilized in 1 patient and improved in 2 patients during treatment with IFX [20]. Gottenberg et al. reported that 15 patients with AA amyloidosis and renal involvement were treated with TNF inhibitors. Baseline characteristic of the 15 patients were different (RA 5, AS 6, JIA 1, psoriatic arthritis (PA) 1, adult Still's disease (ASD) 1, and Chronic infantile neurologic cutaneous and articular (CINCA) syndrome 1). Ten patients received IFX, 4 received ETN, and 1 underwent both types of treatment. Frequency of diarrhea was markedly reduced in 2 of the 3 patients with digestive tract amyloidosis, while amyloidosis progressed in 7 patients and was stabilized in 5 patients. This retrospective study suggested only the possibility that TNF inhibitors were effective for AA amyloidosis [21].

| Authors | Design | Disease | Drugs | Organ dysfunction | Results |
|---|---|---|---|---|---|
| Elkayam et al. 2002 [18] | Case report | RA 1 | IFX | Kidney | Proteinuria improved |
| Verscueren et al. 2003 [19] | Case report | IBD+AS 1 | IFX | Kidney | Proteinuria improved |
| Ortiz-Santamaria et al. 2003 [20] | Case series | RA 5, AS 1 | IFX 6 | Kidney | 3 patients withdrawn, stabilized in 1 patient and improved in 2 patients |
| Gottenberg et al. 2003 [21] | Retrospective study | RA 5, AS 6, JIA1, PA1, ASD1 CINCA 1 | IFX10 ETN4 Both1 | Kidney | Progressed in 7 patients and stabilized in 5 patients |
| Smith et al. 2004 [22] | Case report | RA 1 | ETN | Kidney | Proteinuria improved |
| Ravindran et al. 2004 [23] | Case report | RA with Felty's syndrome 1 | ETN→ IFX | kidney | Proteinuria improved |
| Metyas et al.2004 [28] | Case report | FMF 1 | IFX | Kidney | Proteinuria improved |

**Table 2.** Anti-TNF drugs in the treatment with AA amyloidosis patients

Studies of ETN in AA amyloidosis patients are fewer than those of IFX. In 2004 Smith et al. reported that ETN improved proteinuria in a patient with renal amyloidosis complicating RA for 3 years [22]. In 2004, Ravindran et al. published a report of a case of RA with secondary Sjögren's syndrome and Felty's syndrome complicated by AA amyloidosis and nephrotic syndrome, which was treated with ETN for 1 year and IFX for 1 year. After 1 year, the patient's urinary protein was 6 g over 24 h. The patient changed to monotherapy with IFX. Marked reductions in proteinuria as well as a sustained stabilization of renal function were observed. In addition, a regression of AA amyloid, as quantified by $^{123}$I-labeled SAP scintigraphy was established [23]. It seems that IFX therapy might be more effective than ETN therapy for AA amyloidosis. In fact, while ETN treatment of patients with AA amyloidosis produced a decrease in SAA, there were no significant changes in serum creatinine or proteinuria [24]. In 2009, Kuroda et al. reported the effects of TNF inhibitors on 14 patients with

http://dx.doi.org/10.5772/53315

AA amyloidosis associated with RA. Four patients were treated with IFX and 10 with ETN. Twenty-four hour urinary protein excretion was significantly decreased in 3 patients, stable in 6, and increased in 3 after initiation of anti-TNF therapy. The gastroduodenal biopsies from 9 patients showed significant reductions in amyloid deposits, which were no longer detectable in 2 patients [25].

In 2010, Nakamura et al. evaluated the efficacy of ETN treatment in 14 patients with RA complicated by AA amyloidosis. The AA amyloidosis improved and stabilized after 89.1±27.2 weeks. Proteinuria decreased from 2.24 to 0.57 g/day ($p < 0.01$) and SAA fell from 250 to 26 mg/L. Diarrhea secondary to gastrointestinal AA amyloidosis was less, but serum creatinine levels did not improve.

| Authors | Design | Disease | Drugs | Organ dysfunction | Results |
|---|---|---|---|---|---|
| Bosca et al. 2006 [29] | Case report | Crohn 's disease 1 | IFX | Kidney | Proteinuria improved |
| Perry et al. 2008 [24] | Case series | Inflammatory arthritis 9 | ETN | Kidney | No significant changes in serum creatinine or proteinuria |
| Kuroda et al. 2009 [25] | Case series | RA 14 | IFX 10<br>ETN 4 | Kidney<br>GI tract | Proteinuria improved in 3 patients, remained the same in 6 patients, and increased in 3 patients. Gastroduodenal amyloid deposit reduced in 9 patients. |
| Nowak et al. 2009 [17] | Case report | JIA 1 | ADA | Kidney | Proteinuria improved |
| Nakamura et al. 2010 [26] | Case series | RA 14 | ETN | kidney | After 89.1± 27.2 weeks, proteinuria decreased and diarrhea was less. Serum creatinine level did not improve. |
| Fernandez-Nebro et al. 2010 [27] | Multicenter, controlled, dynamic prospective cohort study | RA 21, SA 8, PA 4, JIA 1, aSD 1, APS 1 | IFX 29<br>ETN 7 | Kidney 94%<br>Liver 8%<br>GI tract 11% | Proteinuria reduced by 59.7 % during the first 24 months. Serum creatinine level did not improve. The level of acute phase reactants diminished but did not reach the normal level. |

**Table 3.** Anti-TNF drugs in the treatment with AA amyloidosis patients

In 2010, Fernandez-Nebro et al. reported a multicenter, controlled, dynamic prospective cohort study of 36 patients with AA amyloidosis who were treated with either IFX (29) or ETN (7). As external controls, 35 non-amyloid patients (RA 18, SA 11, PA 5, JIA1, aSD 0, APS 0) treated with TNF drugs were extracted from the *Base de Datos de Productos Biológicos de la Sociedad Española de Reumatología* registry. Long-term anti-TNF treatment reduced the median levels of proteinuria by 59.7% during the first 24 months, while both mean serum creatinine levels and creatinine clearance levels remained stable. Serum levels of CRP decreased, but did not reach the normal level. In a multivariate Cox regression analysis, the duration of amyloidosis and the level of proteinuria were independent predictors of anti-TNF treatment failure, and the level of proteinuria was the only predictor of mortality in AA amyloidosis. The number of infections was 3 times higher in AA amyloidosis patients [27]. In addition, it has been reported that anti-TNF treatment is effective for clinical improvement in AA amyloidosis associated with FMF [28] or Crohn's disease [29]. Taking these findings together, treatment of AA amyloidosis with TNF inhibitors is promising, although anti-TNF therapy does not always lead to the better clinical outcomes or normalize serum levels of SAA in AA amyloidosis patients. For instance, in an open phase I/II trial of IFX, Elliott et al. reported that IFX reduced serum SAA levels in patients with RA from 245 mg/L to 58 mg/L after 1 week of treatment and to 80 mg/L after 2 weeks [30]. In 1999, Charles et al. reported that IFX therapy after 24 weeks decreased SAA levels from 378 mg/L to 56 mg/L, but did not normalize the levels as in the above report [31].

### 2.2. Anti-IL-1 therapy for AA amyloidosis

IL-1 is a key pro-inflammatory that contributes to pathogenesis of RA. The IL-1 receptor antagonist anakinra (ANA) was thought to be a promising drug for RA, however, it has been reported to be less effective than other biologics for this disease [16]. It has been reported that ANA is effective for Muckle–Wells syndrome caused by a mutation in the gene encoding the protein [32], and we also found several reports that ANA is effective for AA amyloidosis complicating familial cold autoinflammatory syndrome [33], FMF [34], FMA and Behcet's disease [35], and cryopyrin-associated periodic syndrome (CAPS) [36]. In all cases, ANA normalized serum levels of SAA and dramatically improved proteinuria in renal amyloidosis. Unfortunately, these diseases are very rare, thus use of ANA in AA amyloidosis remains limited.

| Authors | Design | Disease | Drugs | Organ dysfunction | Results |
|---|---|---|---|---|---|
| Thornto et al. 2007 [33] | Case report | FCAS 1 | ANA | Kidney | Proteinuria improved |
| Moser et al. 2009 [34] | Case report | FMF 1 | ANA | Kidney | Good outcome after transplantation |
| Bilginer et al. 2010 [35] | Case report | FMF and Behçet's disease 1 | ANA | Kidney | Proteinuria improved |
| Aït-Abdesselam et al 2010 [36] | Case report | CAPS 1 | ANA | Kidney | Proteinuria improved |

**Table 4.** Anti-IL-1 drugs in the treatment with AA dmyloidosis patients

### 2.3. Anti-IL-6 therapy for AA amyloidosis

IL-6 blocking therapy is effected by tocilizumab (TCZ), which is a humanized anti-IL-6 receptor monoclonal antibody of the IgG1 class. TCZ has been used for the treatment of RA [37], JIA [38], and multicentric Castleman's disease [39]. In the EULAR recommendations 2010 for the management of RA, TCZ was noted for demonstrating efficacy in patients who failed treatment with TNF inhibitors (level of evidence 1B) [16]. In 2003, it was reported that 15 patients with active RA were treated with TCZ biweekly for 6 weeks in an open label phase I/II trial [40]. Serum levels of C-reactive protein and SAA were completely normalized at 6 weeks after TCZ therapy, which identified anti-IL-6 therapy as a promising treatment for AA amyloidosis. In 2006, Okuda et al. first reported successful treatment with TCZ in JIA complicated with AA Amyloidosis [41] in a 26-year-old woman with JIA who initially developed severe intractable diarrhea in 2001, after which AA amyloidosis was confirmed by GI tract and mucosal biopsy. In 2003, the patient presented with proteinuria, and amyloid deposits in the kidneys were confirmed by renal biopsy. At the same time, the patient developed steroid induced glaucoma.

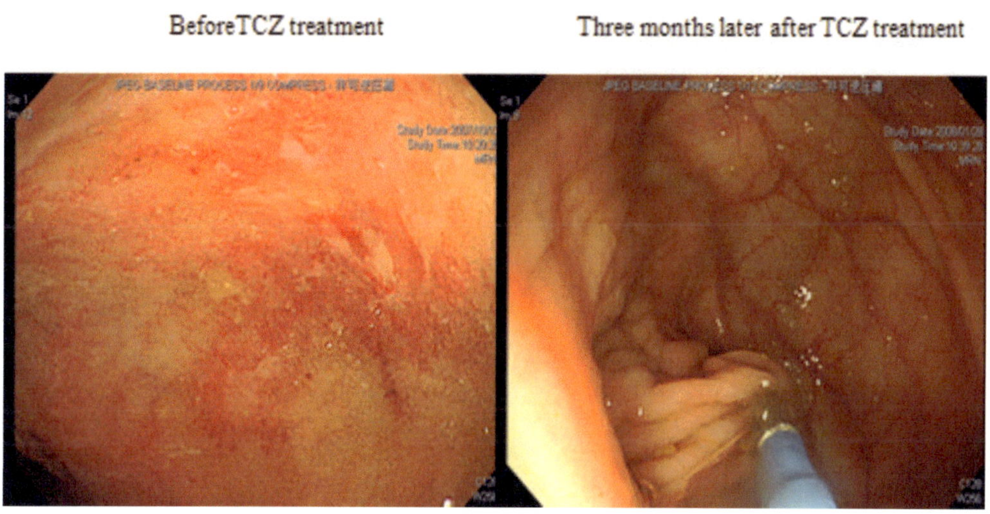


**Figure 2.** Results of endoscopic examination before and after TCZ therapy. Before TCZ therapy the appearance of the mucosa in the colon was edematous and reddish. After 3 months of TCZ therapy, no abnormality was observed. Quoted from : Nishida S., et al. Ann Rheum Dis. 2009 [49] unpublished data.

In patients who showed severe disease activity despite aggressive treatment with MTX at a dosage of 15 mg/week and prednisolone at a dosage of 10 mg/day, TCZ immediately normalized the serum levels of SAA, from 242.7 μg/mL to 2.49 μg/mL after the first dose. Gastrointestinal symptoms such as diarrhea and abdominal pain disappeared after 1 month and proteinuria improved after 2 months. Moreover, gastrointestinal biopsy specimens showed dramatic regression of AA protein deposits. We also experienced successful treatment of AA amyloidosis with TCZ for a 50-year-old woman with RA, who had failed TNF inhibitor including ETN and IFX, and had developed severe diarrhea and weight loss. AA amyloid deposits were confirmed by colon biopsy. TCZ administration immediately normalized serum levels of SAA, stopped the diarrhea, and diminished the disease activity of RA. Notably, 3 months after TCZ treatment, amyloid A protein deposits had completely disappeared (fig.2 and fig.3) [42].

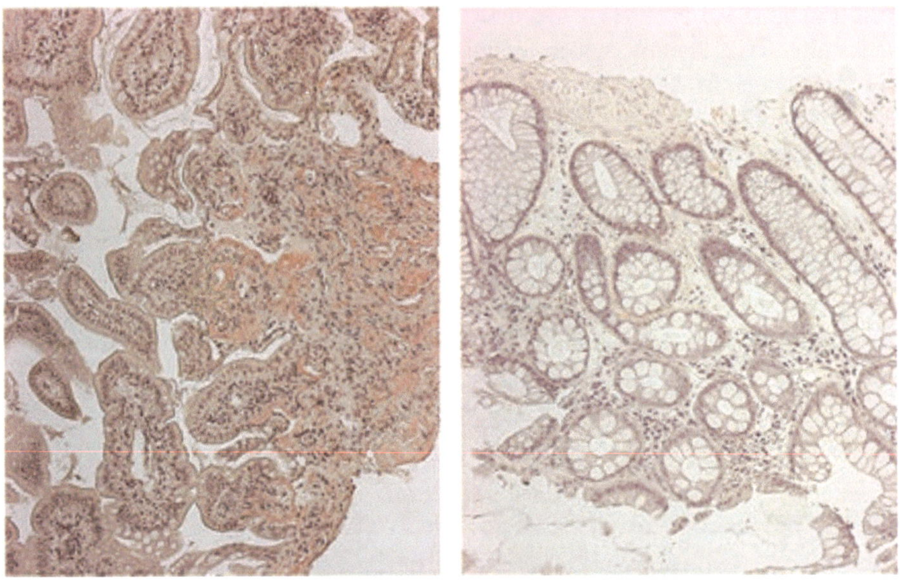


**Figure 3.** Results of colon biopsy before and after TCZ therapy massive amyloid deposits had disappeared 3 months later after TCZ treatment. Quoted from : Nishida S., et al. Ann Rheum Dis. 2009 [49] unpublished data.

| | Design | Disease | Drugs | Organ dysfunction | Results |
|---|---|---|---|---|---|
| Okuda et al. 2006 [41] | Case report | JIA 1 | TCZ | Kidney<br>GI tract | Proteinuria improved<br>GI symptoms disappeared |
| Nishida et al. 2009 [42] | Case report | RA 1 | ETN,IFX → TCZ | GI tract | Severe diarrhea improved |
| Sato et al. 2009 [43] | Case report | RA 1 | TCZ | GI tract | Severe diarrhea improved |
| Inoue et al. 2010 [44] | Case report | RA 1 | TCZ | GI tract | Paralytic ileus improved |
| Kishida et al. 2011 [45] | Case report | JIA with HB 1 | TCZ | Kidney<br>GI tract | Proteinuria improved<br>Amyloid deposits in GI tract disappeared |

**Table 5.** Anti-IL-6 drugs in the treatment with AA amyloidosis patients

In 2009, Sato et al. reported that TCZ relieved severe diarrhea in AA amyloidosis associated with RA. A 53-year-old woman with RA went into hypovolemic shock because of severe watery diarrhea. AA amyloidosis was confirmed by colon biopsy. A 60 mg dosage of prednisolone therapy and glucocorticoid pulse therapy with 1 g dosage of methylprednisolone did not ameliorate the severe diarrhea. After TCZ administration, the life-threatening diarrhea lessened within about 6 h. However, the patient developed a perforation of the small intestine 2 days after TCZ administration. After successful surgery, administration of TCZ resumed and reduced AA amyloid deposits [43]. In 2010, Inoue et al. reported that TCZ resolved paralytic ileus related to AA amyloidosis of the GI tract associated with RA. After 3 courses of TCZ treatment, a colon biopsy revealed no amyloid deposition [44 ]. In addition, Kishida et al. reported that TCZ therapy improved proteinuria and amyloid deposits in duodenal mucosa for a patient with adult-onset Still's disease complicated by AA amyloidosis [45]. These dramatic effects of TCZ on AA amyloidosis provide material for bedside-to-bench research and have indicated that TCZ might be more promising in the treatment of AA amyloidosis than anti-TNF or IL-1 inhibitors, although further clinical studies are needed to further evaluate its efficacy and safety, and the question remains as to how TCZ immediately normalizes the SAA levels.

Next, we summarize animal models of pro-inflammatory cytokines associated with AA amyloidosis.

## 3. AA amyloidosis model mice

AA amyloidosis is the most common form of systemic amyloid disease induced in animals [46]. Mice especially have been used to induce amyloidosis. Several strains (CBA/J, C57B1/6J, C3H/Hej, BALB/cJ) are susceptible [47]. Animal models are considered pivotal for the study of genetic risk factors. The murine model of AA amyloidosis faithfully reproduces the pathogenesis of its human counterpart. Of the major substances used to induce amyloid in animal species, casein has been preferred [47]. Silver nitrate [48], Freund adjuvant [49], and lipopolysaccharide [50] injection also induce AA amyloidosis. Several drugs have been evaluated using the above animal models. For example, in clinical trials, tenidap treatment reduced levels of CRP and SAA in RA patients [51], and in 1996, Husebekk et al. reported that tenidap inhibited amyloid deposits in an AA amyloidosis model using CBA/J mice induced by complete Freund adjuvant [52]. However, they did not examine the levels of IL-1, TNF-$\alpha$, and IL-6.

Triptolide isolated from *Tripterygium wilfordii* has anti-inflammatory effects on adjuvant-induced arthritis in rats and on immune cells including T cells, B cells, and monocyte [53, 54]. Cui et al. reported that triptolide inhibited splenic amyloid deposition in both rapid and chronic induction models of AA amyloidosis induced by casein in ICR mice. Triptolide also immediately decreased SAA and IL-6 levels without changes in IL-1 or TNF-$\alpha$. They suggested that triptolide inhibits experimental murine amyloidosis via suppression of IL-6 [55].

Mihara et al. examined whether the anti-IL-6 receptor antibody MR16-1 inhibited the development of AA-amyloidosis in a transient and chronic mouse model using C57BL/6 mice induced by amyloid enhancing factor (AEF) and complete Freund adjuvant. In the transient model, administration of MR16-1 before the injection of AEF and adjuvant completely prevented amyloid deposition and normalized SAA production. A chronic model was induced by AEF injection into IL-6 transgenic mice. One week later MR16-1 was injected intravenously. MR16-1 decreased amyloid deposition even when injected 1 week after AEF injection, although MR16-1 only partially inhibited SAA and IL-6 levels in IL-6 transgenic mice [56]. Mice that constitutively express the human interleukin 6 (huIL6) proteins from a heritable transgene (H2-Ld-IL-6) begin to develop severe systemic AA amyloidosis. These mice were observed in a hunched posture and moribund state when they were as young as 3 to 5 months of age. The result suggested the possibility that AA amyloidosis is due to genetic rather than environmental factors [57]. In a search, we found no report indicating that the effects of TNF inhibitors in AA Amyloidosis model mice had been examined. IL-1 receptor antagonist partially decreased the mRNA of SAA in C57BL/6 mice using silver nitrate [58]. These studies in mouse models have provided strong evidence to support a pivotal role for IL-6 in the induction of SAA.

Next we describe the molecular mechanisms of the synergistic induction of SAA by IL-1, TNF-$\alpha$, and IL-6.

## 4. Molecular mechanisms of serum amyloid A transcription

The former transcription model reported that the SAA2 gene is induced by NF-κB and CAAT enhancer-binding protein β (C/EBP β) in response to stimulation by IL-1 together with IL-6 [59]. However, this induction model does not fully explain clinical results (fig. 4). Even if IL-6 signal transduction is inhibited, activation of NF-κB signal still remains. However, anti-IL-6 therapy, but not anti-TNF [20, 21, 25-27] or IL-1 therapy [16], normalized the serum levels of SAA in AA amyloidosis patients [41-45]. It remains unclear whether STAT3, which is the main transcription factor of IL-6 signal transduction, plays a role in the transcriptional activation of the SAA gene. We investigated the exact induction mechanism of SAA by proinflammatory cytokines, and especially focused on the SAA1 gene, which is reported as a main amyloidogenic factor in AA amyloidosis [9].

### 4.1. IL-6 plays a critical role in the synergistic induction of the SAA gene by proinflammatory cytokines

We first established SAA isoforms via real time quantitative RT-PCR assay to examine various combination effects of proinflammatory cytokines. IL-6 and IL-1 or IL-6 and TNF-$\alpha$ induced synergistic expression of the SAA1 gene, but not IL-1 and TNF-$\alpha$ (fig. 5A). We confirmed the above results using each specific inhibitor in a triple stimulation with IL-6, IL-1, and TNF-$\alpha$. Only Anti-IL-6R monoclonal antibody (Mab) completely inhibited the synergistic induction of both SAA1 and SAA2 mRNA (fig. 5B). We obtained almost the same results with 3 typical hepatic cell lines, HepG2, Hep3B, and PLC/PRF/5. These results were in good agreement with clinical results of anti-cytokine therapy in inflammatory diseases that indicated that IL-6 plays a pivotal role in the synergistic induction of the SAA1 gene. Next, we sought to identify the signal transduction mechanism to activate the SAA1 gene. IL-6 signal transduction has 2 pathways. One is a MAPK-C/EBPβ pathway and the other is a JAK-STAT pathway [62]. The JAK2 inhibitor AG490, but not the MEK1/2 inhibitor U0126, repressed the SAA1 gene expression in response to IL-1β + IL-6 (fig. 5C) [60]. These data suggested that the JAK-STAT pathway plays an important role in SAA gene induction.

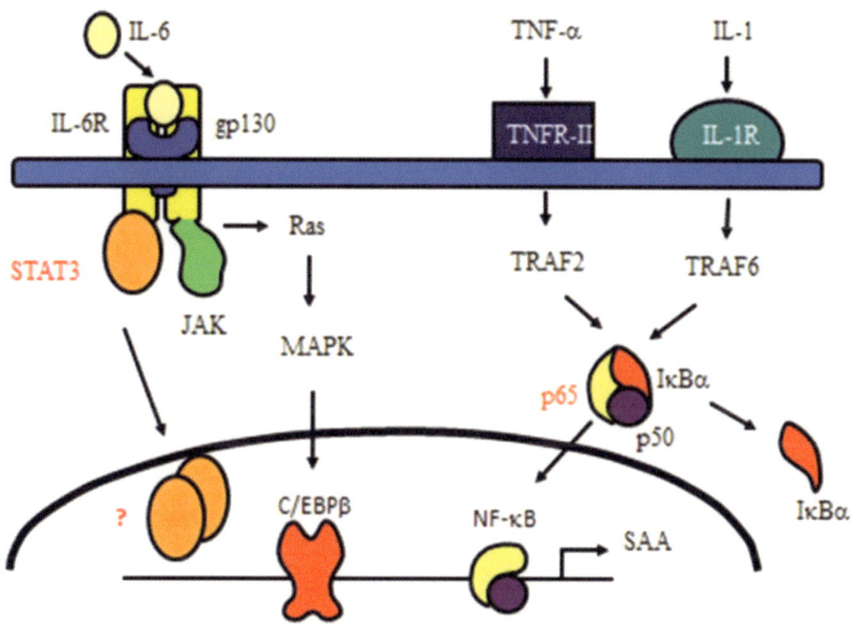


**Figure 4.** Former transcription model of a human SSA gene expression induced by proinflammatory cytokines; Betts et al. J. Biol Chem. 1993 [59]

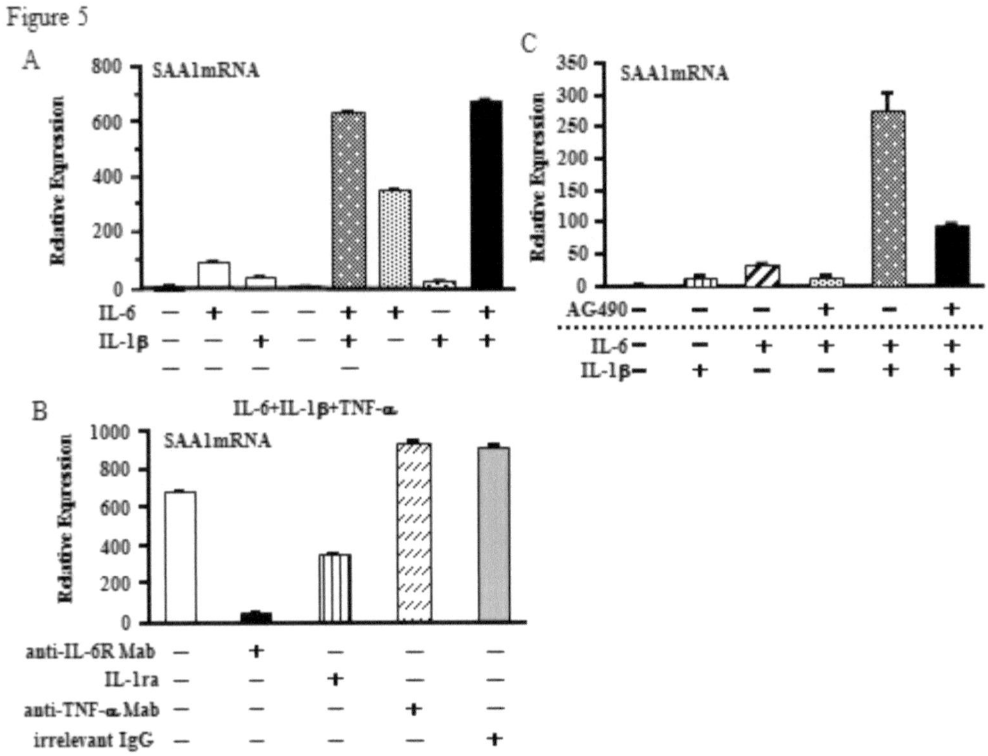


**Figure 5.** A) Combined effects of IL-6 (10 ng/mL), IL-1β (0.1 ng/mL), and/or TNF-α (10 ng/mL) on the induction of SAA 1. (B) Inhibitory effects of anti-IL-6R monoclonal antibody (Mab) (25 μg/μL), IL-1 receptor antagonist (Ra) (100 ng/mL), and anti-TNF-α Mab (4 μg/μL) on the synergistic induction of SAA1 generated by triple stimulation of IL-6, IL-1β, and TNF-α. Each specific reagent was incubated with HepG2 cells for 30 min prior to cytokine stimulation. (C) Effects of Jak2 kinase inhibitor-AG490 (100 μM) on synergistic induction of SAA1 mRNA. HepG2 cells were treated with AG490 or DMSO alone for 30 min before cytokine stimulation. SAA1 mRNA levels in HepG2 cells were measured by real-time quantitative RT-PCR at 6 h after cytokine stimulation. Values are reported as mean (SD) of duplicate measurements.

### 4.2. Essential role of STAT3 for transcriptional activity of the SAA1 gene via the NF-κB RE-containing region after formation of a complex with NF-κB p65.

STAT3 binds to a γ-interferon activation sequence (GAS) such as sequence (-TTNNNGAA), and C-reactive protein (CRP), the acute-phase protein that is active in the response to IL-6, has a STAT3 response element (RE) (-TTCCCGAA) in its promoter [61]. However, the typical STAT3 RE was not found in the human SAA1 promoter. To examine the effect of STAT3 on SAA1 promoter activity, pEF-BOS dominant negative STAT3 Y705F (dn STAT3) or pEF-BOS wild type STAT3 (wt STAT3) HepG2 cells were co-transfected with pGL3-SAA1 promoter luciferase construct (−796/+24) (pGL3-SAA1) [63]. The co-expression of dn STAT3 completely inhibited pGL3-STAT1 expression, whereas the co-expression of wt STAT3 enhanced the transcriptional activity stimulated with IL-1β + IL-6 (fig. 6A). These results indicated that STAT3 plays a critical role in the transcriptional activity of the SAA1 gene. We examined the possibility that STAT3 might act on the transcriptional activity of SAA through the C/EBPβ and NF-κB RE-containing region.

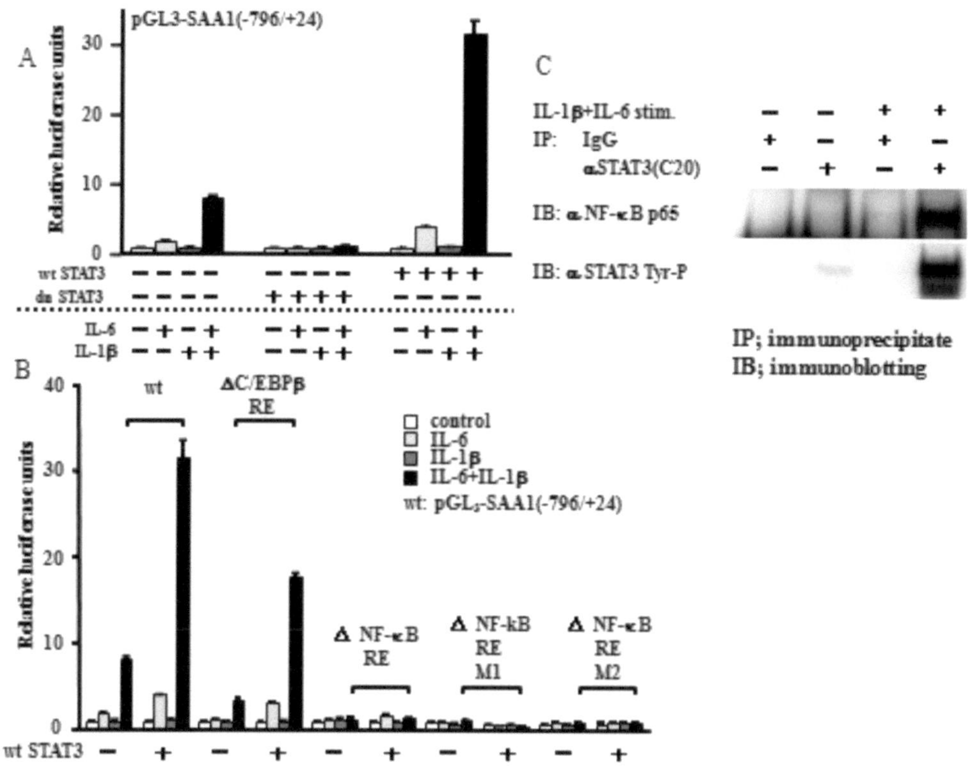


**Figure 6.** A) HepG2 cells were transfected with 0.5 μg of pGL3-SAA1 (–796/+24) alone, or co-transfected with 0.5 μg of pEF-BOS dominant negative STAT3 (dn STAT3) or pEF-BOS wild type STAT3 (wt STAT3), respectively. (B) 0.5 μg of wt STAT3 was co-transfected with 0.5 μg of pGL3-SAA1(–796/+24), pGL3-SAA1 ΔC/EBPβRE, pGL3-SAA1 ΔNF-κB RE, pGL3-SAA1 NF-κB RE M1 (**AGATCTATT**TCC), or M2 (CAGGGACTT**GTAC**). Cytokine stimulation was performed with IL-6 and/or IL-1β for 3 h. The relative luciferase activity is expressed as mean (SD) of triplicate cultures and transfections. (C) Nuclear extracts of HepG2 cells stimulated with IL-1 and IL-6 were immunoprecipitated with the anti-STAT3 C-20 antibody. Western blots were performed as shown. IP: immunoprecipitate, IB: immunoblotting.

In our experimental results, the transcriptional activity of the SAA1 gene was partly decreased by deletion of CEBP-β RE and completely diminished by deletion of NF-κB RE with co-expression of wt STAT3. These results suggest that STAT3 is involved in the transcriptional activity of SAA, most likely through NF-κB RE (fig. 6B). Competitive binding of STAT3 and NF-κB has been found in a rat γ-fibrinogen gene promoter that included a CTGGGAATCCC sequence [64]. It was reported that TCC was important for NF-κB binding and that CTGGGAA was necessary for STAT3 binding. Based on these reports, we created 2 mutant constructs, pGL3-SAA1 NF-κB RE M1 (**AGATCTA**TTTCCC) and M2 (CAGGGACTT**GTA**C). We expected that STAT3 would bind to NF-κB RE M2 but not to NF-κB RE

M1. However, neither transfection with NF-κB RE M1 nor M2 resulted in transcriptional activity, even when WT STAT3 was co-expressed (fig. 6B). We hypothesized that STAT3 forms a complex with NF-κB and augments the transcriptional activity of the human SAA gene. To examine our hypothesis, we performed IP-western blot for STAT3 and NF-κB. Figure 6C clearly shows that STAT3 is associated with NF-κB p65 following IL-1β + IL-6 treatment [63]. However, no specific band of NF-κB p50 was detected. These findings were consistent with those reported by Betts et al. that overexpression of NF-κB p65 but not p50 enhanced the transcriptional activity of human SAA2 in a dose-dependent manner [59], and demonstrating that crosstalk between STAT3 and NF-κB p65 contributes to the transcriptional augmentation of SAA by IL-1β + IL-6 stimulation.

### 4.3. STAT3 acts on the SAA1 promoter by means of a newly discovered *cis*-acting mechanism.

Next, we investigated how STAT3 contributes to the formation of the transcriptional complex comprising NF-κB, C/EBPβ, and STAT3. STAT3 is reportedly associated with p300 [65], which indicates the possibility that heteromeric complex formation of STAT3, NF-κB p65, and p300 is involved in the transcriptional activity of the human SAA gene. To examine this possibility, we performed a chromatin immunoprecipitation (Ch-IP) assay using chromatin isolated from HepG2 cells. STAT3 and p300 were clearly recruited to the SAA1 promoter region (−226 /+24) in response to IL-6 or IL-1β + IL-6, and weakly recruited by IL-1β. NF-κB p65 was recruited by IL-1 or IL-1β + IL-6 and weakly recruited by IL-6 [63] (fig. 7A). When we performed a luciferase assay using pGL3-SAA1 (−226/+24) co-transfected with p300 wt in pCMVβ (wt p300) and wt STAT3, we found that co-expression of wt p300 alone did not augment the luciferase activity of pGL3-SAA1 (−226/+24), but that co-expression of wt p300 with wt STAT3 dramatically enhanced the luciferase activity in a dose-dependent manner (fig. 7B). These results suggest that STAT3 interacts with p300 in the transcriptional activity of the human SAA gene by forming a transcriptional complex with NF−κB p65 and p300 on the SAA promoter region. However, it still remains to be determined how STAT3 binds to the promoter region of the SAA1 gene, because no typical STAT3 RE has been located. To address this, we performed DNA affinity chromatography using a wt SAA1 probe. We hypothesized that the formation of a STAT3-NF-κB p65 complex might confer STAT3 binding affinity to the SAA1 promoter. From our result and study of rat γ-fibrinogen, we focused our attention on the 3' site of NF-κB RE (CAGGGACTTTCCC**CAGGGAC**) as a candidate STAT3 binding site because the sequence contiguous to the NF-κB RE might have influenced the binding affinity of STAT3. To test this hypothesis, we created SAA1 mt NF-κB RE M3 (CAGGGACTTTCCC**AGATCTA**). As expected, the specific bands of STAT3 from the nuclear extracts of HepG2 cells after IL-1β + IL-6 stimulation were decreased by the SAA1 mt NF-κB RE M3 compared to the wt SAA1 probe, although the specific bands of NF-κB p65 were found almost intact, as with the wt SAA1 (fig. 7C). We were able to demonstrate that STAT3 acts on the human SAA promoter via a newly discovered *cis*-acting mechanism, namely, the formation of a heteromeric complex containing STAT3, NF-κB 65, and p300.

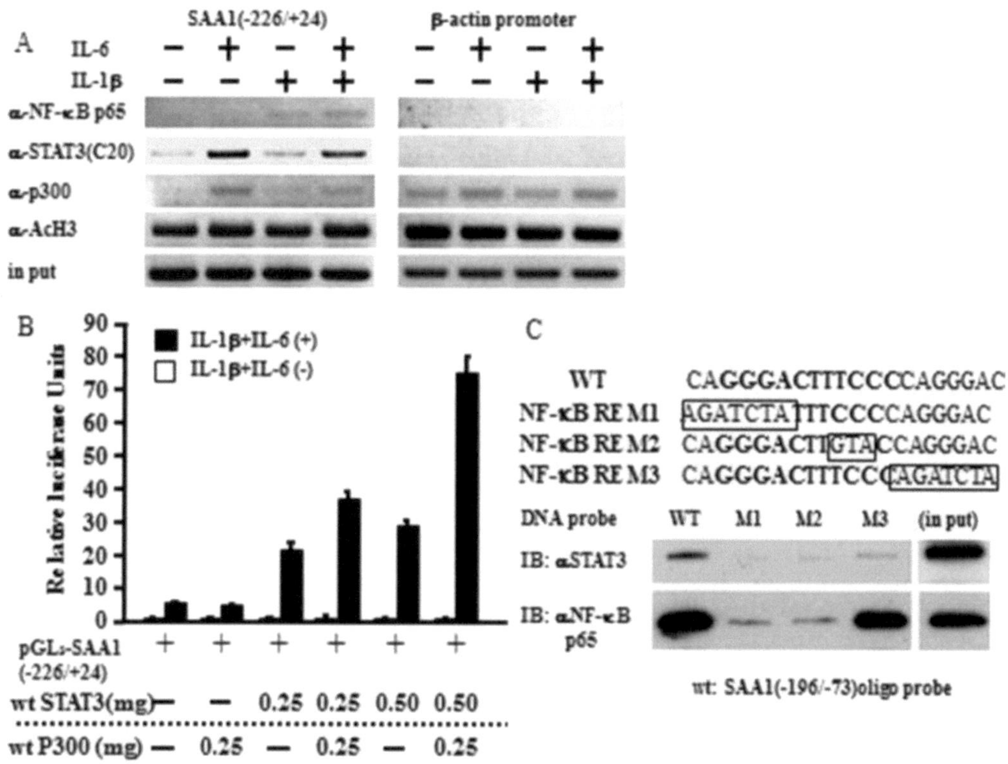


**Figure 7.** A) ChIP assays demonstrate recruitment patterns of STAT3, NF-κB p65 and p300 on the SAA1 promoter (−226/+24) from HepG2 cells treated with IL-6 and/or IL-1 ▪ for 30 min. Anti-AcH3 antibody was used as a positive control for this assay. (B) HepG2 cells were transfected with pGL3-SAA1 (−226/+24) (0.5 μg), 0.25 μg of p300 wild type in pCMVβ (wt p300), and/or 0.25–0.5 μg of wt STAT3. IL-1 and IL-6 stimulation was performed for 3 h. Relative luciferase activity is expressed as the mean (SD) of triplicate cultures and transfections. (C) DNA affinity chromatography was performed with 200 μg of the nuclear extracts from HepG2 cells after cytokine stimulation. The nuclear extracts were mixed with 1 μg of biotinylated DNA probe and 50 μl of streptavidin-Dynabeads was added to the samples, mixed, and collected with a magnet. The trapped proteins were analyzed by western blotting.

We have formulated a schematic model to describe the synergistic induction of the human SAA gene by IL-1β, TNF-α, and IL-6 stimulation (fig. 8A). This model explains the effect of anti-cytokine therapy on the transactivation of SAA. Anti-TNFα or anti-IL-1 therapy reduced NF-κB signaling pathways but they were not eliminated, because the NF-κB signaling pathway is activated by various stimulations, including toll-like receptors and other cytokines [66]. Consequently, the transcriptional complex on the SAA promoter remained after Anti-TNFα or IL-1 therapy (fig. 8B). On the other hand, IL-6 family cytokines, excluding IL-6 but including oncostatin M, IL-11, and LIF, have little influence on the production of acute phase proteins [68]. IL-6 blocking therapy inhibits the activation of STAT3 and C/EBP β, and prevents the formation of the transcriptional complex on the SAA promoter (fig. 8C). It is well known anti-TNF-α decreases serum levels of IL-6 [67], which indicates that the effect of anti-TNF-α therapy represses the serum levels of SAA by decreasing IL-6.

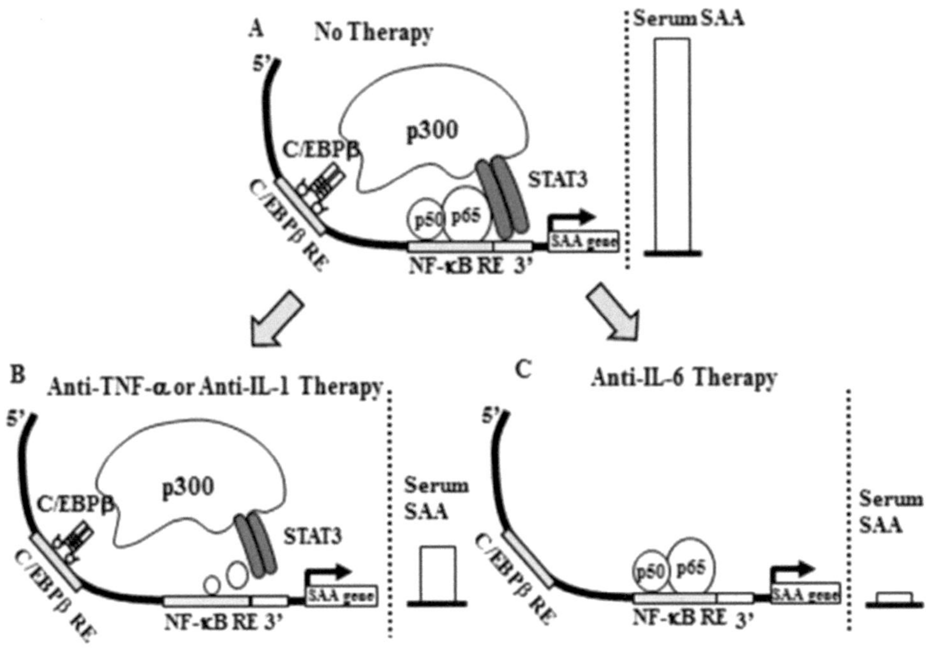


**Figure 8.** Effects of anti-cytokine therapy on the cytokine-driven transcriptional activity of human SAA gene. (A) Cytokine stimulation caused the formation around NF-κB RE of a heteromeric complex with STAT3 and NF-κB p65. STAT3, which is assumed to interact with the 3'-site of NF-κB RE, recruits the co-activator p300, which then coordinate the interaction of NF-κB p65, STAT3, and C/EBP,β thus resulting in the augmentation of transcriptional activity of human SAA gene. (B) anti-TNFα or IL-1 therapy reduce the activity of NF-κB signaling pathway, however, transcriptional complex are still remained. (C) anti-IL-6 therapy inhibits the activation of STAT3 and C/EBP,β, and eliminates the formation of the transcriptional complex on the SAA promoter.

## 5. Conclusion

Patients with AA amyloidosis whose SAA concentrations remain in the low-normal range [14, 15] have been reported to have a better prognosis. From the clinical point of view, our findings indicate that anti-IL-6 therapy is the most rational and promising therapy for AA amyloidosis patients via normalization of SAA level. In addition, our study is a new clinical research approach 'from bedside to bench' and directly lead to a better understanding of the pathogenesis of several inflammatory diseases.

## Acknowledgement

This. study was supported by the Ministry of Education, Culture, Sports, Science and Technology of Japan, the Ministry of Health, Labor and Welfare of Japan, and the Osaka Foundation for Promotion of Clinical Immunology.

## Author details

Keisuke Hagihara, Syota Kagawa, Yuki Kishida and Junsuke Arimitsu

*Address all correspondence to: k.hagihara@imed3.med.osaka-u.ac.jp

Department of Kampo medicine (Traditional Japanese medicine), Osaka University Graduate School of Medicine, Osaka, Japan

## References

[1] Pettersson T, Konttinen YT & Maury CPJ. Treatment strategies for amyloid A amyloidosis. Expert Opinion on Pharmacotherapy 2008;9(12) 2117-2128.

[2] De Beer FC, Mallya RK, Fagan EA, Lanham JG, Hughes GR, Pepys MB. Serum amyloid-A protein concentration in inflammatory diseases and its relationship to the incidence of reactive systemic amyloidosis. Lancet 1982;31(2) 231-234.

[3] Myllykangas-Luosujärvi R, Aho K, Kautiainen H, Hakala M. Amyloidosis in a nationwide series of 1666 subjects with rheumatoid arthritis who died during 1989 in Finland. Rheumatology 1999;38(6) 499-503.

[4] Laiho K, Tiitinen S, Kaarela K, Helin H, Isomäki H. Secondary amyloidosis has decreased in patients with inflammatory joint disease in Finland. Clin Rheumatol 1999;18(2) 122-123.

[5] Hazenberg BP, van Rijswijk MH. Where has secondary amyloid gone? Ann Rheum Dis 2000;59(8) 577-579.

[6] Tunca M, Akar S, Onen F, Ozdogan H, Kasapcopur O, Yalcinkaya F, Tutar E, Ozen S, Topaloglu R, Yilmaz E, Arici M, Bakkaloglu A, Besbas N, Akpolat T, Dinc A, Erken E. Turkish FMF Study Group. Familial Mediterranean fever (FMF) in Turkey: results of a nationwide multicenter study. Medicine 2005;84(1) 1-11.

[7] Touitou I, Sarkisian T, Medlej-Hashim M, Tunca M, Livneh A, Cattan D, Yalçinkaya F, Ozen S, Majeed H, Ozdogan H, Kastner D, Booth D, Ben-Chetrit E, Pugnère D, Michelon C, Séguret F, Gershoni-Baruch R. International Study Group for Phenotype-Genotype Correlation in Familial Mediterranean Fever. Country as the primary risk factor for renal amyloidosis in familial Mediterranean fever. Arthritis Rheum 2007;56(5) 1706-1712.

[8] Greenstein AJ, Sachar DB, Panday AK, Dikman SH, Meyers S, Heimann T, Gumaste V, Werther JL, Janowitz HD. Amyloidosis and inflammatory bowel disease. A 50-year experience with 25 patients. Medicine 1992;71(5) 261-270.

[9] Uhlar CM, Whitehead AS. Serum amyloid A, the major vertebrae acute-phase reactant. Eur J Biochem 1999;265(2):501-23.

[10] Buxbaum JN, Tagoe CE. The genetics of the amyloidoses. Annu Rev Med 2000;51 543-569.

[11] Liepnieks JJ, Kluve-Beckerman B, Benson MD. Characterization of amyloid A protein in human secondary amyloidosis: the predominant deposition of serum amyloid A1. Biochim Biophys Acta 1995;1270(1) 81-86.

[12] Baba S, Masago SA, Takahashi T, Kasama T, Sugimura H, Tsugane S, Tsutsui Y, Shirasawa H. A novel allelic variant of serum amyloid A, SAA1c: genomic evidence, evolution, frequency, and implication as a risk factor for reactive systemic AA-amyloidosis. Hum Mol Genet 1995;4(6) 1083-1087.

[13] Moriguchi M, Terai C, Kaneko H, Koseki Y, Kajiyama H, Uesato M, Inada S, Kamatani N. A novel single nucleotide polymorphism at the 50-flanking region of SAA1 associated with risk of type AA amyloidosis secondary to rheumatoid arthritis. Arthritis Rheum 2001;44(6) 1256-1272.

[14] Gillmore JD, Lovat LB, Persey MR, Pepys MB, Hawkins PN. Amyloid load and clinical outcome in AA amyloidosis in relation to circulating concentration of serum amyloid A protein. Lancet 2001;358(9275) 24-29.

[15] Lachmann HJ, Goodman HJ, Gilbertson JA, Gallimore JR, Sabin CA, Gillmore JD, Hawkins PN. Natural history and outcome in systemic AA amyloidosis. N Engl J Med 2007;356(23) 2361-2371.

[16] Nam JL, Winthrop KL, van Vollenhoven RF, Pavelka K, Valesini G, Hensor EM, Worthy G, Landewé R, Smolen JS, Emery P, Buch MH. Current evidence for the management of rheumatoid arthritis with biological disease-modifying antirheumatic drugs: a systematic literature review informing the EULAR recommendations for the management of RA. Ann Rheum Dis 2010;69(6) 976-986.

[17] Nowak B, Jeka S, Wiland P, Szechiński J. Rapid and complete resolution of ascites and hydrothorax due to nephrotic syndrome caused by renal amyloidosis in a patient with juvenile chronic arthritis treated with adalimumab. Joint Bone Spine 2009;76(2) 217-219.

[18] Elkayam O, Hawkins, PN, Lachmann H, Yaron M & Caspi D. Rapid and complete resolution of proteinuria due to renal amyloidosis in a patient with rheumatoid arthritis treated with infliximab. Arthritis & Rheumatism 2002;46(10) 2571-2573.

[19] Verschueren P, Lensen F, Lerut E, Claes K, De Vos R, Van Damme B, Westhovens R. Benefit of anti-TNF alpha treatment for nephrotic syndrome in a patient with juvenile inflammatory bowel disease associated spondyloarthropathy complicated with amyloidosis and glomerulonephritis. Ann Rheum Dis 2003;62(4) 368-369.

[20] Ortiz-Santamaria V, Valls-Roc M, Sanmarti M & Olive A. Anti-TNF treatment in secondary amyloidosis. Rheumatology 2003;42(11) 1425-1426.

[21] Gottenberg J-E, Merle-Vincent F, Bentaberry F, Allanore Y, Berenbaum F, Fautrel B, Combe B, Durbach A, Sibilia J, Dougados M & Mariette X. Anti-tumor necrosis factor

alpha therapy in fifteen patients with AA amyloidosis secondary to inflammatory arthritides: a followup report of tolerability and efficacy. Arthritis & Rheumatism 2003;48(7) 2019-2024.

[22] Smith GR, Tymms KE, Falk M. Etanercept treatment of renal amyloidosis complicating rheumatoid arthritis. Intern Med J 2004;34(9-10) 570-572.

[23] Ravindran J, Shenker N, Bhalla AK, Lachmann H & Hawkins P. Case report: response in proteinuria due to AA amyloidosis but not Felty's syndrome in a patient with rheumatoid arthritis treated with TNF-alpha blockade. Rheumatology 2004;43(2) 669-672.

[24] Perry ME, Stirling A, Hunter JA. Effect of etanercept on serum amyloid A protein (SAA) levels in patients with AA amyloidosis complicating inflammatory arthritis. Clin Rheumatol 2008;27(7) 923-925.

[25] Kuroda T, Wada Y, Kobayashi D, Murakami S, Sakai T, Hirose S, Tanabe N, Saeki T, Nakano M, Narita I. Effective anti-TNF-alpha therapy can induce rapid resolution and sustained decrease of gastroduodenal mucosal amyloid deposits in reactive amyloidosis associated with rheumatoid arthritis. J Rheumatol 2009;36(11) 2409-2415.

[26] Nakamura T, Higashi S, Tomoda K, Tsukano M, Shono M. Etanercept can induce resolution of renal deterioration in patients with amyloid A amyloidosis secondary to rheumatoid arthritis. Clin Rheumatol 2010;29(12) 1395-1401.

[27] Fernández-Nebro A, Olivé A, Castro MC, Varela AH, Riera E, Irigoyen MV, García de Yébenes MJ, García-Vicuña R. Long-term TNF-alpha blockade in patients with amyloid A amyloidosis complicating rheumatic diseases. Am J Med 2010;123(5) 454-461.

[28] Metyas S, Arkfeld DG, Forrester DM, Ehresmann GR. Infliximab treatment of Familial Mediterranean fever and its effect on secondary AA amyloidosis. J Clin Rheumatol 2004;10(3) 134-137.

[29] Boscá MM, Pérez-Baylach CM, Solis MA, Antón R, Mayordomo E, Pons S, Mínguez M, Benages A. Secondary amyloidosis in Crohn's disease: treatment with tumour necrosis factor inhibitor. Gut 2006;55(2) 294-295.

[30] Elliott MJ, Maini RN, Feldmann M, Long-Fox A, Charles P, Katsikis P, Brennan FM, Walker J, Bijl H, Ghrayeb J, et al. Treatment of rheumatoid arthritis with chimeric monoclonal antibodies to tumor necrosis factor alpha. Arthritis Rheum 1993;36(12) 1681-1690.

[31] Charles P, Elliott MJ, Davis D, Potter A, Kalden JR, Antoni C, Breedveld FC, Smolen JS, Eberl G, deWoody K, Feldmann M, Maini RN. Regulation of cytokines, cytokine inhibitors, and acute-phase proteins following anti-TNF-alpha therapy in rheumatoid arthritis. J Immunol 1999;163(3) 1521-1528.

[32] Hawkins PN, Lachmann HJ, McDermott MF. Interleukin-1-receptor antagonist in the Muckle-Wells syndrome. N Engl J Med 2003;348(25) 2583-2584.

[33] Thornton BD, Hoffman HM, Bhat A, Don BR. Successful treatment of renal amyloidosis due to familial cold autoinflammatory syndrome using an interleukin 1 receptor antagonist. Am J Kidney Dis 2007;49(3) 477-481.

[34] Moser C, Pohl G, Haslinger I, Knapp S, Rowczenio D, Russel T, Lachmann HJ, Lang U, Kovarik J. Successful treatment of familial Mediterranean fever with Anakinra and outcome after renal transplantation. Nephrol Dial Transplant 2009;24(2) 676-678.

[35] Bilginer Y, Ayaz NA, Ozen S. Anti-IL-1 treatment for secondary amyloidosis in an adolescent with FMF and Behçet's disease. Clin Rheumatol 2010;29(2) 209-210.

[36] Aït-Abdesselam T, Lequerré T, Legallicier B, François A, Le Loët X, Vittecoq O. Anakinra efficacy in a Caucasian patient with renal AA amyloidosis secondary to cryopyrin-associated periodic syndrome. Joint Bone Spine 2010;77(6) 616-617.

[37] Nishimoto N, Yoshizaki K, Miyasaka N, Yamamoto K, Kawai S, Takeuchi T, Hashimoto J, Azuma J, Kishimoto T. Treatment of rheumatoid arthritis with humanized anti-interleukin-6 receptor antibody: a multicenter, double-blind, placebo-controlled trial. Arthritis Rheum 2004;50(6) 1761-1769.

[38] Yokota S, Miyamae T, Imagawa T, Iwata N, Katakura S, Mori M, Woo P, Nishimoto N, Yoshizaki K, Kishimoto T. Therapeutic efficacy of humanized recombinant anti-interleukin-6 receptor antibody in children with systemic-onset juvenile idiopathic arthritis. Arthritis Rheum 2005;52(3) 818-825.

[39] Nishimoto N, Kanakura Y, Aozasa K, Johkoh T, Nakamura M, Nakano S, Nakano N, Ikeda Y, Sasaki T, Nishioka K, Hara M, Taguchi H, Kimura Y, Kato Y, Asaoku H, Kumagai S, Kodama F, Nakahara H, Hagihara K, Yoshizaki K, Kishimoto T. Humanized anti-interleukin-6 receptor antibody treatment of multicentric Castleman disease. Blood 2005;106(8) 2627-2632.

[40] Nishimoto N, Yoshizaki K, Maeda K, Kuritani T, Deguchi H, Sato B, Imai N, Suemura M, Kakehi T, Takagi N, Kishimoto T. Toxicity, pharmacokinetics, and dose-finding study of repetitive treatment with the humanized anti-interleukin 6 receptor antibody MRA in rheumatoid arthritis. Phase I/II clinical study. J Rheumatol 2003;30(7) 1426-1435.

[41] Okuda Y, Takasugi K. Successful use of a humanized anti-interleukin-6 receptor antibody, tocilizumab, to treat amyloid A amyloidosis complicating juvenile idiopathic arthritis. Arthritis Rheum 2006;54(9) 2997-3000.

[42] Nishida S, Hagihara K, Shima Y, Kawai M, Kuwahara Y, Arimitsu J, Hirano T, Narazaki M, Ogata A, Yoshizaki K, Kawase I, Kishimoto T, Tanaka T. Rapid improvement of AA amyloidosis with humanised anti-interleukin 6 receptor antibody treatment. Ann Rheum Dis 2009;68(7) 1235-1236.

[43] Sato H, Sakai T, Sugaya T, Otaki Y, Aoki K, Ishii K, Horizono H, Otani H, Abe A, Yamada N, Ishikawa H, Nakazono K, Murasawa A, Gejyo F. Tocilizumab dramati-

cally ameliorated life-threatening diarrhea due to secondary amyloidosis associated with rheumatoid arthritis. Clin Rheumatol 2009;28(9) 1113-1116.

[44] Inoue D, Arima H, Kawanami C, Takiuchi Y, Nagano S, Kimura T, Shimoji S, Mori M, Tabata S, Yanagita S, Matsushita A, Nagai K, Imai Y, Takahashi T. Excellent therapeutic effect of tocilizumab on intestinal amyloid a deposition secondary to active rheumatoid arthritis. Clin Rheumatol 2010;29(10) 1195-1197.

[45] Kishida D, Okuda Y, Onishi M, Takebayashi M, Matoba K, Jouyama K, Yamada A, Sawada N, Mokuda S, Takasugi K. Successful tocilizumab treatment in a patient with adult-onset Still's disease complicated by chronic active hepatitis B and amyloid A amyloidosis. Mod Rheumatol 2011;21(2) 215-218.

[46] Gruys E, Snel FW. Animal models for reactive amyloidosis. Baillieres Clin Rheumatol 1994;8(3) 599-611.

[47] Cohen AS, Shirahama T. Animal model for human disease: spontaneous and induced amyloidosis. Am J Pathol 1972;68(2) 441-444.

[48] Ishihara T. Experimental amyloidosis using silver nitrate--electron microscopic study on the relationship between silver granules, amyloid fibrils and reticuloendothelial system. Acta Pathol Jpn 1973;23(3) 439-464.

[49] Sri Ram J, DeLellis RA, Glenner GG. Amyloid. IV. Is human amyloid immunogenic? Int Arch Allergy Appl Immunol 1968;34(3) 269-282.

[50] Sipe JD. Induction of the acute-phase serum protein SAA requires both RNA and protein synthesis. Br J Exp Pathol 1978;59(3) 305-310.

[51] Blackburn WD Jr, Prupas HM, Silverfield JC, Poiley JE, Caldwell JR, Collins RL, Miller MJ, Sikes DH, Kaplan H, Fleischmann R, et al. Tenidap in rheumatoid arthritis. A 24-week double-blind comparison with hydroxychloroquine-plus-piroxicam, and piroxicam alone. Arthritis Rheum 1995;38(10) 1447-1456.

[52] Husebekk A, Stenstad T. Experimental AA-amyloidosis in mice is inhibited by treatment with the anti-rheumatic drug tenidap. Scand J Immunol 1996;43(5) 551-555.

[53] Chang DM, Chang WY, Kuo SY, Chang ML. The effects of traditional antirheumatic herbal medicines on immune response cells. J Rheumatol 1997;24(3) 436-441.

[54] Qiu D, Zhao G, Aoki Y, Shi L, Uyei A, Nazarian S, Ng JC, Kao PN. Immunosuppressant PG490 (triptolide) inhibits T-cell interleukin-2 expression at the level of purine-box/nuclear factor of activated T-cells and NF-kappaB transcriptional activation. J Biol Chem 1999;274(19) 13443-13450.

[55] Cui D, Hoshii Y, Kawano H, Sugiyama S, Gondo T, Liu Y, Ishihara T. Experimental AA amyloidosis in mice is inhibited by treatment with triptolide, a purified traditional Chinese medicine. Int Immunopharmacol 2007;7(9) 1232-1240.

[56] Mihara M, Shiina M, Nishimoto N, Yoshizaki K, Kishimoto T, Akamatsu K. Anti-interleukin 6 receptor antibody inhibits murine AA-amyloidosis. J Rheumatol 2004;31(6) 1132-1138.

[57] Wall JS, Richey T, Allen A, Donnell R, Kennel SJ, Solomon A. Quantitative tomography of early-onset spontaneous AA amyloidosis in interleukin 6 transgenic mice. Comp Med 2008;58(6) 542-550.

[58] Grehan S, Herbert J, Whitehead AS. Down-regulation of the major circulating precursors of proteins deposited in secondary amyloidosis by a recombinant mouse interleukin-1 receptor antagonist. Eur J Immunol 1997;27(10) 2593-2599.

[59] Betts JC, Cheshire JK, Akira S, Kishimoto T, Woo P. The role of NF-kappa B and NF-IL6 transactivating factors in the synergistic activation of human serum amyloid A gene expression by interleukin-1 and interleukin-6. J Biol Chem 1993;268(34) 25624-25631.

[60] Hagihara K, Nishikawa T, Isobe T, Song J, Sugamata Y, Yoshizaki K. IL-6 plays a critical role in the synergistic induction of human serum amyloid A (SAA) gene when stimulated with proinflammatory cytokines as analyzed with an SAA isoform real-time quantitative RT-PCR assay system. Biochem Biophys Res Commun 2004;314(2) 363-369.

[61] Zhang Z, Fuentes NL, Fuller GM. Characterization of the IL-6 responsive elements in the gamma fibrinogen gene promoter. J Biol Chem 1995;270(41) 24287-24291.

[62] Akira S. IL-6-regulated transcription factors. Int J Biochem Cell Biol 1997;29(12) 1401-1418.

[63] Hagihara K, Nishikawa T, Sugamata Y, Song J, Isobe T, Taga T, Yoshizaki K. Essential role of STAT3 in cytokine-driven NF-kappaB-mediated serum amyloid A gene expression. Genes Cells 2005;10(11) 1051-1063.

[64] Zhang Z, Fuller GM. Interleukin 1beta inhibits interleukin 6-mediated rat gamma fibrinogen gene expression. Blood 2000;96(10) 3466-3472.

[65] Nakashima K, Yanagisawa M, Arakawa H, Kimura N, Hisatsune T, Kawabata M, Miyazono K, Taga T. Synergistic signaling in fetal brain by STAT3-Smad1 complex bridged by p300. Science 1999;284(5413) 479-482.

[66] Li Q, Verma IM. NF-kappaB regulation in the immune system. Nat Rev Immunol 2002;2(10) 725-734.

[67] Feldmann M, Maini RN. Anti-TNF alpha therapy of rheumatoid arthritis: what have we learned? Annu Rev Immunol 2001;19 163-196.

[68] Feldmann M, Brennan FM, Maini RN. Role of cytokines in rheumatoid arthritis. Annu Rev Immunol 1996;14 397-440.

Section 3

# The Advancement of Therapy

Chapter 8

# Treatment of End Stage Heart Failure Related to Cardiac Amyloidosis

Tal Hasin, Eugenia Raichlin, Angela Dispenzieri and Sudhir Kushwaha

Additional information is available at the end of the chapter

http://dx.doi.org/10.5772/55553

## 1. Introduction

Amyloidosis is a disease characterized by deposition of extracellular proteinaceous material known as amyloid in tissues. Amyloidoses are classified according to the protein composition and the clinical characteristics of the disease [1]. Amyloid protein can accumulate at various speeds in multiple organ systems and the disease can have localized or systemic manifestations depending on organ involvement. Amyloidotic cardiomyopathy or cardiac amyloidosis is characterized as a restrictive cardiomyopathy associated with increased ventricular wall thickness caused by the accumulation of amyloid in the heart [2].Cardiac amyloidosis is of special interest since its occurrence usually has a significant impact on morbidity and prognosis.

### 1.2. Subtypes of amyloid disease with cardiac manifestations

At least 27 different precursor proteins for amyloidosis have been identified [3]. Although almost every amyloidogenic protein can deposit in the heart, a few specific types of amyloid have a predilection to involve this organ and are responsible for most clinical presentations. Of the nine proteins that have been shown to potentially involve the heart, two proteins: the immunoglobulin light chain and the serum protein transthyretin are responsible for the two clinically most important types of cardiac amyloidosis. Immunoglobulin light chain is involved in AL amyloidosis and transthyretin (TTR) is involved in both familial- ATTR and senile-SSA amyloid types. Other rare amyloid types that involve the heart (such as apolipoprotein A1) and amyloid types unusual to involve the heart such as secondary amyloid (AA) [4] or hemodialysis associated (Aβ2M) will not be discussed in this chapter. Another more recently described type of cardiac amyloidosis results in isolated atrial deposition. Deposited atrial amyloid resembling natriuretic peptides [5] was initially thought to be of questionable clinical significance. This subtype, found mostly in elderly women, is increasingly associated with atrial fibrillation [6],[7] and remodeling [8] but tends not to be associated with the classical clinical findings of cardiac amyloidosis.

### 1.3. Light chain (AL) Amyloidosis

This is the most common systemic amyloidosis in the United States and the most common cause of cardiac amyloidosis. It occurs equally in men and women usually over the age of 50. The incidence of AL in the United States is between 2000 and 2500 cases a year [9],[10]. This is a systemic disease most commonly involving more than one organ system which may include the kidneys, liver, nerves, and blood vessels. Therefore, most patients have clinical evidence of extra cardiac involvement including proteinuria, peripheral and autonomic neuropathy and evidence of liver and skin involvement. Periorbital purpura is a relatively rare, but characteristic finding. Amyloid can be detected in the heart in almost every case but clinical cardiac involvement is encountered in about half of cases. However, when present, cardiac amyloidosis will usually dominate the clinical presentation and has the greatest impact on survival [11]. The amyloid is derived from monoclonal light chains (intact or fragmented) produced from a population of clonal plasma cells. It is generally thought that organ dysfunction in AL is primarily due to infiltration by the amyloid deposits, but there is increasing evidence for a direct toxic effect of the amyloidogenic light chain [12],[13]. To support this paradigm, after successful chemotherapy patients with AL amyloidosis frequently have improvement in heart failure symptoms associated with decrease in biomarkers despite unchanged echocardiographic findings [14].

There is little overlap with the most common plasma cell dyscrasia- multiple myeloma. Only 10-15% of myeloma patients also develop AL amyloidosis and most AL patients do not develop overt myeloma [9]. These two diseases, however, share several features, that is, excess bone marrow plasma cells and increased monoclonal proteins in the blood and urine. Light chain deposition disease of the heart is a rare condition to be differentiated from AL cardiomyopathy in which cardiac dysfunction may occur due to deposition of immune light chains that do not form amyloid in the myocardium [15],[16]. This condition is related to plasma cell dyscrasias such as multiple myeloma or Waldenstrom's macroglobulinemia and like AL amyloidosis may improve after chemotherapy directed at the underlying bone marrow clone is administered [17].

### 1.4. Transthyretin amyloidosis

Transthyretin (TTR) is a hepatically synthesized plasma protein. The gene is coded on chromosome 18 and includes 4 exons. In the serum the protein circulates as a homotetramer, in which each monomer is comprised of 127 amino acids arranged as 8 antiparallel beta pleated sheet domains [18]. This structure is prone to form beta pleated sheet fibrils, the building blocks for amyloid deposition [19]. Transthyretin can accumulate in the heart to cause cardiac amyloidosis in two clinical syndromes: familial amyloidosis (ATTR) or senile amyloidosis (SSA), the latter of which is more recently been called age-related amyloidosis.

### 1.5. Familial amyloidosis (ATTR)

This disease is most commonly due to a mutation in the TTR protein, and is transmitted as an autosomal dominant trait. To date, about 100 different amyloidogenic TTR point mutations have been described [20]. The prevalence and severity of cardiac disease varies with different mutations. Penetrance may vary resulting in some individuals with a mutated genotype that may not develop clinical disease. Males and females are equally affected. Interestingly the cardiac amyloid deposits consist of both wild type as well as mutant TTR [21]. The disease frequently affects the heart and/or the nervous system. Other manifestations include ocular involvement with opacities of the vitreous humor [18]. A "scalloped pupil" is pathognomonic to the disease but is rarely encountered [22]. Carpal tunnel syndrome is another common feature [18]. Nervous system involvement occurs as a polyneuropathy that usually starts with paresthesias and dysesthesias in the lower extremities and ascends centripetally [23], with possible later motor dysfunction. Autonomic nervous system involvement is common, including dyshidrosis, bowl irregularities, orthostasis, erectile dysfunction, and urinary retention or incontinence. Although the CNS is usually not involved, certain rare mutations are associated with leptomeningeal amyloidosis. In contrast to AL amyloidosis, renal involvement is unusual in TTR associated amyloidosis and neither is liver deposition or macroglossia a prominent feature. Patients may present with neuropathy, cardiomyopathy or a combination of both and specific TTR mutations usually determine the organs of primary involvement [24].

Several common mutations warrant specific consideration. Isoleucine to valine substitution at position 122 (Val122Ile) is among the most common, present in 4% of African Americans [25]. These patients present with severe cardiomyopathy usually by age 60, with little or no neuropathy [26]. Valine to Methionine substitution at position 30 (Val30Met) is probably the most studied TTR mutation worldwide. It is prevalent in a few specific locations (also termed endemic) in Japan [27], Portugal [28] and northern Sweden [29]. In Japan and Portugal patients usually manifest with neuropathy in the mid 30s, and cardiomyopathy is rare, typically occurring after the sixth decade. By contrast the same mutation in Sweden usually manifests later (mid 50s), and has slower progression and lower penetrance [30]. The threonine to alanine substitution at position 60 (Thr60Ala) usually manifests with predominantly cardiac amyloidosis and minimal neuropathy.

### 1.6. Senile amyloidosis (SSA) or age related amyloidosis

This is a non-hereditary form of transthyretin related amyloidosis. It is almost exclusively a disease of the elderly (>70 years old) and occurs more commonly in men. The disease involves deposition of amyloid from normal unmutated transthyretin (wild type). Wild type transthyretin deposits almost exclusively in the heart and when extensive enough is associated with cardiac disease. The only other manifestation may be carpal tunnel syndrome often preceding heart failure by 3-5 years. The finding of some transthyretin amyloid deposition is common in the elderly (up to 25% of autopsies in subjects over the age of 80) and not always associates with clinical cardiac amyloidosis [31].

## 2. Specific features of cardiac amyloidosis

### 2.1. Pathology

Grossly, amyloid can be seen to infiltrate any or all cardiac structures including the myocardium (atrial and ventricular), valves, conduction system, coronary and large arteries [32]. This usually results in thickening of all 4 chambers, biatrial dilatation, normal or mildly dilated right ventricle and normal or small left ventricular cavity. The conduction system is usually involved. Valve infiltration may lead to thickening or nodule formation. Valve regurgitation is generally mild but can be severe.

Microscopically, myocardial cells separate and are distorted by amyloid deposition [33]. Amyloid deposits stain pink with Hematoxylin and Eosin and show an apple-green birefringence when stained with Congo red and viewed under polarized light. By electron microscope the fibrils are non-branching with a consistent diameter of 7.5 to 10 nm [34]. Additionally, the intramyocardial vessels are frequently infiltrated by amyloid [34]. Rarely this small vessel involvement will cause the initial presentation with only minimal myocardial infiltration. Involvement of epicardial vessels is rare but may mimic atherosclerotic plaques. There may be differences in patterns of deposition between AL and SSA amyloid to suggest more vascular involvement in the former [35].

### 2.2. Clinical manifestations

In AL amyloidosis, cardiac manifestations are rare to occur without associated systemic manifestations such as gastrointestinal symptoms or heavy proteinuria [36]. Age at presentation is typically in the fifth to sixth decade, and is rare in patients younger than 30 [36]. ATTR may present with or without neurologic manifestations. SSA usually does not involve other organs, with the exception of carpal tunnel symptom and will manifest usually in an older patient.

Heart failure is the usual cardiac manifestation, typically with preserved left ventricular ejection fraction. Biventricular failure is usually present, but the presenting symptoms are often those of right heart failure including ascites and peripheral edema. This can help differentiate from cardiac hypertrophy due to hypertension alone, where right heart failure is less common on presentation. Other non specific symptoms include fatigue and orthostatic hypotension. Due to the high prevalence of ATTR in the African American population, symptoms of right heart failure in an African American in his/her sixth decade with ventricular wall thickening should alert the physician to suspect familial amyloidosis (transthyretin, Val Ile122) rather than hypertensive heart.

Other cardiac manifestations include arrhythmias and dysrhythmias. Atrial fibrillation is common and may worsen heart failure symptoms. Possible causes of atrial fibrillation are atrial infiltration, elevated left atrial pressure due to the diastolic dysfunction and older age (in SSA amyloidosis). Syncope and sudden death can occur. Differential diagnosis includes orthostatism and arrhythmias. Arrhythmias can include brady-arrhythmias such as caused by conduction delays. Ventricular tachy-arrhythmias are described but sustained VT is uncommon and most cases of monitored sudden death were due to electro-mechanical dissociation [37]. Chest pain due to small vessel disease is a rare (1-2%) presentation of AL amyloidosis [38]. In some of these cases imaging studies may be positive but coronary angiography will demonstrate normal epicardial vessels.

Another clinical aspect is the tendency for thromboembolic events. As stated above atrial fibrillation is a common finding, especially with advanced disease. Atrial standstill can occur due to amyloid infiltration even in the presence of sinus rhythm and contribute to thrombus formation. In AL amyloid nephrotic syndrome can also contribute to hypercoagulopathy and thrombus formation. Although debated, these risks may warrant a relatively liberal use of anticoagulation as discussed below [39]-[41] [42].

### 2.3. Diagnosis

The diagnosis of cardiac amyloidosis can be challenging. A high level of suspicion is needed since diagnosis can often be missed, especially with the transthyretin amyloidosis. Patients may be misdiagnosed with more common causes of heart failure associated with cardiac hypertrophy such as hypertensive cardiomyopathy. Clinical suspicion usually arises during evaluation for right sided heart failure, because other manifestations of cardiac amyloidosis occur less commonly. Systemic manifestations typical of each type of cardiac amyloidosis may be supportive of the diagnosis. Further basic evaluation includes electrocardiography and echocardiography. More advanced evaluation including MRI and radioisotope and hemodynamic studies may also be utilized to substantiate the diagnosis. Definite diagnosis is generally made by cardiac biopsy and pathological evaluation but may not be needed in every case.

### 2.4. Cardiovascular directed physical examination

An irregular rhythm due to atrial fibrillation occurs in 10-15% of the patients. Blood pressure is often low and can further decrease with standing. Manifestations of right heart failure due to restrictive cardiomyopathy will include an elevated jugular venous pressure but Kussmaul's sign is rarely present (in contrast to constrictive pericarditis). The apex beat is frequently impalpable. The first and second heart sounds are usually normal. A left ventricular S3 is rare but a right ventricular S3 may be heard. A fourth heart sound is almost never present, possibly due to atrial dysfunction [9]. On chest examination rales are uncommon but pleural effusion may occur both due to heart failure as well as to amyloid involvement [43]. Hepatomegaly is common, due to either congestion or AL amyloid infiltration (causing a rock-hard organ in the latter case). Peripheral edema may be profound, especially if nephrosis co-exists.

### 2.5. Systemic findings

The diagnosis of systemic amyloid involvement and findings of monoclonal immunoglobulin light chain may suggest AL amyloidosis. In detecting serum light chain, immunofixation is preferred to electrophoresis since the amount of paraprotein may be small. Serum free light chain assay is even more sensitive than immunofixation [44]. The finding of a monoclonal protein is not necessarily pathological and differential diagnosis includes monoclonal gammopathy of uncertain significance (MGUS). A monoclonal protein as an incidental finding (MGUS) can be found in up to 5-10% of patients more than 70 years old [45]. Not all cases are benign and the quantitative serum free light chain assay may predict progression in some cases [46]. The combination of abnormal kappa/lambda ratio and positive immunofixation identified 99% of patients with AL amyloidosis [47]. When considering the serum immunoglobulin free light chain, elevations of either the serum kappa or lambda free light chain in the context of a normal ratio between the two does not suggest a clonal process, like what one sees in AL. Renal failure and non-specific inflammation can cause elevation of both types of light chain, and the normal ratio is preserved. Light chain elevations associated with a clonal process will also include an abnormal ratio. Amyloid deposition can be found in abdominal fat needle aspiration and used for tissue confirmation of systemic amyloidosis [48],[49]. Eventually bone marrow biopsy is necessary to assess the percentage of plasma cells and rule out myeloma and other disorders such as Waldenstrom's macroglobulnemia.

In the case of ATTR amyloidosis systemic evaluation should focus on a thorough neurological evaluation including eye examination. Genetic analysis may be helpful if ATTR is suspected, especially if a familial trait is identified and may be utilized in consulting siblings.

### 2.6. Electrocardiography

Low voltage QRS (<5mm in all limb leads) [50] is one of the hallmarks of the disease. However the lack of low voltage does not rule out the disease and in very rare cases, an unusual presentation with EKG features of left ventricular hypertrophy has been described. Other common observations include pseudoinfarct pattern, repolarization alterations and T-wave abnormalities, and atrial fibrillation [51]. Atrial involvement may lead to delayed atrial conduction and a long PR interval. Interestingly, bundle branch blocks tend to be uncommon [9]

### 2.7. Echocardiography

Usually ventricular wall thickening in the absence of left ventricular cavity dilatation is seen. Ejection fraction is often normal. Trans-mitral Doppler and tissue Doppler frequently suggests elevated left ventricular filling pressure [52],[53]. A decreased transmitral A wave can be due to the direct effect of atrial infiltration and not only the restrictive physiology therefore a normal E wave deceleration time with small A wave can be encountered [54] [55]. Pericardial effusion is common. A typical echocardiographic image is shown in figure 1.

Clues to differentiate LV thickening due to amyloidosis from LV hypertrophy include:

1. Disproportional impairment of longitudinal motion. Subendocardial fibers are particularly susceptible to damage in amyloidosis. Since these are longitudinal, the longitudinal contraction of the heart is impaired early in the disease process. This can be diagnosed using tissue Doppler as well as strain and strain rate [56],[57].

2. Involvement of other cardiac structures including RV free wall thickening, prominent biatrial dilatation and valvular thickening.

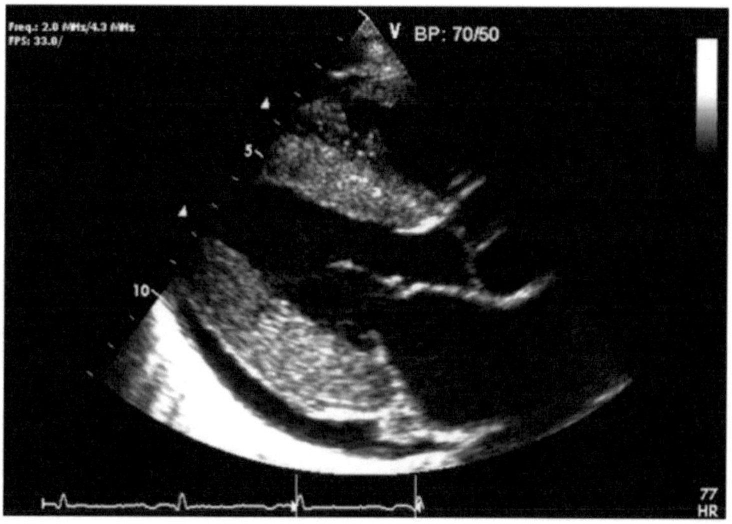


**Figure 1. Representative echocardiographic image in a patient with cardiac amyloidosis.** Parasternal long axis echocardiographic view showing granular myocardium with increased left and right ventricular wall thickness in a 77 year old with cardiac amyloidosis. Note the pericardial effusion.

3. Absence of high voltage QRS on surface EKG despite the appearance of a thickened left ventricle. The opposite may occur with decreased voltage as ventricular mass is increased [58].

In about 5% of patients cardiac amyloidosis can mimic hypertrophic cardiomyopathy echocardiographically [59],[60]. Unlike true hypertrophic cardiomyopathy ventricular hypertrophy on the EKG limb leads is almost never seen and systolic anterior motion of the mitral leaflet is uncommon, although chordal anterior motion may be present.

Echocardiographically distinguishing the different types of cardiac amyloidosis is challenging. Ventricular cavity is usually smaller and ventricular walls thicker in SSR compared to AL amyloidosis [61]. One clue to differentiate ATTR and AL amyloidosis may be that QRS voltage may be higher due to the amount of ventricular thickening in ATTR as compared to AL amyloidosis [62]. Subtle differences in strain and strain rate were described between the two [57]. These are possibly related to the toxic effects of the light chains in AL, absent in ATTR amyloidosis [12].

### 2.8. Magnetic Resonance Imaging (MRI)

Gadolinium tends to accumulate in the amyloid infiltrated cardiac interstitium. Therefore a distinctive pattern in cardiac MRI can be highly suggestive of the diagnosis. This consists of faster washout than usual from blood and myocardium, and later a diffuse, predominantly subendocardial delayed gadolinium uptake pattern [63]-[68]. A representative MRI is shown in figure 2. Less commonly a focal distribution with variable trans-mural extension is seen, more often in the mid-ventricle [69]. The analysis of gadolinium kinetics may have prognostic value as well as diagnostic utility [70]. The use of gadolinium may be restricted by the potential harm of causing nephrogenic systemic fibrosis in patients with renal impairment (especially in AL amyloidosis) and therefore the possible utility in substantiating the diagnosis should be carefully weighed against this possible risk.

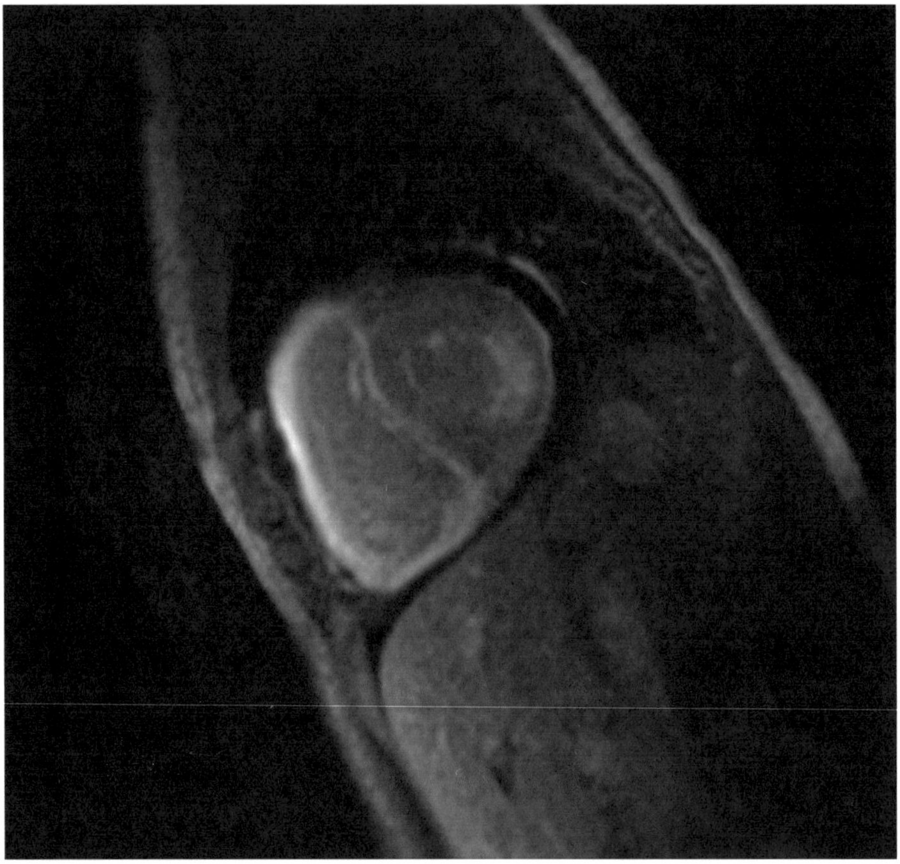

**Figure 2. Magnetic resonance image in cardiac amyloidosis.** Cardiac MRI showing a short axis myocardial delayed enhancement image obtained 10 minutes following gadolinium administration demonstrating diffuse abnormal enhancement (white) of the right ventricular free and inferior walls as well as focal abnormal enhancement of the inferolateral left ventricular myocardium in a subendocardial distribution. The diffuse abnormal enhancement involving both right and left ventricles is characteristic of cardiac amyloid deposition.

## 2.9. Radioisotope imaging

Serum amyloid P binds in a calcium dependent way to amyloid and 123I-labeled serum amyloid P component has been used to identify amyloid deposits. However its use in the heart is hampered by blood pool uptake [71] and it is available only in a few highly specialized centers. 99m-Tc-aprotinin may be fairly specific for cardiac amyloidosis but experience with this tecnique is limited [72].

### 2.10. Hemodynamics

Amyloid cardiomyopathy physiology is typically restrictive. Left ventricular end diastolic pressure (LVEDP) is typically elevated with a dip and plateau waveform. Since the left ventricle does not dilate the patients are usually sensitive to volume loading and even small reductions in contractility may cause significant reduction in stroke volume. However hemodynamics displayed by catheterization are not always typical. Among 38 patients with ATTR cardiac amyloidosis one had an RV pressure curve dip and plateau, 34% had elevated wedge pressure. Interestingly 29% patients did not display hemodynamic diastolic abnormalities at rest [73].

Differentiation from constrictive pericarditis may necessitate a simultaneous right and left hemodynamics study. Early observations suggested that unlike constrictive pericarditis, in amyloidosis LVEDP is elevated at least 7mmHg above right ventricular end diastolic pressure [74]. Later reports have argued this is not always the case and amyloidosis can masquerade constriction hemodynamics [75]. Pulmonary systolic pressure >50mmHg is another parameter thought to be less likely in pure constriction and if occurs may suggest restrictive physiology such that occurs with amyloidosis. Currently accepted parameters that best differentiate constriction from restrictive cardiomyopathy include exacerbated interventricular dependence (demonstrated by increased inspiratory rise in RV pressure and fall in LV pressure as measured by the systolic area index) and dissociation between intrathoracic and intracardiac pressures [76] [77].

### 2.11. The role of cardiac biopsy

In treating a patient with suspected cardiac amyloidosis, the clinician may be faced with the dilemma whether to perform a cardiac biopsy, most commonly in the setting of TTR. A careful risk benefit evaluation is warranted for every case since, while this procedure may provide useful diagnostic information [78],[79], the risks are not negligible. Myocardial biopsy has a good negative predictive value (since cardiac involvement is widespread). Biopsy of the myocardium (or any involved tissue) provides information on the type of amyloid. The most accurate technique appears to be molecular analysis of the amyloid fibrils using mass spectrometry [80]. In patients with a confirmed diagnosis of systemic amyloidosis via biopsy proof of another tissue, ventricular wall thickening and low or normal voltage EKG, the diagnosis of cardiac amyloidosis is probable and biopsy should be avoided. If the patient is hypertensive and there is uncertainty regarding cardiac involvement, biopsy may be useful. The most accessible tissue to biopsy is that abdominal fat, which has sensitivities for AL of about 80% and for TTR of about 40%. If suspicion of amyloidosis is high, and there is no other organ involvement, cardiac biopsy may be needed to confirm the diagnosis. Since small amounts of amyloid deposition are a common finding in the very elderly [81] caution should be taken when interpreting the results in this population, especially if the amyloid deposits are sparse and the echocardiographic appearance is not convincing. In an elderly patient with clinical and echocardiographic findings consistent of cardiac amyloidosis and free light chain in the serum the differential will include coincidental SSA amyloid and MGUS versus AL amyloid. If other tissue is not available or yields negative results, endomyocardial biopsy with typing using laser capture mass spectrometry or immunochemistry or immunogold electron microscopy may be needed to differentiate ATTR from AL.

### 2.12. Prognostic markers

The type of amyloidosis by itself is an important determinant of survival and every type should be considered separately when discussing prognostic issues. Patients with AL amyloidosis generally carry the worst prognosis and most of the current research on prognostic evaluation is focused on this group. Clinical features such as low ejection fraction and low voltage pattern were associated with increased mortality [82]. Cardiac biomarkers may be elevated in patients with AL and are being utilized to estimate prognosis. Cardiac troponins may be elevated due to myocyte death or injury and elevated levels predict worse prognosis in AL patients [83]. Elevated brain natriuretic peptide (BNP) may reflect both congestive HF as well as compression by adjacent amyloid deposits [84],[85] and has also been associated with worse survival. Staging using serum levels of BNP or its n-terminal portion (NT-proBNP) together with serum troponin is used to aid in risk assessment and prognosis in AL amyloidosis [86],[87]. More recently, a risk stratification score using cardiac troponin, NT-proBNP and uric acid was developed to assess early death among AL patients [88]. Even more recently, an additional risk score that includes NT-proBNP, troponin T, and serum immunoglobulin free light chain adds further prognostic discrimination[89].

### 2.13. Prognosis

In the absence of treatment, the natural history of AL amyloidosis is dismal (80% two year mortality) [90]. Although prognosis has improved over the years with the advancement of treatment [88], mortality remains high, especially in the presence of heart failure symptoms (median survival 4-6 months) [11]. The course in ATTR amyloidosis is generally more indolent, with 92% 1 year survival [62] and heart failure may be easier to control. Genotypes differ in prognosis, and patients with the Val30Met mutation tend for better prognosis compared to other mutations [24]. Senile amyloidosis is also associated with better survival compared to AL amyloidosis, despite older age of presentation and thicker myocardium by echocardiography [61]. In one report median survival was 60 months, compared to 5.4 months for AL amyloidosis [91]. Similar results were shown in a larger series comparing the 3 major cardiac amyloidosis syndromes [73].

## 3. Treatment

### 3.1. Disease specific treatment

Cardiac dysfunction in AL amyloidosis may be caused by direct toxicity of the circulating serum free light chains, in addition to the deposited amyloid tissue [13]. Therefore, treatment of the underlying plasma cell dyscrasia in AL amyloid involving chemotherapy [92] can cause a reduction in the cardiac biomarker NT-proBNP and improve survival [14],[93]. A range of chemotherapies ranging from low dose melphalan and dexamethasone to high dose melphalan with autologous hematopoietic stem cell transplantation are among the most commonly used therapies. One of the more promising, but least well studied drugs, that is directed against the plasma cell clone is bortezomib. Bortezomib is a proteasome inhibitor and utilizing it, a hematological response can be achieved more rapidly (in about a month) in high percentages of patients [94],[95], but clinical trials using this drug have typically excluded those AL patients with the most significant cardiac dysfunction. Other treatments using thalidomide or lenalidomide may also be effective, but these drugs have been shown to exacerbate cardiac failure in a percentage of patients [96]. Despite the advancement in hematological treatment, mortality in patients with severe heart failure is still high [97]. Moreover, worsening of cardiac function may occur during the course of treatment and an ejection fraction below 40% is considered a contraindication to high dose chemotherapy with autologous hematopoietic stem cell transplantation. The complexity and potential deterioration of cardiac function during treatment warrants cardiologist involvement during evaluation for chemotherapy and during follow-up after treatment in every case, even if cardiac involvement seems minor.

Stabilization of the tetrameric structure of transthyretin using small molecule ligands is under investigation [98] and may assist patients with TTR associated amyloidosis. The non-steroidal anti-inflammatory drug Diflunisal has been found to have this effect [99],[100] but chronic use is limited due to possible worsening of fluid overload and renal function. Tafamidis is a novel transthyretin kinetic stabilizer which has been recently investigated clinically [101]. In a randomized trial this agent was well tolerated and showed a trend for delaying peripheral neurologic impairment in patients with ATTR [102]. While showing promise, this agent is not yet in routine clinical use.

### 3.2. Conventional heart failure treatment

It is important to differentiate AL from ATTR amyloid. While in AL amyloid "conventional" heart failure treatment including beta blockers and angiotensin pathway inhibitors is usually not well tolerated, these medications may be better tolerated in ATTR patients who do not suffer from significant autonomic neuropathy. Calcium channel blockers with negative inotropic effects have no role in AL amyloid and may cause harm [103] [104]. Compared to other causes of heart failure there is no evidence for remodeling effects from beta blockers and therefore they are not indicated for patients in sinus rhythm [105]. They may be used to slow atrial fibrillation response if needed, but take care if your patient decompensates after institution. Amiodarone and digoxin may be preferred for rate control. Due to their impaired cardiac function (and restrictive LV filling), some of these patients require mild tachycardia to maintain cardiac output. There is also no role for digoxin for patients in sinus rhythm but it also may help slow atrial fibrillation response. Possible increased toxicity by increased binding of digoxin to amyloid fibrils has been reported [106] and therefore lower dosing and caution is probably justified when using this medication. Angiotensin pathway inhibitors (both angiotensin converting enzyme inhibitors and receptor blockers) may provoke hypotension (possibly due to impaired sympathetic nervous system function and reduced and relatively fixed stroke volume) and therefore should be administered only if being used to treat hypertension [32]. Patients with SSA amyloid tend to tolerate these medications better than patients with AL amyloid. Diuretics and salt restriction remains the mainstay of medical treatment in cardiac amyloidosis. Careful titration is utilized since reduced preload with reduced ventricular filling pressures can decrease cardiac output and cause hypotension. Higher doses may be needed if albumin is low as a result of nephrotic syndrome (with AL). If absorption is impaired due to anasarca, intravenous treatment may be necessary sometimes in association with IV albumin.

Ancillary treatment in patients with autonomic neuropathy includes compression stockings and alpha adrenergic agonists such as midodrine [107]. Fludrocortisone is usually less well tolerated due to its sodium retaining effects and worsening of edema. Patients with erectile dysfunction can be aided by phosphodiasterase inhibitors [108].

The question of anticoagulation is complex since both a thrombotic tendency as well as a bleeding tendency (especially in AL) may occur. ATTR patients tend to bleed less than AL patients. Due to an increased risk, anticoagulation with warfarin is probably indicated when atrial fibrillation occurs, even in the absence of other risk factors. The decision is more complex in patients with sinus rhythm. Because of an increased tendency for thrombotic events and the occurrence of atrial stand-still, anticoagulation should be considered. Though this must be counterbalanced by the increased risk of bleeding, especially from the GI tract. The head and neck purpura may also be a challenge to manage among patients on anticoagulation. Atrial thrombi were indeed identified in patients with AL amyloid in sinus rhythm [39]. A small transmitral A wave (<20cm/s) can suggest impaired atrial function with more tendency to form thrombi and can be used as another clue to decision making. Transesophageal echocardiography may help to identify patients in sinus rhythm with higher risk for thrombosis such as those with spontaneous echo contrast or low left atrial appendage velocities. A cutoff of <40cm/sec was initially suggested [109] but this may be considerably lower (reported as 13±5cm/sec for patients with and 27±15cm/sec for patients without thrombosis) [41].

### 3.3. Arrhythmia, pacing and defibrillators

Maintenance of sinus rhythm seems important in the stiff restrictive amyloidotic hearts, possibly due to the importance of the atrial kick and avoiding tachycardia. Therefore careful consideration should be given to electrical cardioversion for atrial flutter or fibrillation. Amiodarone can be useful to help maintain sinus rhythm. If pacing is needed strong consideration should be given to biventricular pacing since RV pacing and the resulting dysynergy may decrease stroke volume.

Sudden death is common in patients with cardiac amyloidosis. Early studies using holter monitoring suggested a high incidence of ventricular arrhythmia [110]. However, it is presently thought that the cause of death is less often rapid ventricular arrhythmias but may include electromechanical dissociation [111] and advanced heart block. Among 19 patients with either non-sustained ventricular tachycardia or high grade ventricular arrhythmia treated with an ICD only 2 received appropriate shocks for sustained VT, while 6 died of electromechanical dissociation [112]. Thus, there seems to be little role for implantable pacemakers in cardiac amyloid patients, unless a sustained ventricular arrhythmia was documented.

Amiodarone has been used to try and prevent arrhythmias and sudden death although there is no clear evidence of benefit.

## 4. Advanced heart failure treatment

### 4.1. Cardiac transplantation in AL amyloidosis

The negative impact of cardiac involvement on survival, the rapidly deteriorating clinical manifestations and the potential for hematologic treatment led clinicians as early as the 1980's to consider cardiac transplantation in AL amyloid. While initial reports based on individual cases generated optimism [113],[114], subsequent experience highlighted suboptimal outcomes [115] calling for careful and specialized patient selection and management, including disease modifying hematological treatment such as bone marrow transplant. In selected patients with both cardiac and renal failure, combined heart kidney transplant may be offered [116]. All these considerations necessitate that transplant for this complex population is carried out in highly specialized centers with high volumes.

### 4.2. Patient selection

Patient selection for patients with cardiac amyloidosis is usually a complex decision that is to be based on careful evaluation involving multiple disciplines. Considerations include the routine assessment utilized in "ordinary" cardiac transplant including factors such as age, frailty, the advancement of cardiomyopathy and co-morbidities. Additional evaluation specific to the AL includes evaluating whether other organs are involved, ruling out multiple myeloma, and collaboration with a hematologist regarding chemotherapy. Baseline evaluation before considering heart transplant includes therefore bone marrow aspirate and biopsy, echocardiogram, serum and 24-hour urine monoclonal protein studies, serum immunoglobulin free light chain assay, a chemistry panel including creatinine, liver function tests and renal clearance estimates (table 1). Major involvement of other organ systems will render the patients as less optimal candidates. This includes evidence of peripheral neuropathy, autonomic neuropathy, gastrointestinal symptoms (diarrhea), hepatic involvement, and renal failure. Patients with significant proteinuria (>500 mg/day) are usually considered higher risk due to kidney involvement. Hepatic involvement may be suspected with elevated alkaline phosphatase and hepatomegaly and a liver biopsy may be needed to differentiate it from right heart failure. Since amyloidosis is a vascular disease, the mere presence of vascular involvement in the liver would not render a patient ineligible for cardiac transplant. The acronym DANGER was suggested for evaluation of tissue involvement and adverse outcome in the context of pre-transplant evaluation for AL amyloid. It includes *Diarrhea*, *Autonomic nervous* involvement, poor *Nutritional status*, *Gastrointestinal involvement* (bleeding), *Elimination* (renal) or *Respiratory* dysfunction[117]. Recurrent pleural effusion (more common in AL amyloidosis) is also an ominous sign for bad prognosis [43].

| | |
|---|---|
| Routine cardiac transplantation evaluation with the following additional studies: | • Serum protein electrophoresis<br>• Urine protein electrophoresis (24-hour urine)<br>• Factor X and thrombin time (special coagulation studies)<br>• Bone marrow biopsy with aspirate, labeling index and smear<br>• Labeling index in peripheral blood with number of circulating plasma cells<br>• Serum carotene<br>• $\beta_2$-microglobulin<br>• C-reactive protein<br>• 24-hour urine creatinine clearance<br>• 48-hour stool collection for fat<br>• Subcutaneous fat aspirate<br>• Metastatic bone survey with single views of humeri and femurs |
| Pulmonary assessment will proceed as follows: | Recurrent pleural effusions, refractory to treatment will necessitate:<br>• Chest CT<br>• Possible lung biopsy dependent on CT findings |
| Liver assessment will proceed as follows: | • If alkaline phosphatase <1.5-fold upper limit of normal (350), then proceed with transplant evaluation<br>• If alkaline phosphatase 1.5- to 3-fold upper limit of normal, then proceed to liver biopsy:<br>1. If there is portal tract amyloid deposition, then there is an absolute contraindication<br>2. If vascular amyloid only, then proceed with transplant evaluation<br>• If alkaline phosphatase is ≥3.0-fold upper limit of normal (750), absolute then there is an contraindication to HT |
| Renal assessment will proceed as follows: | Lothalamate clearance should exceed 50 ml/min/1.73 $m^2$<br>• If urinary albumin is <250 mg/24 hours, then proceed with transplant evaluation<br>• If urinary albumin is 250 to 1,000 mg/24 hours, then proceed to renal biopsy<br>1. If vascular amyloid only, is present then proceed with transplant evaluation<br>2. If interstitial or glomerular amyloid is present, then there is an absolute contraindication to cardiac transplant |
| Blood/marrow plasma cell labeling index assessment will proceed as follows: | Plasma cell labeling index<br>• If plasma cell labeling index is ≥2%, then exclude from consideration for transplant evaluation<br>• If plasma cell labeling index is ≥1%, then proceed to metastatic bone survey to exclude myeloma-associated bony lesions |

http://dx.doi.org/10.5772/55553

| | |
|---|---|
| | • If plasma cell labeling index is <1%, then proceed with transplant evaluation |
| | Peripheral blood labeling index |
| | • If peripheral blood plasma cell labeling index is "/>1%, then absolute contraindication to cardiac transplant |
| | Plasmacytosis |
| | • If plasma cell differential on marrow aspirate is <10%, then proceed with transplant evaluation |
| | • If plasma cell differential on marrow aspirate is 10% to 20%, then do metastatic bone survey to exclude myeloma-associated bony lesions |
| | • If plasma cell differential on marrow aspirate, marrow biopsy or cytoplasmic immunoglobulin–positive plasma cells are ≥20%, then contraindication to there is an absolute cardiac transplant |
| Intestinal assessment will proceed as follows: | • 48-hour stool collection for fecal fat to rule out malabsorption |
| | • Serum carotene if low level could indicate malabsorption |
| | • Endoscopic and flexible sigmoidoscopic evaluation with biopsy |
| | 1. If vascular amyloid deposition only, then proceed with transplant evaluation |
| | 2. If mucosal amyloid deposition, then there is an absolute contraindication to cardiac transplantation |
| Adopted from Lacy MQ et al. 2008. | |

**Table 1.** Pre-transplant evaluation of AL amyloid patients.

### 4.3. High dose chemotherapy with autologous hematopoietic stem cell transplant (ASCT) after heart transplant in patients with AL

Since the clinical course of these patients is usually rapidly progressive once heart failure occurs, death rates on the transplant list tend to be high. Cardiac transplant alone does not halt the ongoing amyloid deposition and although it results in temporary improvement, this is followed by an overall poor prognosis [114],[115]. Unless therapy directed at the underlying plasma cell clone is effective, the amyloid may also recur in the transplanted heart at a later stage, despite initial clinical improvement of heart failure [118]. Therefore, the treatment strategy should be to follow the heart transplant with chemotherapy, usually within 6 months to a year after the heart transplant to allow for healing from the surgery and tapering down of the immunosuppression. Initial experience was described in 5 patients, of whom 2 died of progressive amyloid and 3 survived [119]. With increasing experience with patient selection and treatment results are improving [120] and in selected patients prognosis may be comparable to non-amyloid patients [117]. This strategy has been shown to be feasible and associated with improved survival with carefully selected patients [121]. Although there are some reports of late recurrence of cardiac amyloidosis [122] despite ASCT this is considered still the strategy that offers the best chance for long term good outcomes.

Since the disease is rapidly progressive and patients will generally wait 4-6 months after heart transplant to be fit for ASCT. Therefore timing of heart transplant is especially crucial in this patient setting since patients might miss the window of opportunity for hematologic treatment. Extended donor criteria have been advocated and may be utilized to facilitate a timely transplant in selected cases [123]. Another approach would be to consider heart transplant after successful hematological treatment including ASCT [124], but this strategy is fraught with more hazard, because of the high risk of death among ASCT AL patients with cardiac amyloid bad enough to require cardiac transplantation.. Newer chemotherapeutic agents that are better tolerated may be used to achieve partial remission [95] and may halt the progression of cardiac symptoms by decreasing serum levels of light chains with potential toxic myocardial effects, and thereby facilitate survival on the waiting list for heart transplant.

### 4.4. Outcomes of heart transplant in AL cardiac amyloidosis

Survival in transplanted patients with amyloidosis is generally poorer when compared to patients without amyloidosis. Five year survival rates reported from the European registry were 38%, with prevalent progression of the systemic disease [125]. Analyzing results of the United Network of Organ Sharing for 69 patients with amyloid heart disease, 1 year actuarial survival was 74.6% compared to 81.6% for all other heart transplanted patients and 5 year survival was 54% versus 63.3% respectively. The authors included all types of amyloid and did not detail treatment for the underlying disease [126]. Data from other registries suggests poorer prognosis for patients transplanted with AL amyloidosis compared to other types of cardiac amyloidosis [127]. As described above, survival may be improved if bone marrow transplantation is performed after cardiac transplant. In carefully selected patients survival utilizing this strategy can reach about 60% in five years which is comparable to the general heart transplant population [121],[128],[129].

### 4.5. Cardiac transplantation for transthyretin related amyloidosis

Heart transplant for significant cardiomyopathy related to transthyretin amyloid deposition has been successfully deployed with overall good outcomes. Specific considerations include possible associated neuropathy and need for combined heart-liver transplant in ATTR amyloidosis and the advanced age of presentation in SSA amyloidosis.

### 4.6. Patient selection

In ATTR cardiac amyloidosis a major determinant of pre-transplant evaluation and candidacy is the presence and severity of associated neuropathy. Autonomic disturbances should be evaluated specifically including orthostatic hypotension, gastrointestinal and urinary tract dysfunction. Other factors of importance include the body mass index, patient age and degree of disability. Generally patients with SSA are not offered transplant due to their advanced age, however if presenting early, transplantation may be successfully performed [130].

### 4.7. Combined heart and liver transplant in ATTR cardiac amyloidosis

Since the abnormal transthyretin is primarily synthesized by the liver, liver transplantation is a reasonable treatment for ATTR. Liver transplantation in ATTR can halt, and in some cases is associated with regression of amyloid deposits [131],[132]. This is especially true for certain mutations (such as Val30Met) where liver transplantation can halt neurological symptoms and improve general symptoms (gastrointestinal, nutritional, orthostasis and dyshidrosis) however this mutation less commonly causes cardiac disease [132]. Paradoxical acceleration of cardiac involvement after liver transplantation may occur in patients with mutation variants other than Val30Met [133]-[135], due to wild-type transthyretin deposition in addition to the background amyloid fibrils [136]-[138]. Therefore combined heart and liver transplantation rather heart transplant alone is considered in patients with significant cardiac involvement [139],[140]. Combined heart and liver transplantation can be performed in selected patients with results similar to heart transplant for other indications [141]. The indications for combined heart liver transplant include patients with heart failure symptoms and without advanced neurological involvement and patients with non Val30Met mutations who are candidates for liver transplant and have echocardiographic evidence of cardiomyopathy.

The liver in these patients otherwise functions normally and generally the explanted liver can be used for another patient requiring liver transplantation (domino transplant) [142]. Amyloid deposition from the implanted liver is thought to occur very slowly. Rare cases of recurrence of amyloid deposition in the liver recipient have been reported 8-10 years after the transplant [143]-[145].

The surgical approach to combined heart-liver transplant has changed over the years. Initially transplantation of the heart and maintaining the patient on cardio-pulmonary bypass during the liver transplant was used. Subsequent concerns about substantial coagulopathy and increased bleeding changed the strategy to performing liver implantation after separation from cardiopulmonary bypass [139],[146],[147]. Later, improved surgical and anesthetic techniques during liver transplant and the potential benefits to the transplanted heart to remain on cardio-pulmonary bypass during liver implantation led to revising this strategy. This technique was suggested to provide a considerably shortened liver ischemia time and decreased blood transfusion compared to the sequential approach [148]. Staged heart and liver transplantation where initial cardiac transplant is later followed by liver transplant from a different donor can be used, especially for patients that are hemodynamically unstable after cardiac reperfusion [149],[150]. However the preferred method is a single donor transplant, due to the avoidance of a second major operation early after cardiac transplant as well as certain possible immunological advantages. In cases of elevated pre-formed anti-HLA antibodies, there might be an advantage to a surgical strategy where liver transplant is performed initially, followed by sequential heart transplant. The liver is thought to sequester pre-formed anti-HLA antibodies and "protect" the heart in this scenario. This approach necessitates maximal coordination to avoid a prolonged ischemic time for the implanted heart but was successful at least in one case [151].

Interestingly, heart rejection is infrequent in combined heart-liver compared to heart alone transplantation [141]. A possible explanation may be an induction of partial tolerance. The liver has been demonstrated to shed soluble HLA antigens [152],[153]. Soluble HLA antigens may lead to tolerance of the specific allotype and permit acceptance of other transplanted organs [154]. Less intensive immunosuppression may be needed in these cases and a reduced tendency for allograft vasculopathy has been recently demonstrated [155]. Overall, potentially due to the supportive contribution of these considerations and despite a larger and more complex operation results for the heart and liver transplant are comparable to those in other heart transplant patients [125].

### 4.8. Cardiac assist devices in patients with cardiac amyloidosis

Left ventricular assist devices (LVAD) are currently implanted for patients with advanced heart failure and improve survival and quality of life. The number of devices implanted and medical centers involved in device implantation is rapidly increasing and newer continuous flow devices replacing the older pulsatile ones and allowing for improved durability [156]. While traditional indications for LVAD support were dilated cardiomyopathies (either ischemic or non-ischemic), LVAD implantation has been successfully administered to patients with primarily restrictive physiology. Early reports of include implantation and successful support for one patient with amyloidosis with the Jarvik-2000 device [157]. A case series recently described successful support with the HeartMate II device in patients with restrictive cardiomyopathy, several of whom had cardiac amyloidosis [158]. Candidates had transthyretin related cardiac amyloidosis since the immune suppression, coagulopathy and systemic involvement in AL amyloidosis renders them less optimal candidates for this line of treatment.

In selecting patients with cardiac amyloidosis for LVAD some important considerations should be considered. Since the assist device will not support the right ventricle, specific consideration should be given to assess the right ventricular function. Detailed directed echocardiographic evaluation as well as hemodynamic catheterization are critical to establishing candidacy. The right ventricle is anticipated to be involved in the infiltrative disease and RV dilatation may not occur despite significant dysfunction. Total artificial heart implant may be considered if right ventricular function is poor suggesting that LVAD support alone may not be sufficient. However the long-term durability of these devices has not been evaluated and therefore implantation in patients not eligible for heart transplant (such as for older patients with SSA) may be problematic. Another important consideration is the degree of systemic involvement, particularly neuropathy. This will influence considerably their ability to recuperate from the operation and the remaining degree of physical limitation and dysfunction. Patients with LVAD support often display orthostatism and this may worsen if the patient had pre-existing autonomic dysfunction due to amyloid. Overall, with careful patient selection, meticulous operative technique (with extra care for cannula positioning in the small cavity) and dedicated post-operative follow-up, assist devices can be deployed in patients with cardiac amyloidosis with success rates comparable to conventional indications [158].

## Author details

Tal Hasin[1], Eugenia Raichlin[2], Angela Dispenzieri[3] and Sudhir Kushwaha[3]

1 Departement of Cardiology, Rabin Medical Center, Petach- Tikva, Israel

2 Division of Cardiology, Department of Internal Medicine, University of Nebraska Medical Center, Omaha NE, USA

3 Divisions of Hematology and Cardiology, Mayo Clinic, Rochester MN, USA

## References

[1] Westermark, P, Benson, M. D, Buxbaum, J. N, et al. A primer of amyloid nomenclature. Amyloid (2007). , 14, 179-83.

[2] Maron, B. J, Towbin, J. A, Thiene, G, et al. Contemporary definitions and classification of the cardiomyopathies: an American Heart Association Scientific Statement from the Council on Clinical Cardiology, Heart Failure and Transplantation Committee; Quality of Care and Outcomes Research and Functional Genomics and Translational Biology Interdisciplinary Working Groups; and Council on Epidemiology and Prevention. Circulation (2006). , 113, 1807-16.

[3] Sipe, J. D, Benson, M. D, Buxbaum, J. N, et al. Amyloid fibril protein nomenclature: 2010 recommendations from the nomenclature committee of the International Society of Amyloidosis. Amyloid (2010). , 17, 101-4.

[4] Dubrey, S. W, Cha, K, Simms, R. W, Skinner, M, & Falk, R. H. Electrocardiography and Doppler echocardiography in secondary (AA) amyloidosis. The American journal of cardiology (1996). , 77, 313-5.

[5] Pucci, A, Wharton, J, Arbustini, E, et al. Atrial amyloid deposits in the failing human heart display both atrial and brain natriuretic peptide-like immunoreactivity. The Journal of pathology (1991). , 165, 235-41.

[6] Goette, A, & Rocken, C. Atrial amyloidosis and atrial fibrillation: a gender-dependent "arrhythmogenic substrate"? European heart journal (2004). , 25, 1185-6.

[7] Rocken, C, Peters, B, Juenemann, G, et al. Atrial amyloidosis: an arrhythmogenic substrate for persistent atrial fibrillation. Circulation (2002). , 106, 2091-7.

[8] Leone, O, Boriani, G, Chiappini, B, et al. Amyloid deposition as a cause of atrial remodelling in persistent valvular atrial fibrillation. European heart journal (2004). , 25, 1237-41.

[9] Falk, R. H. Diagnosis and management of the cardiac amyloidoses. Circulation (2005)., 112, 2047-60.

[10] Simms, R. W, Prout, M. N, & Cohen, A. S. The epidemiology of AL and AA amyloidosis. Bailliere's clinical rheumatology (1994)., 8, 627-34.

[11] Kyle, R. A, & Gertz, M. A. Primary systemic amyloidosis: clinical and laboratory features in 474 cases. Seminars in hematology (1995)., 32, 45-59.

[12] Brenner, D. A, Jain, M, Pimentel, D. R, et al. Human amyloidogenic light chains directly impair cardiomyocyte function through an increase in cellular oxidant stress. Circulation research (2004)., 94, 1008-10.

[13] Liao, R, Jain, M, Teller, P, et al. Infusion of light chains from patients with cardiac amyloidosis causes diastolic dysfunction in isolated mouse hearts. Circulation (2001)., 104, 1594-7.

[14] Palladini, G, Lavatelli, F, Russo, P, et al. Circulating amyloidogenic free light chains and serum N-terminal natriuretic peptide type B decrease simultaneously in association with improvement of survival in AL. Blood (2006)., 107, 3854-8.

[15] Gallo, G, Goni, F, Boctor, F, et al. Light chain cardiomyopathy. Structural analysis of the light chain tissue deposits. The American journal of pathology (1996). , 148, 1397-406.

[16] Buxbaum, J. N, Genega, E. M, Lazowski, P, et al. Infiltrative nonamyloidotic monoclonal immunoglobulin light chain cardiomyopathy: an underappreciated manifestation of plasma cell dyscrasias. Cardiology (2000)., 93, 220-8.

[17] Nakamura, M, Satoh, M, Kowada, S, et al. Reversible restrictive cardiomyopathy due to light-chain deposition disease. Mayo Clinic proceedings Mayo Clinic (2002). , 77, 193-6.

[18] Benson, M. D, & Kincaid, J. C. The molecular biology and clinical features of amyloid neuropathy. Muscle & nerve (2007)., 36, 411-23.

[19] Hou, X, Aguilar, M. I, & Small, D. H. Transthyretin and familial amyloidotic polyneuropathy. Recent progress in understanding the molecular mechanism of neurodegeneration. The FEBS journal (2007)., 274, 1637-50.

[20] Connors, L. H, Lim, A, Prokaeva, T, Roskens, V. A, & Costello, C. E. Tabulation of human transthyretin (TTR) variants, (2003). Amyloid 2003;, 10, 160-84.

[21] Yazaki, M, Tokuda, T, Nakamura, A, et al. Cardiac amyloid in patients with familial amyloid polyneuropathy consists of abundant wild-type transthyretin. Biochemical and biophysical research communications (2000)., 274, 702-6.

[22] Lessell, S, Wolf, P. A, Benson, M. D, & Cohen, A. S. Scalloped pupils in familial amyloidosis. The New England journal of medicine (1975)., 293, 914-5.

[23] Ando, Y, Nakamura, M, & Araki, S. Transthyretin-related familial amyloidotic polyneuropathy. Archives of neurology (2005). , 62, 1057-62.

[24] Rapezzi, C, Perugini, E, Salvi, F, et al. Phenotypic and genotypic heterogeneity in transthyretin-related cardiac amyloidosis: towards tailoring of therapeutic strategies? Amyloid (2006). , 13, 143-53.

[25] Jacobson, D. R, Pastore, R. D, Yaghoubian, R, et al. Variant-sequence transthyretin (isoleucine 122) in late-onset cardiac amyloidosis in black Americans. The New England journal of medicine (1997). , 336, 466-73.

[26] Falk, R. H. The neglected entity of familial cardiac amyloidosis in African Americans. Ethnicity & disease (2002). , 12, 141-3.

[27] Ikeda, S, Nakazato, M, Ando, Y, & Sobue, G. Familial transthyretin-type amyloid polyneuropathy in Japan: clinical and genetic heterogeneity. Neurology (2002). , 58, 1001-7.

[28] Conceicao, I, & De Carvalho, M. Clinical variability in type I familial amyloid polyneuropathy (Val30Met): comparison between late- and early-onset cases in Portugal. Muscle & nerve (2007). , 35, 116-8.

[29] Suhr, O. B, Svendsen, I. H, Andersson, R, Danielsson, A, Holmgren, G, & Ranlov, P. J. Hereditary transthyretin amyloidosis from a Scandinavian perspective. Journal of internal medicine (2003). , 254, 225-35.

[30] Hellman, U, Alarcon, F, Lundgren, H. E, Suhr, O. B, Bonaiti-pellie, C, & Plante-bordeneuve, V. Heterogeneity of penetrance in familial amyloid polyneuropathy, ATTR Val30Met, in the Swedish population. Amyloid (2008). , 15, 181-6.

[31] Westermark, P, Sletten, K, Johansson, B, & Cornwell, G. G. rd. Fibril in senile systemic amyloidosis is derived from normal transthyretin. Proceedings of the National Academy of Sciences of the United States of America (1990). , 87, 2843-5.

[32] Falk, R. H, & Dubrey, S. W. Amyloid heart disease. Prog Cardiovasc Dis (2010). , 52, 347-61.

[33] Pellikka, P. A, & Holmes, D. R. Jr., Edwards WD, Nishimura RA, Tajik AJ, Kyle RA. Endomyocardial biopsy in 30 patients with primary amyloidosis and suspected cardiac involvement. Archives of internal medicine (1988). , 148, 662-6.

[34] Shirahama, T, & Cohen, A. S. High-resolution electron microscopic analysis of the amyloid fibril. The Journal of cell biology (1967). , 33, 679-708.

[35] Sharma, P. P, Payvar, S, & Litovsky, S. H. Histomorphometric analysis of intramyocardial vessels in primary and senile amyloidosis: epicardium versus endocardium. Cardiovascular pathology : the official journal of the Society for Cardiovascular Pathology (2008). , 17, 65-71.

[36] Dubrey, S. W, Cha, K, Anderson, J, et al. The clinical features of immunoglobulin light-chain (AL) amyloidosis with heart involvement. QJM : monthly journal of the Association of Physicians (1998)., 91, 141-57.

[37] Chamarthi, B, Dubrey, S. W, Cha, K, Skinner, M, & Falk, R. H. Features and prognosis of exertional syncope in light-chain associated AL cardiac amyloidosis. The American journal of cardiology (1997)., 80, 1242-5.

[38] Mueller, P. S, Edwards, W. D, & Gertz, M. A. Symptomatic ischemic heart disease resulting from obstructive intramural coronary amyloidosis. The American journal of medicine (2000)., 109, 181-8.

[39] Dubrey, S, Pollak, A, Skinner, M, & Falk, R. H. Atrial thrombi occurring during sinus rhythm in cardiac amyloidosis: evidence for atrial electromechanical dissociation. British heart journal (1995)., 74, 541-4.

[40] Feng, D, Edwards, W. D, Oh, J. K, et al. Intracardiac thrombosis and embolism in patients with cardiac amyloidosis. Circulation (2007)., 116, 2420-6.

[41] Feng, D, Syed, I. S, Martinez, M, et al. Intracardiac thrombosis and anticoagulation therapy in cardiac amyloidosis. Circulation (2009)., 119, 2490-7.

[42] Zubkov, A. Y, Rabinstein, A. A, Dispenzieri, A, & Wijdicks, E. F. Primary systemic amyloidosis with ischemic stroke as a presenting complication. Neurology (2007)., 69, 1136-41.

[43] Berk, J. L, Keane, J, Seldin, D. C, et al. Persistent pleural effusions in primary systemic amyloidosis: etiology and prognosis. Chest (2003)., 124, 969-77.

[44] Abraham, R. S, Katzmann, J. A, Clark, R. J, Bradwell, A. R, Kyle, R. A, & Gertz, M. A. Quantitative analysis of serum free light chains. A new marker for the diagnostic evaluation of primary systemic amyloidosis. American journal of clinical pathology (2003)., 119, 274-8.

[45] Kyle, R. A, Therneau, T. M, Rajkumar, S. V, Larson, D. R, Plevak, M. F, & Melton, L. J. rd. Long-term follow-up of 241 patients with monoclonal gammopathy of undetermined significance: the original Mayo Clinic series 25 years later. Mayo Clinic proceedings Mayo Clinic (2004)., 79, 859-66.

[46] Rajkumar, S. V, Kyle, R. A, Therneau, T. M, et al. Presence of monoclonal free light chains in the serum predicts risk of progression in monoclonal gammopathy of undetermined significance. British journal of haematology (2004)., 127, 308-10.

[47] Katzmann, J. A, Abraham, R. S, Dispenzieri, A, Lust, J. A, & Kyle, R. A. Diagnostic performance of quantitative kappa and lambda free light chain assays in clinical practice. Clinical chemistry (2005)., 51, 878-81.

[48] Ansari-lari, M. A, & Ali, S. Z. Fine-needle aspiration of abdominal fat pad for amyloid detection: a clinically useful test? Diagnostic cytopathology (2004)., 30, 178-81.

[49] Guy, C. D, & Jones, C. K. Abdominal fat pad aspiration biopsy for tissue confirmation of systemic amyloidosis: specificity, positive predictive value, and diagnostic pitfalls. Diagnostic cytopathology (2001). , 24, 181-5.

[50] Reisinger, J, Dubrey, S. W, Lavalley, M, Skinner, M, & Falk, R. H. Electrophysiologic abnormalities in AL (primary) amyloidosis with cardiac involvement. Journal of the American College of Cardiology (1997). , 30, 1046-51.

[51] Murtagh, B, Hammill, S. C, Gertz, M. A, Kyle, R. A, Tajik, A. J, & Grogan, M. Electrocardiographic findings in primary systemic amyloidosis and biopsy-proven cardiac involvement. The American journal of cardiology (2005). , 95, 535-7.

[52] Klein, A. L, Hatle, L. K, Burstow, D. J, et al. Doppler characterization of left ventricular diastolic function in cardiac amyloidosis. Journal of the American College of Cardiology (1989). , 13, 1017-26.

[53] Abdalla, I, Murray, R. D, Lee, J. C, Stewart, W. J, Tajik, A. J, & Klein, A. L. Duration of pulmonary venous atrial reversal flow velocity and mitral inflow a wave: new measure of severity of cardiac amyloidosis. J Am Soc Echocardiogr (1998). , 11, 1125-33.

[54] Plehn, J. F, Southworth, J, & Cornwell, G. G. rd. Brief report: atrial systolic failure in primary amyloidosis. The New England journal of medicine (1992). , 327, 1570-3.

[55] Modesto, K. M, Dispenzieri, A, Cauduro, S. A, et al. Left atrial myopathy in cardiac amyloidosis: implications of novel echocardiographic techniques. European heart journal (2005). , 26, 173-9.

[56] Koyama, J, Davidoff, R, & Falk, R. H. Longitudinal myocardial velocity gradient derived from pulsed Doppler tissue imaging in AL amyloidosis: a sensitive indicator of systolic and diastolic dysfunction. J Am Soc Echocardiogr (2004). , 17, 36-44.

[57] Ogiwara, F, Koyama, J, Ikeda, S, Kinoshita, O, & Falk, R. H. Comparison of the strain Doppler echocardiographic features of familial amyloid polyneuropathy (FAP) and light-chain amyloidosis. The American journal of cardiology (2005). , 95, 538-40.

[58] Carroll, J. D, Gaasch, W. H, & Mcadam, K. P. Amyloid cardiomyopathy: characterization by a distinctive voltage/mass relation. The American journal of cardiology (1982). , 49, 9-13.

[59] Sedlis, S. P, Saffitz, J. E, Schwob, V. S, & Jaffe, A. S. Cardiac amyloidosis simulating hypertrophic cardiomyopathy. The American journal of cardiology (1984). , 53, 969-70.

[60] Hemmingson, L. O, & Eriksson, P. Cardiac amyloidosis mimicking hypertrophic cardiomyopathy. Acta medica Scandinavica (1986). , 219, 421-3.

[61] Ng, B, Connors, L. H, Davidoff, R, Skinner, M, & Falk, R. H. Senile systemic amyloidosis presenting with heart failure: a comparison with light chain-associated amyloidosis. Archives of internal medicine (2005). , 165, 1425-9.

[62] Dubrey, S. W, Cha, K, & Skinner, M. LaValley M, Falk RH. Familial and primary (AL) cardiac amyloidosis: echocardiographically similar diseases with distinctly different clinical outcomes. Heart (1997). , 78, 74-82.

[63] Kwong, R. Y, & Falk, R. H. Cardiovascular magnetic resonance in cardiac amyloidosis. Circulation (2005). , 111, 122-4.

[64] Sparrow, P, Amirabadi, A, Sussman, M. S, Paul, N, & Merchant, N. Quantitative assessment of myocardial T2 relaxation times in cardiac amyloidosis. Journal of magnetic resonance imaging : JMRI (2009). , 30, 942-6.

[65] Migrino, R. Q, Christenson, R, Szabo, A, Bright, M, Truran, S, & Hari, P. Prognostic implication of late gadolinium enhancement on cardiac MRI in light chain (AL) amyloidosis on long term follow up. BMC medical physics (2009).

[66] Hosch, W, Kristen, A. V, Libicher, M, et al. Late enhancement in cardiac amyloidosis: correlation of MRI enhancement pattern with histopathological findings. Amyloid (2008). , 15, 196-204.

[67] Maceira, A. M, Joshi, J, Prasad, S. K, et al. Cardiovascular magnetic resonance in cardiac amyloidosis. Circulation (2005). , 111, 186-93.

[68] Ruberg, F. L, Appelbaum, E, Davidoff, R, et al. Diagnostic and prognostic utility of cardiovascular magnetic resonance imaging in light-chain cardiac amyloidosis. The American journal of cardiology (2009). , 103, 544-9.

[69] Perugini, E, Rapezzi, C, Piva, T, et al. Non-invasive evaluation of the myocardial substrate of cardiac amyloidosis by gadolinium cardiac magnetic resonance. Heart (2006). , 92, 343-9.

[70] Maceira, A. M, Prasad, S. K, Hawkins, P. N, Roughton, M, & Pennell, D. J. Cardiovascular magnetic resonance and prognosis in cardiac amyloidosis. Journal of cardiovascular magnetic resonance : official journal of the Society for Cardiovascular Magnetic Resonance (2008).

[71] Hazenberg, B. P, Van Rijswijk, M. H, Piers, D. A, et al. Diagnostic performance of 123I-labeled serum amyloid P component scintigraphy in patients with amyloidosis. The American journal of medicine (2006). e, 15-24.

[72] Glaudemans, A. W, Slart, R. H, Zeebregts, C. J, et al. Nuclear imaging in cardiac amyloidosis. European journal of nuclear medicine and molecular imaging (2009). , 36, 702-14.

[73] Rapezzi, C, Merlini, G, Quarta, C. C, et al. Systemic cardiac amyloidoses: disease profiles and clinical courses of the 3 main types. Circulation (2009). , 120, 1203-12.

[74] Swanton, R. H, Brooksby, I. A, Davies, M. J, Coltart, D. J, Jenkins, B. S, & Webb-peploe, M. M. Systolic and diastolic ventricular function in cardiac amyloidosis. Studies in six cases diagnosed with endomyocardial biopsy. The American journal of cardiology (1977)., 39, 658-64.

[75] Kern, M. J, Lorell, B. H, & Grossman, W. Cardiac amyloidosis masquerading as constrictive pericarditis. Catheterization and cardiovascular diagnosis (1982)., 8, 629-35.

[76] Hurrell, D. G, Nishimura, R. A, Higano, S. T, et al. Value of dynamic respiratory changes in left and right ventricular pressures for the diagnosis of constrictive pericarditis. Circulation (1996)., 93, 2007-13.

[77] Talreja, D. R, Nishimura, R. A, Oh, J. K, & Holmes, D. R. Constrictive pericarditis in the modern era: novel criteria for diagnosis in the cardiac catheterization laboratory. Journal of the American College of Cardiology (2008)., 51, 315-9.

[78] Gertz, M. A, Grogan, M, Kyle, R. A, & Tajik, A. J. Endomyocardial biopsy-proven light chain amyloidosis (AL) without echocardiographic features of infiltrative cardiomyopathy. The American journal of cardiology (1997)., 80, 93-5.

[79] Arbustini, E, Merlini, G, Gavazzi, A, et al. Cardiac immunocyte-derived (AL) amyloidosis: an endomyocardial biopsy study in 11 patients. American heart journal (1995)., 130, 528-36.

[80] Vrana, J. A, Gamez, J. D, Madden, B. J, Theis, J. D, & Bergen, H. R. rd, Dogan A. Classification of amyloidosis by laser microdissection and mass spectrometry-based proteomic analysis in clinical biopsy specimens. Blood (2009)., 114, 4957-9.

[81] Cornwell, G. G. rd, Westermark P. Senile amyloidosis: a protean manifestation of the aging process. Journal of clinical pathology (1980)., 33, 1146-52.

[82] Kristen, A. V, Perz, J. B, Schonland, S. O, et al. Non-invasive predictors of survival in cardiac amyloidosis. European journal of heart failure (2007)., 9, 617-24.

[83] Dispenzieri, A, Kyle, R. A, Gertz, M. A, et al. Survival in patients with primary systemic amyloidosis and raised serum cardiac troponins. Lancet (2003)., 361, 1787-9.

[84] Nordlinger, M, Magnani, B, Skinner, M, & Falk, R. H. Is elevated plasma B-natriuretic peptide in amyloidosis simply a function of the presence of heart failure? The American journal of cardiology (2005)., 96, 982-4.

[85] Takemura, G, Takatsu, Y, Doyama, K, et al. Expression of atrial and brain natriuretic peptides and their genes in hearts of patients with cardiac amyloidosis. Journal of the American College of Cardiology (1998)., 31, 754-65.

[86] Dispenzieri, A, Gertz, M. A, Kyle, R. A, et al. Serum cardiac troponins and N-terminal pro-brain natriuretic peptide: a staging system for primary systemic amyloidosis. Journal of clinical oncology : official journal of the American Society of Clinical Oncology (2004)., 22, 3751-7.

[87] Dispenzieri, A, Gertz, M. A, Kyle, R. A, et al. Prognostication of survival using cardiac troponins and N-terminal pro-brain natriuretic peptide in patients with primary systemic amyloidosis undergoing peripheral blood stem cell transplantation. Blood (2004). , 104, 1881-7.

[88] Kumar, S. K, Gertz, M. A, Lacy, M. Q, et al. Recent improvements in survival in primary systemic amyloidosis and the importance of an early mortality risk score. Mayo Clinic proceedings Mayo Clinic (2011). , 86, 12-8.

[89] Kumar, S, Dispenzieri, A, Lacy, M. Q, et al. Revised prognostic staging system for light chain amyloidosis incorporating cardiac biomarkers and serum free light chain measurements. Journal of clinical oncology : official journal of the American Society of Clinical Oncology (2012). , 30, 989-95.

[90] Kyle, R. A, Gertz, M. A, Greipp, P. R, et al. A trial of three regimens for primary amyloidosis: colchicine alone, melphalan and prednisone, and melphalan, prednisone, and colchicine. The New England journal of medicine (1997). , 336, 1202-7.

[91] Kyle, R. A, Spittell, P. C, Gertz, M. A, et al. The premortem recognition of systemic senile amyloidosis with cardiac involvement. The American journal of medicine (1996). , 101, 395-400.

[92] Palladini, G, & Merlini, G. Transplantation vs. conventional-dose therapy for amyloidosis. Current opinion in oncology (2011). , 23, 214-20.

[93] Skinner, M, Sanchorawala, V, Seldin, D. C, et al. High-dose melphalan and autologous stem-cell transplantation in patients with AL amyloidosis: an 8-year study. Annals of internal medicine (2004). , 140, 85-93.

[94] Reece, D. E, Sanchorawala, V, Hegenbart, U, et al. Weekly and twice-weekly bortezomib in patients with systemic AL amyloidosis: results of a phase 1 dose-escalation study. Blood (2009). , 114, 1489-97.

[95] Kastritis, E, Anagnostopoulos, A, Roussou, M, et al. Treatment of light chain (AL) amyloidosis with the combination of bortezomib and dexamethasone. Haematologica (2007). , 92, 1351-8.

[96] Dispenzieri, A, Dingli, D, Kumar, S. K, et al. Discordance between serum cardiac biomarker and immunoglobulin-free light-chain response in patients with immunoglobulin light-chain amyloidosis treated with immune modulatory drugs. American journal of hematology (2010). , 85, 757-9.

[97] Palladini, G, Russo, P, Lavatelli, F, et al. Treatment of patients with advanced cardiac AL amyloidosis with oral melphalan, dexamethasone, and thalidomide. Annals of hematology (2009). , 88, 347-50.

[98] Almeida, M. R, Gales, L, Damas, A. M, Cardoso, I, & Saraiva, M. J. Small transthyretin (TTR) ligands as possible therapeutic agents in TTR amyloidoses. Current drug targets CNS and neurological disorders (2005). , 4, 587-96.

[99] Sekijima, Y, Dendle, M. A, & Kelly, J. W. Orally administered diflunisal stabilizes transthyretin against dissociation required for amyloidogenesis. Amyloid (2006)., 13, 236-49.

[100] Tojo, K, Sekijima, Y, Kelly, J. W, & Ikeda, S. Diflunisal stabilizes familial amyloid polyneuropathy-associated transthyretin variant tetramers in serum against dissociation required for amyloidogenesis. Neuroscience research (2006)., 56, 441-9.

[101] Bulawa, C. E, Connelly, S, Devit, M, et al. Tafamidis, a potent and selective transthyretin kinetic stabilizer that inhibits the amyloid cascade. Proceedings of the National Academy of Sciences of the United States of America (2012)., 109, 9629-34.

[102] Coelho, T, & Maia, L. F. Martins da Silva A, et al. Tafamidis for transthyretin familial amyloid polyneuropathy: A randomized, controlled trial. Neurology (2012)., 79, 785-92.

[103] Gertz, M. A, Falk, R. H, Skinner, M, Cohen, A. S, & Kyle, R. A. Worsening of congestive heart failure in amyloid heart disease treated by calcium channel-blocking agents. The American journal of cardiology (1985).

[104] Pollak, A, & Falk, R. H. Left ventricular systolic dysfunction precipitated by verapamil in cardiac amyloidosis. Chest (1993)., 104, 618-20.

[105] Selvanayagam, J. B, Hawkins, P. N, Paul, B, Myerson, S. G, & Neubauer, S. Evaluation and management of the cardiac amyloidosis. Journal of the American College of Cardiology (2007)., 50, 2101-10.

[106] Rubinow, A, Skinner, M, & Cohen, A. S. Digoxin sensitivity in amyloid cardiomyopathy. Circulation (1981)., 63, 1285-8.

[107] Freeman, R. Clinical practice. Neurogenic orthostatic hypotension. The New England journal of medicine (2008)., 358, 615-24.

[108] Obayashi, K, Ando, Y, Terazaki, H, et al. Effect of sildenafil citrate (Viagra) on erectile dysfunction in a patient with familial amyloidotic polyneuropathy ATTR Val30Met. Journal of the autonomic nervous system (2000)., 80, 89-92.

[109] Santarone, M, Corrado, G, Tagliagambe, L. M, et al. Atrial thrombosis in cardiac amyloidosis: diagnostic contribution of transesophageal echocardiography. J Am Soc Echocardiogr (1999)., 12, 533-6.

[110] Falk, R. H, Rubinow, A, & Cohen, A. S. Cardiac arrhythmias in systemic amyloidosis: correlation with echocardiographic abnormalities. Journal of the American College of Cardiology (1984)., 3, 107-13.

[111] Hess, E. P, & White, R. D. Out-of-hospital cardiac arrest in patients with cardiac amyloidosis: presenting rhythms, management and outcomes in four patients. Resuscitation (2004)., 60, 105-11.

[112] Kristen, A. V, Dengler, T. J, Hegenbart, U, et al. Prophylactic implantation of cardioverter-defibrillator in patients with severe cardiac amyloidosis and high risk for

sudden cardiac death. Heart rhythm : the official journal of the Heart Rhythm Society (2008)., 5, 235-40.

[113] Hall, R, & Hawkins, P. N. Cardiac transplantation for AL amyloidosis. BMJ (1994)., 309, 1135-7.

[114] Hosenpud, J. D, Uretsky, B. F, Griffith, B. P, Connell, O, Olivari, J. B, & Valantine, M. T. HA. Successful intermediate-term outcome for patients with cardiac amyloidosis undergoing heart transplantation: results of a multicenter survey. The Journal of heart transplantation (1990)., 9, 346-50.

[115] Hosenpud, J. D, Demarco, T, Frazier, O. H, et al. Progression of systemic disease and reduced long-term survival in patients with cardiac amyloidosis undergoing heart transplantation. Follow-up results of a multicenter survey. Circulation (1991). III, 338-43.

[116] Audard, V, Matignon, M, Weiss, L, et al. Successful long-term outcome of the first combined heart and kidney transplant in a patient with systemic Al amyloidosis. American journal of transplantation : official journal of the American Society of Transplantation and the American Society of Transplant Surgeons (2009)., 9, 236-40.

[117] Kristen, A. V, Sack, F. U, Schonland, S. O, et al. Staged heart transplantation and chemotherapy as a treatment option in patients with severe cardiac light-chain amyloidosis. European journal of heart failure (2009)., 11, 1014-20.

[118] Dubrey, S, Simms, R. W, Skinner, M, & Falk, R. H. Recurrence of primary (AL) amyloidosis in a transplanted heart with four-year survival. The American journal of cardiology (1995)., 76, 739-41.

[119] Gillmore, J. D, Goodman, H. J, Lachmann, H. J, et al. Sequential heart and autologous stem cell transplantation for systemic AL amyloidosis. Blood (2006)., 107, 1227-9.

[120] Sack, F. U, Kristen, A, Goldschmidt, H, et al. Treatment options for severe cardiac amyloidosis: heart transplantation combined with chemotherapy and stem cell transplantation for patients with AL-amyloidosis and heart and liver transplantation for patients with ATTR-amyloidosis. European journal of cardio-thoracic surgery : official journal of the European Association for Cardio-thoracic Surgery (2008). , 33, 257-62.

[121] Dey, B. R, Chung, S. S, Spitzer, T. R, et al. Cardiac transplantation followed by dose-intensive melphalan and autologous stem-cell transplantation for light chain amyloidosis and heart failure. Transplantation (2010)., 90, 905-11.

[122] Luk, A, Ahn, E, Lee, A, Ross, H. J, & Butany, J. Recurrent cardiac amyloidosis following previous heart transplantation. Cardiovascular pathology : the official journal of the Society for Cardiovascular Pathology (2010). e, 129-33.

[123] Maurer, M. S, Raina, A, Hesdorffer, C, et al. Cardiac transplantation using extended-donor criteria organs for systemic amyloidosis complicated by heart failure. Transplantation (2007). , 83, 539-45.

[124] Mignot, A, Bridoux, F, Thierry, A, et al. Successful heart transplantation following melphalan plus dexamethasone therapy in systemic AL amyloidosis. Haematologica (2008). e, 32-5.

[125] Dubrey, S. W, Burke, M. M, Hawkins, P. N, & Banner, N. R. Cardiac transplantation for amyloid heart disease: the United Kingdom experience. The Journal of heart and lung transplantation : the official publication of the International Society for Heart Transplantation (2004). , 23, 1142-53.

[126] Kpodonu, J, Massad, M. G, Caines, A, & Geha, A. S. Outcome of heart transplantation in patients with amyloid cardiomyopathy. The Journal of heart and lung transplantation : the official publication of the International Society for Heart Transplantation (2005). , 24, 1763-5.

[127] Roig, E, Almenar, L, Gonzalez-vilchez, F, et al. Outcomes of heart transplantation for cardiac amyloidosis: subanalysis of the spanish registry for heart transplantation. American journal of transplantation : official journal of the American Society of Transplantation and the American Society of Transplant Surgeons (2009). , 9, 1414-9.

[128] Sattianayagam, P. T, Gibbs, S. D, Pinney, J. H, et al. Solid organ transplantation in AL amyloidosis. American journal of transplantation : official journal of the American Society of Transplantation and the American Society of Transplant Surgeons (2010). , 10, 2124-31.

[129] Lacy, M. Q, Dispenzieri, A, Hayman, S. R, et al. Autologous stem cell transplant after heart transplant for light chain (Al) amyloid cardiomyopathy. The Journal of heart and lung transplantation : the official publication of the International Society for Heart Transplantation (2008). , 27, 823-9.

[130] Fuchs, U, Zittermann, A, Suhr, O, et al. Heart transplantation in a 68-year-old patient with senile systemic amyloidosis. American journal of transplantation : official journal of the American Society of Transplantation and the American Society of Transplant Surgeons (2005). , 5, 1159-62.

[131] Holmgren, G, Ericzon, B. G, Groth, C. G, et al. Clinical improvement and amyloid regression after liver transplantation in hereditary transthyretin amyloidosis. Lancet (1993). , 341, 1113-6.

[132] Herlenius, G, Wilczek, H. E, Larsson, M, & Ericzon, B. G. Ten years of international experience with liver transplantation for familial amyloidotic polyneuropathy: results from the Familial Amyloidotic Polyneuropathy World Transplant Registry. Transplantation (2004). , 77, 64-71.

[133] Dubrey, S. W, Davidoff, R, Skinner, M, Bergethon, P, Lewis, D, & Falk, R. H. Progression of ventricular wall thickening after liver transplantation for familial amyloidosis. Transplantation (1997). , 64, 74-80.

[134] Pomfret, E. A, Lewis, W. D, Jenkins, R. L, et al. Effect of orthotopic liver transplantation on the progression of familial amyloidotic polyneuropathy. Transplantation (1998). , 65, 918-25.

[135] Stangou, A. J, Hawkins, P. N, Heaton, N. D, et al. Progressive cardiac amyloidosis following liver transplantation for familial amyloid polyneuropathy: implications for amyloid fibrillogenesis. Transplantation (1998). , 66, 229-33.

[136] Yazaki, M, Mitsuhashi, S, Tokuda, T, et al. Progressive wild-type transthyretin deposition after liver transplantation preferentially occurs onto myocardium in FAP patients. American journal of transplantation : official journal of the American Society of Transplantation and the American Society of Transplant Surgeons (2007). , 7, 235-42.

[137] Liepnieks, J. J, & Benson, M. D. Progression of cardiac amyloid deposition in hereditary transthyretin amyloidosis patients after liver transplantation. Amyloid (2007). , 14, 277-82.

[138] Ihse, E, Stangou, A. J, Heaton, N. D, et al. Proportion between wild-type and mutant protein in truncated compared to full-length ATTR: an analysis on transplanted transthyretin T60A amyloidosis patients. Biochemical and biophysical research communications (2009). , 379, 846-50.

[139] Grazi, G. L, Cescon, M, Salvi, F, et al. Combined heart and liver transplantation for familial amyloidotic neuropathy: considerations from the hepatic point of view. Liver transplantation : official publication of the American Association for the Study of Liver Diseases and the International Liver Transplantation Society (2003). , 9, 986-92.

[140] Arpesella, G, Chiappini, B, Marinelli, G, et al. Combined heart and liver transplantation for familial amyloidotic polyneuropathy. The Journal of thoracic and cardiovascular surgery (2003). , 125, 1165-6.

[141] Raichlin, E, Daly, R. C, Rosen, C. B, et al. Combined heart and liver transplantation: a single-center experience. Transplantation (2009). , 88, 219-25.

[142] Inomata, Y, Zeledon, M. E, Asonuma, K, et al. Whole-liver graft without the retrohepatic inferior vena cava for sequential (domino) living donor liver transplantation. American journal of transplantation : official journal of the American Society of Transplantation and the American Society of Transplant Surgeons (2007). , 7, 1629-32.

[143] Stangou, A. J, Heaton, N. D, & Hawkins, P. N. Transmission of systemic transthyretin amyloidosis by means of domino liver transplantation. The New England journal of medicine (2005).

[144] Goto, T, Yamashita, T, Ueda, M, et al. Iatrogenic amyloid neuropathy in a Japanese patient after sequential liver transplantation. American journal of transplantation :

official journal of the American Society of Transplantation and the American Society of Transplant Surgeons (2006). , 6, 2512-5.

[145] Barreiros, A. P, Geber, C, Birklein, F, Galle, P. R, & Otto, G. Clinical symptomatic de novo systemic transthyretin amyloidosis 9 years after domino liver transplantation. Liver transplantation : official publication of the American Association for the Study of Liver Diseases and the International Liver Transplantation Society (2010).

[146] Befeler, A. S, Schiano, T. D, Lissoos, T. W, et al. Successful combined liver-heart transplantation in adults: report of three patients and review of the literature. Transplantation (1999). , 68, 1423-7.

[147] Nardo, B, Beltempo, P, Bertelli, R, et al. Combined heart and liver transplantation in four adults with familial amyloidosis: experience of a single center. Transplantation proceedings (2004). , 36, 645-7.

[148] Hennessey, T, Backman, S. B, Cecere, R, et al. Combined heart and liver transplantation on cardiopulmonary bypass: report of four cases. Canadian journal of anaesthesia = Journal canadien d'anesthesie (2010). , 57, 355-60.

[149] Barreiros, A. P, Post, F, Hoppe-lotichius, M, et al. Liver transplantation and combined liver-heart transplantation in patients with familial amyloid polyneuropathy: a single-center experience. Liver transplantation : official publication of the American Association for the Study of Liver Diseases and the International Liver Transplantation Society (2010). , 16, 314-23.

[150] Pilato, E. Dell'Amore A, Botta L, Arpesella G. Combined heart and liver transplantation for familial amyloidotic neuropathy. European journal of cardio-thoracic surgery : official journal of the European Association for Cardio-thoracic Surgery (2007). , 32, 180-2.

[151] Daly, C. R, Topilsky, Y, Joyce, L, et al. Combined Heart and Liver Transplant: Protection of the Cardiac Graft from Antibody Rejection by Initial Liver Implantation. transplantation journal (in print) (2012).

[152] Davies, H. S, Pollard, S. G, & Calne, R. Y. Soluble HLA antigens in the circulation of liver graft recipients. Transplantation (1989). , 47, 524-7.

[153] Mcmillan, R. W, Gelder, F. B, Zibari, G. B, Aultman, D. F, Adamashvili, I, & Mcdonald, J. C. Soluble fraction of class I human histocompatibility leukocyte antigens in the serum of liver transplant recipients. Clinical transplantation (1997). , 11, 98-103.

[154] Vogel, W, Steiner, E, Kornberger, R, et al. Preliminary results with combined hepatorenal allografting. Transplantation (1988). , 45, 491-3.

[155] Topilsky, Y, Raichlin, E, Hasin, T, et al. Combined Heart and liver Transplant Attenuates Cardiac Allograft Vasculopathy Compared to Isolated Heart Transplantation. transplantation journal (in print) (2012).

[156] Kirklin, J. K, Naftel, D. C, Kormos, R. L, et al. The Fourth INTERMACS Annual Report: 4,000 implants and counting. The Journal of heart and lung transplantation : the official publication of the International Society for Heart Transplantation (2012). , 31, 117-26.

[157] Siegenthaler, M. P, & Martin, J. van de Loo A, Doenst T, Bothe W, Beyersdorf F. Implantation of the permanent Jarvik-2000 left ventricular assist device: a single-center experience. Journal of the American College of Cardiology (2002). , 39, 1764-72.

[158] Topilsky, Y, Pereira, N. L, Shah, D. K, et al. Left ventricular assist device therapy in patients with restrictive and hypertrophic cardiomyopathy. Circulation Heart failure (2011). , 4, 266-75.

Chapter 9

# Diagnosis and Treatment of AA Amyloidosis with Rheumatoid Arthritis: State of the Art

Takeshi Kuroda, Yoko Wada and Masaaki Nakano

Additional information is available at the end of the chapter

http://dx.doi.org/10.5772/54332

## 1. Introduction

Amyloidosis is a term applied to a heterogeneous group of rare diseases characterized by extracellular deposition of amyloid, causing target-organ dysfunction and a wide range of clinical symptoms [1]. These symptoms depend on the organ involved, and include nephrotic syndrome, hepatosplenomegaly, congestive heart failure, carpal tunnel syndrome, gastrointestinal (GI) symptoms and macroglossia [2]. Amyloidosis is classified clinically into several types depending on the precursor of the amyloid fibril. The disease involves amyloid fibrils formed in vivo by more than 25 different types of protein [3]. Reactive amyloid A (AA) amyloidosis is the representative systemic condition that develops in patients with chronic inflammatory diseases such as rheumatoid arthritis (RA), juvenile idiopathic arthritis, ankylosing spondylitis, inflammatory bowel disease, familial periodic fever syndrome, and chronic infections [4,5,6,7]. In some parts of the world, heredofamilial causes and infections are responsible for a larger proportion of cases of AA amyloidosis. In Turkey, familial Mediterranean fever (FMF) is the cause of more than 60 percent of cases [8]. Other conditions that may be associated with AA amyloidosis include neoplasms, particularly renal cell carcinoma [9], non-Hodgkin lymphoma [10], Castleman's disease [11], and cystic fibrosis [12]. Therapy with biologic agents including anti-tumor necrosis factor (anti-TNF) and anti-interleukin-6 (IL-6) is now employed routinely for the management of RA in patients for whom traditional disease-modifying antirheumatic drugs (DMARDs) have failed. In parallel with this shift of treatment strategy, the treatment of amyloidosis has also changed. Recently, we have revealed that the use of biologic agents for these patients can reduce the risk of death [13]. This article discusses current concepts of AA amyloidosis occurring mainly secondarily to RA, and addresses various strategies for prophylaxis, diagnosis, and therapy of this important complication in the light of changes in clinical management, especially hemodialysis (HD).

## 2. Prevalence

Epidemiological data for AA amyloidosis, extrapolated from autopsy records in Western nations, has indicated that its prevalence varies from about 0.5% to 0.86% according to environmental risk factors and geographic clustering [14,15]. The incidence of AA amyloidosis in RA is still undefined, but is considered to be underestimated. In Europe, 5- 20% of patients with RA develop amyloidosis, the highest incidence being in Finland [16], where reevaluation of autopsy materials for the period 1952-1991 yielded a 30% incidence of AA amyloidosis compared with a figure of 18% detected by routine testing, indicating that a significant proportion of cases may not be detected by standard histologic analysis [17]. Japanese autopsy reports have revealed that about 30% of autopsied RA patients have amyloid deposits [18]. Some Japanese medical centers have reported the incidence of amyloidosis in consecutive patients undergoing GI biopsy. The frequency of amyloidosis in RA has been reported to vary between 5% and 13.3% in cases confirmed by biopsy, and from 14% to 26% in cases confirmed at autopsy [19,20,21,22]. More than 95% of patients with AA amyloidosis are considered to have renal involvement, end-stage kidney disease (ESKD) being found in 10% of cases at the time of diagnosis [23]. Although the subclinical phase of AA amyloidosis is defined by the formation of amyloid deposits in tissue without any clinical manifestation, it is very difficult to distinguish between the clinical and subclinical phases. Obviously, it is difficult to evaluate the natural history of amyloid deposition and to know the length of this phase and its final outcome. In contrast, the prevalence of clinical amyloidosis is likely to be lower; at least half of amyloidosis patients have subclinical disease, and AA amyloidosis is clinically overt in only 25-50%, even after longer periods of follow-up sampling. Considering this discrepancy between the prevalence rates of clinical and subclinical AA amyloidosis, the wide variation in the prevalence of AA amyloidosis secondary to RA may be due partly to marked geographic differences worldwide, possibly including genetic factors, and to the lack of unified statistical studies of AA amyloidosis among races and districts. In view of these factors, the prevalence of AA amyloidosis associated with RA is probably higher than that estimated so far.

## 3. Pathogenesis of amyloid fibril formation and genetic background

Precise details of the mechanism of amyloid fibril formation are unknown, and may differ among the various types of amyloid [24, 25]. Factors that contribute to fibrillogenesis include a variant or unstable protein structure, extensive beta-conformation of the precursor protein, association with components of the serum or extracellular matrix, and physical properties including the pH of the tissue site. Extracellular matrix components include the amyloid P component, amyloid enhancing factor (AEF), apolipoprotein E (ApoE), and glycosaminoglycans (GAGs). Amyloidosis is classified clinically into several types according to the precursor of the amyloid fibril and the type of amyloid fibril protein. Any complete definition of amyloidosis includes the amyloid fibril protein precursor, the protein type or variant, and the clinical setting at diagnosis [3]. AA amyloidosis complicates many chronic inflammatory diseases and has been studied most widely in experimental animal models. AA amyloid also occurs spontaneously in various animal species, and can be induced by chronic inflammatory stimuli. The best-known model of this disease is amyloid induction by injection of casein/azocasein in certain genetically susceptible strains of mice. AA fibril formation can be accelerated by an AEF in murine models present at high concentration in the spleen, by basement membrane heparan sulfate proteoglycan, or by seeding with AA or heterologous fibrils [26,27] (AEF has not yet been detected in humans). Therefore, sustained overproduction of SAA is a prerequisite for the development of AA amyloidosis. The mechanism of amyloidosis is initiated by overproduction of SAA as a consequence of acute and chronic inflammation. Next, SAA is internalized by macrophages, followed by intracellular proteolysis, and subsequent release of amyloidogenic peptides into the extracellular space, apparently preceding fibril formation [28]. AA amyloidosis is caused by organ deposition of AA fibrils, which are formed from an N-terminal cleavage fragment of SAA [29]. SAA is a 104-amino-acid protein produced in the liver under transcriptional regulation by proinflammatory cytokines, and transported by a high-density lipoprotein (HDL), HDL3, in plasma [30,31,32,33]. SAA is encoded by a family of SAA genes, which are responsive to proinflammatory cytokines [34,35]. A major factor responsible for the development of AA amyloidosis is increased synthesis and subsequent degeneration of SAA under conditions of chronic inflammation. AA amyloidosis is a rare but serious complication of diseases that stimulate a sustained and substantial acute-phase response, and foremost of which is RA. In RA, there is increased synthesis of SAA accompanied by inflammation, which may be due to elevated levels of proinflammatory cytokines. The increased cytokine levels are correlated with synovitis, which may stimulate synoviocytes to produce SAA [28,36,37] (Figure 1). These mechanisms lead to elevated levels of SAA in joint fluid relative to serum [37], sometimes reaching up to 1,000 times the baseline level [23], thus facilitating the development of AA amyloidosis. However, a high concentration of SAA alone is not sufficient for development of amyloidosis. Several genetic factors have been evaluated, and recent studies have focused on SAA polymorphism as a genetic background factor linked to amyloidogenesis. Allelic variants include acute phase SAAs (SAA1 and SAA2) and SAA4, and post-translational modifications of these gene products. SAA3 is a pseudogene with no product, and the serum concentration of SAA4 does not change during an acute-phase response [31]. The acute-phase proteins SAA1 and SAA2 are apolipoproteins, primarily associated with specific HDL, and are expressed extrahepatically in the absence of HDL [38]. SAA1 and SAA2 are inducible by interleukin (IL)-1, IL-6, tumor necrosis factor (TNF)-alpha, lipopolysaccharide (LPS), and several transcription factors, notably SAA activating factor (SAF-1) [39,40]. Both SAA1 and SAA2 are polymorphic proteins, and amyloid fibrils are considered to be formed in tissues from both SAAs1 and 2, but predominantly from SAA1 in humans [41]. Synthesis of amyloid protein from SAAs1 and 2 is strongly induced by inflammatory cytokines such as IL-6 in the liver, in parallel with the disease activity of RA [42]. SAA1 is the most important precursor for tissue AA deposition, because this isotype is predominant in plasma, and AA proteins are derived largely from it. SAA1 has three alleles, designated SAA1.1, SAA1.3, and SAA1.5, defined by amino acid substitutions at positions 52 and 57 of the molecule [3]. SAA2 has two alleles, SAA2.1 and 2.2. The frequency of these alleles varies among populations, and may be associated with the occurrence of AA amyloidosis in diseases such as RA, and also with the level of SAA in blood, efficacy of clearance, susceptibility to proteolytic cleavage by specific metalloproteinases, disease severity, and response to treatment [43]. The SAA1 alleles 1.1 and 1.3 have been proposed as positive risk factors in Caucasian and Japanese patients, respectively [44,45,46,47,48,49,50,51]. While the SAA1.1 allele was found to have a negative association with amyloidosis in Japanese subjects, it showed a positive association in Caucasians. Similarly, SAA1.3 showed an inverse association between Japanese and Caucasians. Recent new data have indicated that the -13T/C single nucleotide polymorphism in the 50-flanking region of SAA1 is a better marker of AA amyloidosis than the exon-3-based haplotype in both Japanese and American Caucasian populations [49,52,53]. Polymorphism of ApoE has been investigated as a potentially relevant genetic background factor, as this molecule is generally involved in the process of amyloid deposition [30]. According to several recent reports, ApoE4 is positively related to the development of AA amyloidosis in patients with RA [54]. Amyloid fibrils associate with other moieties, including GAGs, serum amyloid P component (SAP) and ApoA-II, which are related to the onset of amyloidosis [32, 55]. Recently, aging has also been shown to be a risk factor for AA amyloidosis associated with RA [56]. The fibrils bind Congo red and exhibit green birefringence when viewed by polarization light microscopy, although the deposits can also be recognized in hematoxylin and eosin-stained sections [57, 58]. Electron microscopy demonstrates deposits of amyloid fibril protein in tissues as rigid, non-branching fibrils approximately 8 to 10 nm wide and of varying length, with a 2.5 to 3.5 nm filamentous subunit arranged with a slow twist along the long axis of the fibril [59]. When isolated and analysed by X-ray diffraction, the fibrils exhibit a characteristically abnormal beta-sheet pattern [60]. Typing of amyloid deposits can be done by conventional immunohistochemical staining.

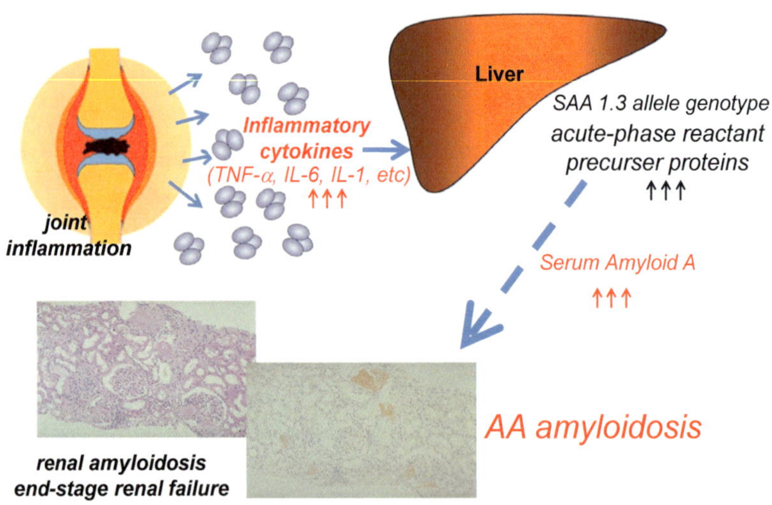


**Figure 1. Pathogenesis of AA amyloidosis secondary to RA.** RA begins with joint synovitis, and serum amyloid A protein (SAA) is synthesized in the liver chiefly as a result of stimulation with proinflammatory cytokines. Genetic background factors such as the SAA 1.3 allele genotype are a risk factor for amyloidosis. Amyloid fibrils are deposited in tissues of various organs, leading to organ failure. TNF-alpha: tumor necrosis factor-alpha, IL-6: interleukin-6, IL-1: interleukin-1, SAA1.3: one of the SAA1 gene polymorphisms.

# 4. Diagnosis

A cohort study of patients with RA has shown that deposits of fat AA fibrils are not uncommon (16.3%) [61]. Any patient with long-standing active inflammatory disease, such as RA, who develops proteinuria or intractable diarrhea must first be investigated for AA amyloidosis. No blood test is specially diagnostic for amyloidosis. Results of tests confirming the presence of chronic inflammatory disease, such as an increased erythrocyte sedimentation rate (ESR), or elevated levels of C-reactive protein (CRP) and SAA, are not necessarily discriminatory because most patients with chronic inflammation do not develop amyloidosis. The next step for diagnosis is to perform a biopsy and histopathological examination. In order to begin intensive treatment as early as possible before organ function worsens, it is important to choose a high-sensitivity biopsy site and employ a safe technique. In general, subcutaneous fat, spleen, adrenal gland, liver, labial salivary gland, and sites in the alimentary canal ranging from the tongue and gingiva to the rectum, are frequent sites of AA amyloid deposition [62,63,64,65,66,67,68,69,70,71]. Many non-invasive techniques are useful for assessing organ involvement, but cannot establish whether the findings are related to amyloid. The definitive diagnostic test is biopsy of either an accessible tissue expected to contain amyloid, or a clinically affected organ. GI, rectal and subcutaneous fat biopsies are the procedures of choice, because the methodology is simple [19,72,73,74]. Aspiration biopsy of abdominal fat is recommended for screening in outpatient clinics because it is easy to perform in that setting, requires no specialty consultation or technical experience, has a high yield, and results in only minimal side effects [61]. As experience has shown that the amount of amyloid in fat tissue is low, the operator should aspirate as large a sample as possible. If possible, GI and rectal biopsies are also recommended because their sensitivity is high and they can also be performed at hospitals in an outpatient setting. Generally, the GI is a more sensitive site for biopsy than subcutaneous fat [19,63]. The detection rate is higher in the duodenal bulb and second portion of the small intestine than in the stomach. Additionally, the incidence of amyloidosis in GI biopsies is highly correlated with that in renal biopsies [20]. If GI biopsy reveals amyloid deposition, the presence of renal amyloidosis should be considered [20]. However, a more recent study has revealed that the amounts of amyloid deposition in GI and renal biopsies are not correlated. GI amyloid-positive areas are larger than renal amyloid-positive areas [75]. If a fat biopsy proves negative, biopsy of the clinically involved site is suggested for patients with a limited number of affected organs. More organ-specific biopsies, such as heart, kidney and liver, are recommended. However, such biopsy sites carry a relatively higher risk than GI, rectal or subcutaneous fat biopsies. In such cases, clinicians should weigh the risks and benefits of biopsy. In Japan, however, GI biopsy is commonly performed for screening, rather than fat biopsy. If amyloidosis is strongly suspected clinically in association with marked inflammation, annual screening biopsy is recommended. However, it should be considered that rheumatologist put treatment for inflammation before organ biopsies. The many reports of renal biopsy results for RA patients have suggested that renal amyloidosis is the most serious complication. In RA patients, renal biopsy can sometimes be hazardous because of difficulties in maintaining a fixed body position, osteoporosis, or advanced age [76]. Renal involvement tends to determine the clinical course in such patients. Renal biopsy can also reveal underlying renal disorders such as mesangial proliferative glomerulonephritis (MesPGN), membranous nephropathy (MN), and thin basement membrane disease (TBMD). Pathological information on such underlying conditions is sometimes very important for the treatment of concomitant amyloidosis. Amyloid cardiomyopathy and autonomic neuropathy have been extremely rare in previously reported series [68], but should be keep in mind when interpreting biopsy results. The third step is histological diagnosis of amyloidosis, which can be established by light microscopy using special staining for amyloid. Alkaline Congo red has long been the standard method of staining for amyloid [57,58, 65]. Deposits of amyloid bind Congo red and exhibit apple-green birefringence when viewed by polarization light microscopy. This provides definitive diagnosis of amyloidosis. However, Dylon stain is more sensitive, and is therefore more useful for the detection of small amounts of amyloid [70, 71]. The use of Dylon stain, also known as direct fast scarlet, has recently become more popular. However, it requires more careful observation because of a tendency for over-staining (Figure 2). Thioflavin T is also more sensitive than Congo red, but less specific [77,78,79]. Although it yields a more intense fluorescent reaction, over-staining often hinders accurate diagnosis. If biopsy samples show a positive reaction, the type of amyloidosis should then be determined. Immunohistochemistry with fluorescent antibodies specific for precursor proteins, such as light chain lambda, kappa, SAA, etc., is a reliable diagnostic complement. Additional testing of serum and urine samples for monoclonal immunoglobulins, and of serum for free light chains, should be performed to exclude AL amyloidosis. Amino acid sequencing and mass spectroscopy of amyloid deposits have been utilitized to identify the precursor protein in some cases, but these techniques are not used routinely. Electron microscopy demonstrates straight, unbranched amyloid fibrils 8 to10 nm in width. Scintigraphy using radiolabeled SAP can identify the distribution of amyloid, and provide an estimate of the total body burden of fibrillar deposits [80]. SAP scintigraphy provides for a good tool for noninvasive diagnosis and for evaluation of the response to therapy over time [23]. The fourth step is to initiate treatment. If AA amyloid is revealed in any organ, the treatment should be focused on systemic amyloidosis, while giving due attention to any underlying chronic inflammatory diseases. If AA amyloidosis is related to tuberculosis or FMF, treatment of these underlying diseases should also be started. It is important to introduce specific therapies for individual diseases in such cases.

## 5. Quantification of amyloid deposition from biopsy specimens

Amyloidosis is usually diagnosed by histological examination of biopsy samples. However, its quantitative evaluation can be difficult. Some previous studies have tried to clarify the correlation between amyloid load and clinical features, and some trials of image analysis of GI biopsy and/or renal biopsy specimens have been attempted. Amyloid-positive areas in such biopsy specimens were determined on Congo-red-stained sections. One whole-tissue section was photographed, and then the borders of the amyloid-positive areas were traced, excluding any tissue-free spaces. Several studies have examined correlations between amyloid load and clinical parameters, and amyloid load in both GI and renal biopsy specimens were found to be highly correlated with kidney function [75,81,82]. Recently, some studies have also employed SAA measurements from GI biopsy samples or abdominal fat obtained by needle aspiration to quantify AA [83, 84, 85]. Such quantification of AA from biopsy samples is useful for screening of AA amyloidosis and can be used for follow-up of the disease. Additionally, amyloid load in fat tissue reflects disease severity and can predict the survival of patients with the use of a grading system [86]. These reports have suggested that amyloid load reflects organ damage or disease severity.

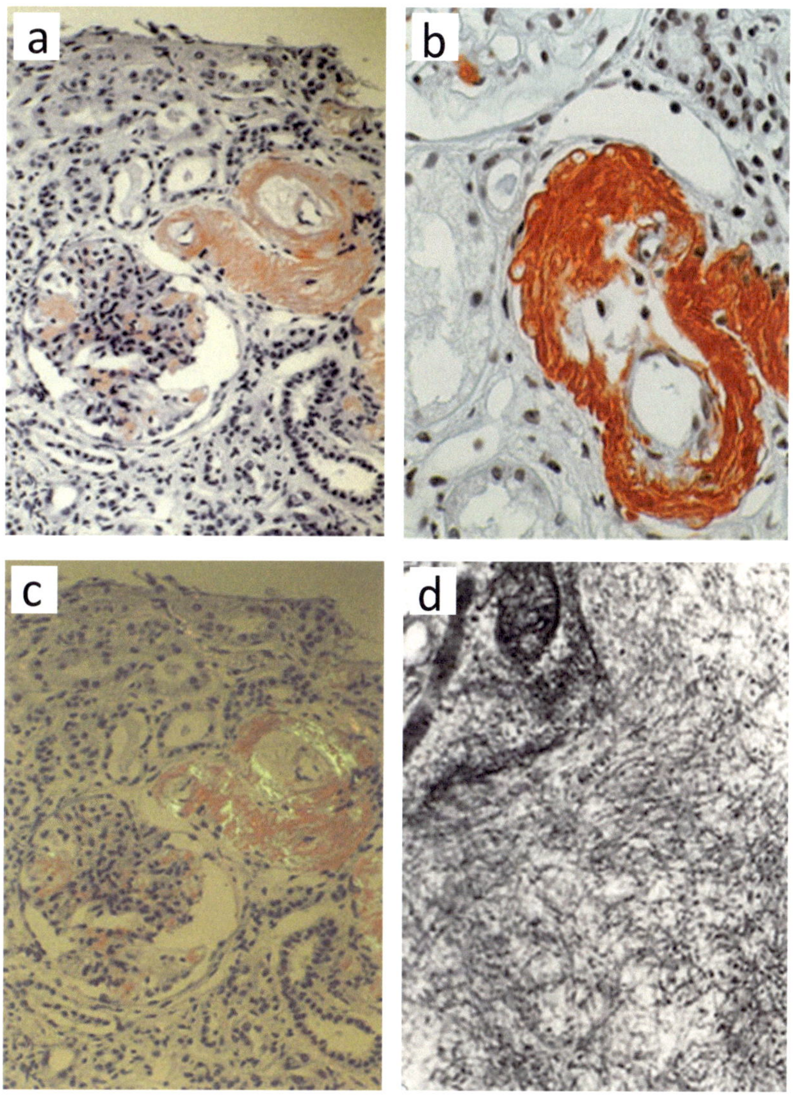


**Figure 2. Histological diagnosis of renal amyloidosis.** Amyloid substance is reactive with Congo red stain (a) and Dylon stain (b), and shows apple-green fluorescence under a polarizing microscope (c). Electron microscopy shows thin amyloid fibrils with a diameter of about 10 nm in AA and AL amyloidosis

## 6. Clinical features

The clinical features of amyloidosis are compatible with the infiltration of amyloid deposits. AA amyloidosis is a serious disease with a significant mortality due to ESKD, heart failure, bowel perforation, or GI bleeding [72,85]. Common clinical features of AA amyloidosis include proteinuria, loss of kidney function, and GI disorders. A clinical diagnosis of amyloidosis is usually suspected if proteinuria, renal insufficiency, or intractable diarrhea is present. Attention should also be paid to long-lasting and high inflammatory disease activity. Although AA amyloid can sometimes be detected in patients with arthritis in the absence of other clinical features, the clinical importance of such "silent" deposits remains to be determined. Renal involvement is a well-known complication of amylodiosis with RA. It is usually manifested as proteinuria or nephrotic syndrome with a variable degree of renal impairment that may progress to ESKD. If proteinuria worsens to about 0.5 g/day, amyloidosis should be suspected even if other reasons are plausible. In RA, several underlying renal disorders accompanying renal amyloidosis have been observed [87], including MesPGN, MN, TBMD, and interstitial nephritis [87]. Crescentic glomerulonephritis is a rare underlying disease in RA patients, and can result in rupture of the fragile glomerular basement membrane due to amyloid deposition [88]. Usually, MesPGN and interstitial nephritis are associated with mild to moderate proteinuria, and MN with severe proteinuria. TBMD shows no proteinuria, and usually hematuria alone is evident. Histological investigation frequently demonstrates renal amyloidosis concomitant with these underlying diseases [87]. In renal tissue, primary amyloid deposition may be limited to the blood vessels or tubules. Such patients present with renal failure but little or no proteinuria [89]. These deposits lead to narrowing of the vascular lumina [90]. Glomerular deposits are more common, and are associated with a poor renal outcome in patients with AA amyloidosis associated with RA. One report has described that 27 patients with renal amyloidosis due to RA had glomerular deposits, and that 85% of them showed progression to ESRD during a five-year observation period. However, patients with vascular and tubular amyloid deposits showed no deterioration of kidney function [91]. Such patients with vascular and tubular amyloid deposits usually present with slowly progressive chronic kidney disease with little or no proteinuria, and their prognosis appears to be more favorable [91]. Several studies have demonstrated a relationship between kidney function parameters and histopathological findings in patients with RA. The area of amyloid deposition in renal biopsy specimens was highly correlated with kidney function [81]. Additionally, if amyloid deposits in renal biopsy specimens progressed to some extent, the deterioration of kidney function became irreversible [82]. Because there are currently no methods for correlating the results of renal amyloid biopsy with outcome or therapeutic results, the clinical value of such investigations is still unclear. Standardization of renal amyloid biopsy parameters has been attempted, including biochemical classification, histopathologic classification, scoring of renal amyloid deposition, and association with other histopathologic lesions and grading [92]. The kidneys are usually enlarged slightly when nephrotic, but show a decrease in size as ESKD ensues. GI symptoms, such as alternating periods of constipation and diarrhea or bleeding, may frequently suggest early localization of amyloid deposits and warrant further investigation. Abdominal distention and appetite loss are also frequently observed. Diminished peristalsis and malabsorption are common results of amyloid deposition, and can lead to nausea, vomiting, diarrhea, or hypoalbuminemia [93]. Endoscopy may demonstrate erosion, ulceration, mucosal weakness, or micro-polyposis, but sometimes no abnormality is evident in patients with mild amyloid deposition [64,94]. Fatal pancreatitis can sometimes occur at the end-stage of renal disease, and this is due to vascular obstruction by amyloid deposits in the pancreas [95]. Liver involvement can be manifested as weight loss, fatigue, and abdominal pain. About one-fourth of patients with amyloidosis have hepatic disease. Clinical signs may include only mild hepatomegaly with elevation of the serum alkaline phosphatase level [96]. In the cardiovascular system, amyloid deposition is limited to the heart. In cases of unexplained heart failure, only small amounts of amyloid deposition are observed around the vascular walls. In contrast, in AL amyloidosis, massive cardiac involvement is invariably evident. In AL amyloidosis, intracardiac thrombosis and embolism are frequently observed in those with arterial fibrillation with cardiac amyloidosis [97]. For these patients, anticoagulation therapy should be considered for the protection of left ventricular dysfunction and atrial mechanical dysfunction [98]. Unlike the situation in AL amyloidosis, cardiac involvement in reactive AA amyloidosis is not so common, affecting only about 10% of patients, and clinically overt heart failure is usually present in the terminal phase of the disease course, in addition to ESKD [99]. Restrictive cardiomyopathy or ischemic heart disease is rarely the cause of death [100]. Hypertension is frequent, and hypotension is rare in such patients, except in those with ESKD. Optimal control of hypertension is necessary for these patients. Hypothyroidism due to amyloid deposition is sometimes observed [101]. In AA amyloidosis, involvement of the musculoskeletal system is rare. Usually, most of the symptoms are due to RA itself, and amyloid deposits do not elicit musculoskeletal symptoms. Central nervous system involvement is also unusual. Infiltration of subcutaneous fat is generally asymptomatic, but provides a convenient site for biopsy.

## 7. Management and treatment

Clinicians should remain vigilant for early signs of amyloidosis. For this purpose, patients with chronic rheumatic disorders, including those with elevated levels of inflammatory markers despite adequate symptom control by specific therapy, should undergo periodic urinalysis or assessments of 24-hour urinary protein excretion. If proteinuria exceeds 1(+) or increases to 0.5 g/day, screening for amyloidosis should be performed to search for amyloid deposits [43]. Occasionally, GI symptoms, such as alternating periods of constipation and diarrhea or bleeding, may suggest early localization of amyloid deposits and warrant further investigation. If possible, GI endoscopy is recommended, because of its diagnostic yield. If a positive biopsy result is obtained after Congo red staining, accurate immunohistochemical characterization of amyloid as the AA type is mandatory. Although isolated amyloid fibrils are stable *in vitro*, AA amyloid deposits exist in a state of dynamic turnover, which suggests that AA amyloidosis should not be regarded as an end-stage, irreversible process. Once

| Control SAA synthesis |
|---|
| 1) Tight control of disease activity of RA |
| a) DMARDs: MTX as the anchor drug |
| b) Immunosupressant: cyclophosphamide, azathiopurine, tacrolimus, MMF |
| c) Biologics: anti-TNF, anti-IL-6, rituximab, abatacept |
| d) Tofacitinib |
| e) Antifibril drug: eprosidate |
| Supportive treatment |
| 1) Cardiac |
| a) Congestive heart failure*: Salt restriction, Diuretics, antihypertensive agent |
| b) Arrhythmia: Pacemaker, Automatic implantable cardiac defibrillator, antiarrythmics |
| 2) Renal |
| a) Nephrotic syndrome: Salt restriction, Maintain dietary protein, ACE inhibiter, ARB |
| b) Renal failure: Dialysis (HD, CAPD): Programmed initiation** |
| 3) Gastrointestinal |
| a) Diarrhea: Steroid, codeine phosphate, lactate bacteria, octreotide, parenteral nutrition, anti-IL-6 |
| 4) Others |
| a) DMSO: resoluble amyloid deposits (very limited) |
| b) HB carrier : Etanercept with anti-viral agents is relatively safe. |
| *If co-existence of renal failure, CHDF (Continuous hemodiafiltration) is effective. |
| ** To avid the trouble for the HD initiation, programmed initiation is recommended. |

**Table 1.** Treatment for AA amyloidosis. SAA serum amyloid A protein, RA rheumatoid arthritis, DMARDs disease-modifying antirheumatic, Drugs, MTX methotrexate, MMF mycophenolate mofetil, TNF tumor necrosis factor, IL-6 interleukin-6, ACE angiotensin converting enzyme, ARB angiotensin receptor blocker, HD hemodialysis, CAPD continuous ambulatory peritoneal dialysis, DMSO dimethyl sulfoxide

amyloidosis has developed, the SAA concentration over the course of the disease represents the main factor affecting renal progression and survival [23,102]. A previous study has revealed a relationship between turnover and regression of amyloid deposits and the corresponding clinical benefit, in terms of both organ function and survival [23]. The natural history of AA amyloidosis is typically progressive, leading to organ failure and death, in patients whose underlying inflammatory disease remains active. By contrast, patients in whom the serum SAA concentration falls to within the reference range as a result of anti-inflammatory therapy show regression of amyloid deposits, stabilisation or recovery of amyloidotic organ function, and excellent long-term survival [103]. The therapeutic approach to AA involves treatment of the RA inflammatory process. It is important to control the level of SAA protein. It appears that reduction of the SAA level to less than 10 mg/L allows resorption of the deposits and prevents further accumulation [102]. Frequent monitoring of SAA, when available, is therefore recommended in patients with AA amyloidosis as a guide to treatment strategy and follow-up. Alternatively, quantification of CRP may provide a valid marker for monitoring the effective suppression of underlying inflammation in these patients. The therapeutic strategy is shown in Table 1. It may be assumed that tight control of RA with DMARDs such as methotrexate (MTX), or immunosuppressant such as cyclophosphamide, azathioprine, tacrolimus, mycophenolate mofetil, or their combinations would have a similar impact. A small retrospective study has indicated that cyclophosphamide may confer a significant survival benefit in patients with RA and renal AA amyloidosis [104]. In that study, six of 15 patients received monthly pulse cyclophosphamide following confirmation of renal involvement. These treated patients survived longer than those administered non-alkylating drugs. Trends toward decreased proteinuria and maintenance of renal function have also been noted in patients treated with cyclophosphamide. Similar results have been confirmed in a cohort study reported from Japan [105]. Prospective studies are required to properly assess the role and toxicity of this agent in this setting. If treatments for the organ damage, such as immunosuppressive agents or anti-cytokine therapy, are unavailable, medium-dose steroid (prednisolone 10~40 mg daily) is effective. Eprodisate is a glycosaminoglycan (GAG) mimetic that binds to the GAG binding site on serum amyloid A to prevent its interaction with GAG, thus arresting amyloidosis [100]. A recent report has indicated that eprodisate is a useful antifibril compound for treatment of AA amyloidosis, significantly delaying progression to HD or ESKD [107]. When considering supplementary treatment, cardiac amyloidosis is a major therapeutic problem. Loop diuretics are the main therapeutic agents for management of volume overload. However, many patients with cardiac amyloidosis have concomitant renal amyloidosis, making it difficult to maintain a balance between edema and intravascular contraction. Antihypertensive treatment is also important. Rheumatologists should be mindful of hypertension to maintain an optimal blood pressure in treated patients. With regard to renal impairment in patients with RA and amyloidosis, the serum creatinine (Cr) level is relatively low because of reduced muscle volume. Gender, long-lasting inflammation and RA, together with a low level of serum protein, may be associated with a decrease of muscle volume, and these in turn affect the level of serum Cr. This may partly explain why the serum Cr level is not elevated in comparison with creatinine clearance (Ccr) in patients with RA-associated amyloidosis [108]. Measurement of cystatin C and calculation of the estimated glomerular filtration rate (eGFR) are also useful [109]. Even if the serum Cr level is normal, such patients may still have renal damage. If patients are in a nephrotic state, angiotensin converting enzyme (ACE) inhibitor and/or angiotensin II receptor antagonist (ARB) are effective for reducing the level of urinary protein. For patients with renal failure, dialysis is needed. The prognosis of those who require dialysis is not good, although some data suggest a survival benefit among patients with AA amyloidosis [72]. The poor prognosis of these patients is due mainly to a large number of sudden deaths immediately after introduction of HD therapy [110,111]. Additionally, unplanned initiation of HD is significantly associated with poor survival. Therefore, properly planned initiation of HD is highly recommended. To circumvent the problem of HD initiation while ensuring its safety, the procedure for planned introduction is shown in Figure 4.

Programmed initiation of HD will improve the prognosis of patients with ESKD [112]. Continuous ambulatory peritoneal dialysis (CAPD) can also be considered for patients with ESKD, as it has an advantage in preserving the functionality of the kidneys and avoiding hypotension associated with HD. However, in RA patients, disability of the hands due to chronic inflammation, and also the risk of peritonitis, should be considered [113]. Kidney transplantation has been performed successfully for a number of patients with renal failure and AA amyloidosis, but only on a very limited basis [114]. In the near future, kidney transplantation may become a recommended therapy for such patients. For treatment of GI symptoms, mostly intractable diarrhea, medium- to high-dose steroid (prednisolone 10~40 mg daily) is effective. Parenteral nutrition is also effective for this condition. Immunosuppressive therapies may be associated with serious infection in patients with amyloidosis. Advanced age is an important risk factor for infection in patients with RA. Some of the increased risk may be related to steroid usage. Additionally, such patients generally show low protein levels or hypoalbuminemia. These factors may lead to serious infection and/or opportunistic infection. It is possible that infection may exacerbate elevation of the SAA level and lead to additional organ damage. Preventive therapy against infection should always be borne in mind. Dimethyl sulfoxide (DMSO) has been proposed as a therapeutic agent for solubilization of AA deposits, and a number of patients have been treated with DMSO in an uncontrolled trial. There appeared to be salutary effects in some patients, but the accompanying body odor made the treatment unacceptable [115]. Recently, treatment with DMSO has been very limited. Earlier diagnosis of amyloidosis leads to better treatment and an improved chance of recovery.

## 8. Treatment with biologics

Recent studies have indicated the therapeutic benefit of anti-TNF or anti-IL-6 agents for AA amyloidosis secondary to inflammatory arthritides, including RA [82,103, 116, 117,118,119]. These agents strongly inhibit the production of SAA. If possible, for the treatment of reabsorption of amyloid deposits, and, possibly, recovery of target organ function, treatment with biologics has been recommended. A recent report has indicated that etanercept was effective in a patient with cardiac amyloidosis associated with RA [119]. Biologics are known to be contraindicated for patients with heart failure [120], but may be effective if the heart failure is well controlled. The anti-IL-6 agent tocilizumab has an excellent inhibitory effect on disease activity and joint destruction, and is therapeutically beneficial for the symptoms of AA amyloidosis, especially intractable diarrhea [121]. Recently, we were revealed that treatment of these patients with biologic agents can reduce risk of death. In that study, a total of 133 patients were evaluated and 52 were treated with biologics such as the anti-TNF agents infliximab and etanercept, as well as tocilizumab, with a follow-up of more than 6 years (Figure 3). However, the use of biologics may not significantly influence the HD-free survival rate [13]. Although there are no data for the effect of abatacept on AA amyloidosis, it may be effective in theory. Janus kinase inhibitor also appears to be favorable for the treatment of AA amyloidosis associated with RA [122]. Rituximab therapy also appears effective for reduction of acute-phase protein and stabilization of kidney function and proteinuria in patients with RA-associated amyloidosis [123]. The use of biologics is not part of the conventional treatment approach, and they are chosen according to the conditions in individual patients, such as kidney and pulmonary function. If there is any risk of infection, short-acting biologics are desirable. Especially, in patients receiving tocilizumab, infection may be difficult to find, and rheumatologists therefore need to be vigilant. Treatment with biologic agents is prohibited in certain circumstances, such as severe infections or demyelinating diseases. The treatment of patients with coexisting RA and hepatitis B poses a difficult therapeutic challenge because of the risk that treatment of the RA could aggravate the hepatic disease and increase viremia. In general, the use of biologics such as anti-TNF and anti-IL-6 is contraindicated in patients who are hepatitis B virus (HBV) carriers or have chronic hepatitis B. Reactivation of HBV infection is a well-recognized complication in cancer patients with chronic HBV (hepatitis B surface antigen [HBsAg]-positive) undergoing cytotoxic chemotherapy, and prophylactic antiviral therapy before chemotherapy is recommended in such individuals. Additionally, HBV reactivation in patients with resolved HBV infection (HBsAg-negative and HBs antibody [anti-HBs]-positive and/or hepatitis B core antibody [anti-HBc]-positive) during or after cytotoxic therapy has recently been reported [124,125]. Rheumatologists also need to pay attention to HBV reactivation. However, in clinical practice, it is necessary to use anti-TNF in these patients. The existing data suggest that treatment of such patients with etanercept and tocilizmab co-administered with lamivudine or entecavir is safe [126,127].

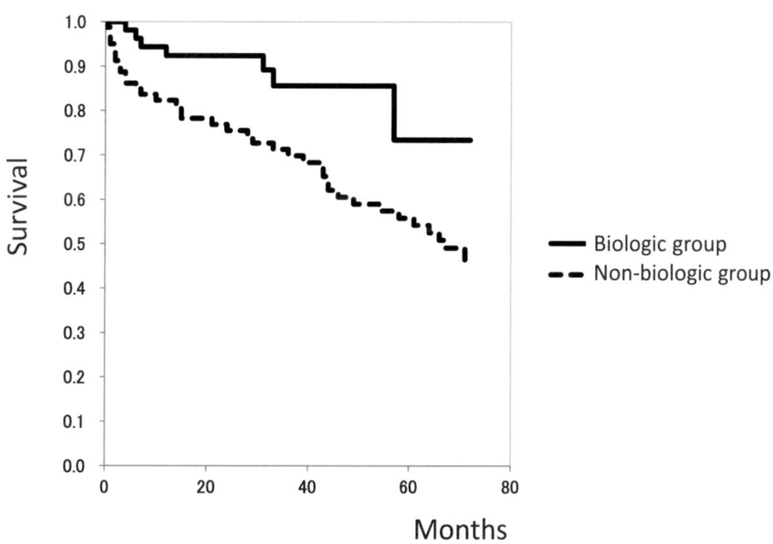


**Figure 3. Survival of patients receiving biologic or non-biologic therapy.** Fifty-three patients were treated with biologic agents (biologic group) and 80 patients were not (non-biologic group). Survival of patients with and without biologics treatment was assessed using the Kaplan-Meier method. Survival was significantly higher in the biologic group than in the non-biologic group (p=0.012).

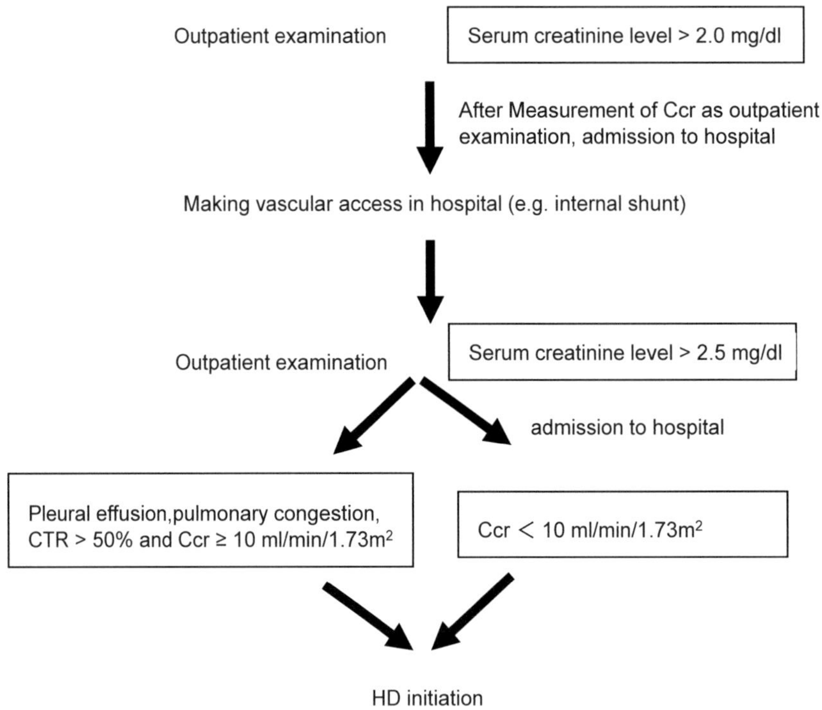


**Figure 4. Program for initiation of hemodialysis.** Schematic representation of the program used for our patients with end-stage kidney disease due to reactive amyloidosis associated with rheumatoid arthritis. Ccr: creatinine clearance, CTR: cardiothoracic ratio

## 9. Outcome

Survival after the diagnosis of AA amyloidosis secondary to RA seems to be 4–5 years [110,128]. Recently, however, a median survival period of more than 10 years after diagnosis has been reported [23]. Survival seems to depend on the timing of diagnosis, and this may partly explain the great individual variation in observed survival time, leading to the notion that an active diagnostic attitude for AA amyloidosis should be adopted in patients with RA. Treatment strategy is also important. Infection and renal failure are generally common causes of death in RA patients with AA amyloidosis [129,130]. A higher risk of severe infection is a substantial problem in the management of such patients. Potent immunosuppressive treatment may sometimes result in infection, and in such cases, prophylactic treatment with an antituberculosis agent is recommended. As for P. jirovecii pneumonia (PCP),prophylactic treatment is less common except for outbrake of PCP [131]. Increased production of SAA is a strong risk factor for ESKD and death, but this may be ameliorated by anti-inflammatory treatment. A relationship between SAA concentration, kidney function and whole-body amyloid burden has been revealed. Outcome has been shown to be favorable in

http://dx.doi.org/10.5772/54332

patients with AA amyloidosis when the SAA concentration is maintained below 10 mg/L [23]. Additionally, the use of biologics is expected improve the prognosis for these patients [13]. Factors associated with poor prognosis are well known to include age at onset of RA and amyloidosis, female gender, a reduced serum albumin concentration, ESKD, the level of disease activity including serum levels of CRP and IgG, and the SAA concentration during follow-up [130]. Steroid dosage, and markers of kidney function that are correlated with kidney disease, such as BUN, Cr, and Ccr, at the time of detection of amyloidosis are also important factors predictive of survival [110]. The results of dialysis for AA amyloidosis are extremely poor, and trouble with the initiation of HD in fact worsens the prognosis, due to a rapid decline of kidney function in the year preceding dialysis. Reported median survival after initiation of HD is more than 1 year [132], or more than 5 years [133]. These reports indicate that strict treatment and care will improve the clinical outcome. It is possible that the use of biologics may improve the HD-free survival rate, but accumulation of further cases is required. Amyloidotic cardiac involvement has been shown to be a poor prognostic factor [134,135]. Heart failure is a severe complication in these patients, who also usually develop concomitant multiple organ failure, as well as renal failure, in the later phase of the RA disease course. To improve the outcome of these patients, frequent examinations for infection and acute inflammatory reactants such as CRP and SAA are necessary.

## 10. Conclusion

The best approach to treatment of amyloidosis is to prevent progression by controlling the serum level of SAA. In AA amyloidosis, proteinurea, renal dysfunction and GI symptoms are diagnostically informative. It is important not to overlook these symptoms, and to confirm the presence of amyloidosis by organ biopsy. Treatment with biologic agents plays a key role, especially for decreasing the production of SAA, along with prophylactic administration of anti-tuberculosis and anti-fungal agents. Monitoring of adverse events such as infection is an important part of the standard strategy associated with biologics treatment, and checks for chronic inflammatory disorders should be conducted routinely. Rheumatologists should carefully consider the use of biologics in patients with difficult background conditions such as hepatitis B. Such efforts should help to improve the outcome of patients with AA amyloidosis, achieve stabilization or regression of amyloid deposits, and prolong survival.

## Acknowledgements

This work was supported in part by a Grant-in-Aid for scientific research from the Japanese Ministry of Health, Labor, and Welfare. The authors thank Professor Shinichi Nishi, M.D., Kobe University, for the photographs of renal tissue.

## Author details

Takeshi Kuroda[1], Yoko Wada[1] and Masaaki Nakano[2]

1 Division of Clinical Nephrology and Rheumatology, Niigata University Graduate School of Medical and Dental Sciences, Chuo-ku, Niigata City, Japan

2 Department of Medical Technology, School of Health Sciences, Faculty of Medicine, Niigata University, Chuo-ku, Niigata City, Japan

## References

[1] Mueller OS. Amyloidosis. Current rheumatology diagnosis & treatment. 2nd ed. USA: Mc Graw Hill; 2007.

[2] Kyle RA. Amyloidosis: a convoluted story. Br. J Haematol. 2001; 114(3) 529-538.

[3] Sipe JD, Benson MD, Buxbaum JN, Ikeda S, Merlini G, Saraiva MJ, Westermark P. Amyloid fibril protein nomenclature: 2010 recommendations from the nomenclature committee of the International Society of Amyloidosis. Amyloid. 2010; 17(3-4) 101-104.

[4] Missen GA, Taylor JD. Amyloidosis in rheumatoid arthritis. J pathol Bact. 1956;71(1) 179-192.

[5] Scheinberg MA, Hubscher O, Morteo OG, Benson MD. Serum amyloid protein levels in south american children with rheumatoid arthritis: a co-operative study. Ann Rheum Dis.1980;39(3) 228–230.

[6] van Eijk IC, de Vries MK, Levels JH, Peters MJ, Huizer EE, Dijkmans BA, van der Horst-Bruinsma IE, Hazenberg BP, van de Stadt RJ, Wolbink GJ, Nurmohamed MT. Improvement of lipid profile is accompanied by atheroprotective alterations in high-density lipoprotein composition upon tumor necrosis factor blockade: a prospective cohort study in ankylosing spondylitis. Arthritis Rheum. 2009;60(5) 1324-1330.

[7] Greenstein AJ, Sachar DB, Panday AK, Dikman SH, Meyers S, Heimann T, Gumaste V, Werther JL, Janowitz HD. Amyloidosis and inflammatory bowel disease. A 50-year experience with 25 patients. Medicine (Baltimore). 1992;71(5) 261-270.

[8] Ensari C, Ensari A, Tümer, Ertug E. Clinicopathological and epidemiological analysis of amyloidosis in Turkish patients. Nephrol Dial Transplant. 2005;20(8) 1721-1725.

[9] Pras M, Franklin EC, Shibolet S, Frangione B. Amyloidosis associated with renal cell carcinoma of the AA type. Am J Med. 1982;73(3) 426-428.

[10] Piskin O, Alacacioglu I, Ozkal S, Ozcan MA, Demirkan F, Hayri Ozsan G, Kargi A, Undar B. A patient with diffuse large B-cell non-Hodgkin's lymphoma and AA type amyloidosis. J BUON. 2008;13(1) 113-116.

[11] Ogita, M, Hoshino, J, Sogawa, Y, Sawa N, Katori H, Takemoto F, Ubara Y, Hara S, Miyakoshi S, Takaichi K. Multicentric Castleman disease with secondary AA renal amyloidosis, nephrotic syndrome and chronic renal failure, remission after high-dose melphalan and autologous stem cell transplantation. Clin Nephrol. 2007; 68(3) 171-176.

[12] Skinner, M, Pinnette, A, Travis, WD, Shwachman H, Cohen AS. Isolation and sequence analysis of amyloid protein AA from a patient with cystic fibrosis. J Lab Clin Med. 1988;112(4) 413-417.

[13] Kuroda T, Tanabe N, Kobayashi D, Sato H, Wada Y, Murakami S, Saeki T, Nakano M, Narita I. Treatment with biologic agents improves the prognosis of patients with rheumatoid arthritis and amyloidosis. J Rheumatol. 2012;39(7):1348-1354.

[14] Simms RW, Prout MN, Cohen AS. The epidemiology of AL and AA amyloidosis. Baillieres Clin Rheumatol 1994; 8(3) 627–634.

[15] Hazenberg BP, Van Rijswijk MH. Where has secondary amyloid gone? Ann Rheum Dis. 2000; 59(8) 577–579.

[16] Lender M, Wolf E. Incidence of amyloidosis in rheumatoid arthritis. Scand J Rheumatol. 1972;1(3) 109-112.

[17] Koivuniemi R, Paimela L, Suomalinen R, Tornroth T, Leirisalo-Repo M. Amyloidosis is frequently undetected in patients with rheumatoid arthritis. Amyloid. 2008;15(4) 262–268.

[18] Toyoshima H, Kusaba T, Yamaguchi M. Cause of death in autopsied RA patients. Rheumachi. 1993;33(3) 209-214.

[19] Kobayashi H, Tada S, Fuchigami T, Okuda Y, Takasugi K, Matsumoto T, Iida M, Aoyagi K, Iwashita A, Daimaru Y, Fujishima M. Secondary amyloidosis in patients with rheumatoid arthritis: diagnostic and prognostic value of gastroduodenal biopsy. Br J Rheumatol. 1996;35(1) 44–49.

[20] Kuroda T, Tanabe N, Sakatsume M, Nozawa S, Mitsuka T, Ishikawa H, Tohyama CT, Nakazono K, Murasawa A, Nakano M, Gejyo F. Comparison of gastroduodenal, renal and abdominal fat biopsies for diagnosing amyloidosis in rheumatoid arthritis. Clin Rheumatol. 2002;21(2) 123–128.

[21] Wakhlu A, Krisnani N, Hissatia P, Aggarwal A, Misra R. Prevalence of secondary amyloidosis in Asian north Indian patients with rheumatoid arthritis. J Rheumatol. 2003;30(5) 948–951.

[22] Okuda Y, Takasugi K. Diagnostic and prognostic study of secondary amyloidosis complication rheumatoid arthritis. Amyloid and Amyloidosis. Parthenon Publishing Group. New York. 1998.

[23] Lachmann HJ, Goodman HJ, Gilbertson JA, Gallimore JR, Sabin CA, Gillmore JD, Hawkins PN. Natural history and outcome in systemic AA amyloidosis. N Engl J Med. 2007;356(23) 2361-2371.

[24] Bolloti V, Mangione P, Merline G. Immunoglobulin light chain amyloidosis the archtype of structural and pathologic variability. J Struct Biol. 2000;130(2-3) 280-289.

[25] Lansbury PT. Evolition of amyloid:What normal protein foldint may tell us about fibrinogenesis and disease. Proc Natl Acad Sci USA. 1999;96(7) 3342-3344.

[26] Westermark GT, Westermark P. Serum amyloid A and protein AA: molecular mechanisms of a transmissible amyloidosis. FEBS Letter. 2009;583(16) 2685-2690.

[27] Yoshida T, Zhang P, Fu X, Higuchi K, Ikeda S. Slaughtered aged cattle might be one dietary source exhibiting amyloid enhancing factor activity. Amyloid. 2009;16(1) 25-31.

[28] Röcken C, Menard R, Bühling F, Vöckler S, Raynes J, Stix B, Krüger S, Roessner A, Kähne T. Proteolysis of serum amyloid A and AA amyloid proteins by cysteine proteases: cathepsin B generates AA amyloid proteins and cathepsin L may prevent their formation. Ann Rheum Dis. 2005;64(6) 808-815.

[29] Cunnane G. Amyloid precursors and amyloidosis in inflammatory arthritis. Curr Opin Rheumatol. 2001;13(1) 67–73.

[30] Malle E, Steinmetz A, Raynes JG. Serum amyloid A (SAA): an acute phase protein and apolipoprotein. Atherosclerosis. 1993;102(2) 131–146.

[31] Uhlar CM, Whitehead AS. Serum amyloid A, the major vertebrate acute-phase reactant. Eur J Biochem. 1999;265(2) 501–523.

[32] Gallo G, Wisniewski T, Choi-Miura NH, Ghiso J, Frangione B. Potential role of apolipoprotein-E in fibrillogenesis. Am J Pathol. 1994;145(3) 526–530.

[33] Marhaug G, Husby G. Serum amyloid A protein in high density lipoprotein fraction of human acute phase serum. Lancet. 1982;2(8313) 1463.

[34] Kelly JW. Alternative conformations of amyloidogenic proteins govern their behavior. Curr Opin Struct Biol. 1996; 6(1) 11-17.

[35] Dobson CM. Protein folding and disease: a view from the first Horizon Symposium. Nat Rev Drug Discov. 2003:2(2) 154-160.

[36] Vallon R, Freuler F, Desta-Tsedu N, Robeva A, Dawson J, Wenner P, Engelhardt P, Boes L, Schnyder J, Tschopp C, Urfer R, Baumann G. Serum amyloid A (apoSAA) expression is up-regulated in rheumatoid arthritis and induces transcription of matrix metalloproteinases. J Immunol. 2001;166(4) 2801-2807.

[37] Ray A, Schatten H, Ray BK. Activation of Sp1 and its functional co-operation with serum amyloid A-activating sequence binding factor in synoviocyte cells trigger synergistic action of interleukin-1 and interleukin-6 in serum amyloid A gene expression. J Biol Chem. 1999;274(7) 4300-4308.

[38] O'Hara, R, Murphy, EP, Whitehead, AS, FitzGerald O, Bresnihan B. Local expression of the serum amyloid A and formyl peptide receptor-like 1 genes in synovial tissue is associated with matrix metalloproteinase production in patients with inflammatory arthritis. Arthritis Rheum. 2004; 50(6) 1788-1799.

[39] Thorn, CF, Lu, ZY, Whitehead, AS. Regulation of the human acute phase serum amyloid A genes by tumour necrosis factor-alpha, interleukin-6 and glucocorticoids in hepatic and epithelial cell lines. Scand J Immunol. 2004;59(2) 152-158.

[40] Ray, A, Shakya, A, Kumar, D, Benson MD, Ray BK. Inflammation-responsive transcription factor SAF-1 activity is linked to the development of amyloid A amyloidosis. J Immunol. 2006; 177(4) 2601-2609.

[41] Thorn CF, Whitehead AS. Differential glucocorticoid enhancement of the cytokine-driven transcriptional activation of the human acute phase serum amyloid A genes, SAA1 and SAA2. J Immunol. 2002;169(1) 399-406.

[42] Nakamura T, Higashi S, Tomoda K, Tsukano M, Baba S, Shono M. Significance of SAA1.3 allele genotype in Japanese patients with amyloidosis secondary to rheumatoid arthritis. Rheumatology (Oxford). 2006;45(1) 43-49.

[43] Obici, L, Raimondi, S, Lavatelli, F, Bellotti V, Merlini G. Susceptibility to AA amyloidosis in rheumatic diseases: a critical overview. Arthritis Rheum. 2009; 61(10) 1435-1440.

[44] Baba S, Takahashi T, Kasama T, Fujie M, Shirasawa H. Identification of two novel amyloid A protein subsets coexisting in an individual patient of AA-amyloidosis. Biochim Biophys Acta. 1992;1180(2) 195–200.

[45] Baba S, Takahashi T, Kasama T, Shirasawa H. A novel polymorphism of human serum amyloid A protein, SAA1 gamma, is characterized by alanines at both residues 52 and 57. Arch Biochem Biophys. 1993;303(2) 361–366.

[46] Xu Y, Yamada T, Satoh T, Okuda Y.. Measurement of serum amyloid A1 (SAA1), a major isotype of acute phase SAA. Clin hem Lab Med. 2006;44(1) 59–63.

[47] Moriguchi M, Terai C, Koseki Y, Uesato M, Nakajima A, Inada S, Nishinarita M, Uchida S, Nakajima A, Kim SY, Chen CL, Kamatani N. Influence of genotypes at SAA1 and SAA2 loci on the development and the length of latent period of secondary AA-amyloidosis in patients with rheumatoid arthritis. Hum Genet. 1999;105(4) 360–366.

[48] Utku U, Dilek M, Akpolat I, Bedir A, Akpolat T. SAA1 alpha/alpha alleles in Behcet's disease related amyloidosis. Clin Rheumatol. 2007;26(6) 927–929.

[49] Yamada T, Okuda Y, Takasugi K, Wang L, Marks D, Benson MD, Kluve-Beckerman B. An allele of serum amyloid A1 associated with amyloidosis in both Japanese and Caucasians. Amyloid. 2003;10(1) 7–11.

[50] Nakamura T. Amyloid A amyloidosis secondary to rheumatoid arthritis: an uncommon yet important complication. Curr Rheumatol Rev. 2007;3(3) 231–241.

[51] Baba S, Masago SA, Takahashi T, Kasama T, Sugimura H, Tsugane S, Tsutsui Y, Shirasawa H. A novel allelic variant of serum amyloid A, SAA1gamma: genomic evidence, evolution, frequency, and implication as a risk factor for reactive systemic AA-amyloidosis. Hum Mol Genet. 1995;4(6) 1083–1087.

[52] Moriguchi M, Kaneko H, Terai C, Koseki Y, Kajiyama H, Inada S, Kitamura Y, Kamatani N. Relative transcriptional activities of SAA1 promoters polymorphic at position -13T(T/C): potential association between increased transcription and amyloidosis. Amyloid. 2005;12(1) 26–32.

[53] Ajiro J, Narita I, Sato F, Saga D, Hasegawa H, Kuroda T, Nakano M, Gejyo F. SAA1 gene polymorphisms and the risk of AA amyloidosis on Japanese patients with rheumatoid arthritis. Mod Rheumatol. 2006;16(5) 294–299.

[54] Hasegawa H, Nishi S, Ito S, Saeki T, Kuroda T, Kimura H, Watababe T, Nakano M, Gejyo F, Arakawa M. High prevalence of serum apolipoprotein E4 isoprotein in rheumatoid arthritis patients with amyloidosis. Arthritis Rheum. 1996;39(10) 1728–1732.

[55] Coker AR, Purvis A, Baker D, Pepys MB, Wood SP. Molecular chaperone properties of serum amyloid P component. FEBS Letter. 2000;473(2) 199–202.

[56] Okuda Y, Yamada T, Matsuura M, Takasugi K, Goto M. Ageing: a risk factor for amyloid A amyloidosis in rheumatoid arthritis. Amyloid. 2011;18(3) 108-111.

[57] Elghetany MT, Saleem A, Barr K. The Congo red stain revisited. Ann Clin Lab Sci. 1989;19(3) 190–195.

[58] Puchtler H, Waldrop FS, Meloan SN. A review of light, polarization and fluorescence microscopic methods for amyloid. Appl Pathol. 1985;3(1-2) 5–17.

[59] Shirahama T, Cohen AS. High-resolution electron microscopic analysis of the amyloid fibril. J Cell Biol. 1967;33(3) 679–708.

[60] Sipe JD, McAdam KP, Torain BF, Glenner GG. Conformational flexibility of the serum amyloid precursor SAA. Br J Exp Pathol. 1976;57(5) 582-592.

[61] Gomez-Casanovas E, Sanmarti R, Sole M, Cañete JD, Muñoz-Gómez J. The clinical significance of amyloid fat deposit in rheumatoid arthritis. A systemic long-term follow up study using abdominal fat aspiration. Arthritis Rheum. 2001;44(1) 66–72.

[62] Hachulla E, Janin A, Flipo RM, Saïle R, Facon T, Bataille D, Vanhille P, Hatron PY, Devulder B, Duquesnoy B. Labial salivary gland biopsy is a reliable test for the diag-

nosis of primary and secondary amyloidosis. A prospective clinical and immunohistologic study in 59 patients. Arthritis Rheum. 1993;36(5) 691-697.

[63] Tada S, Iida M, Iwashita A, Matsui T, Fuchigami T, Yamamoto T, Yao T, Fujishima M. Endoscopic and biopsy findings of the upper digestive tract in patients with amyloidosis. Gastrointest Endosc. 1990;36(1) 10-14.

[64] Falk RH, Comenzo RL, Skinner M. The systemic amyloidoses. N Engl J Med. 1997;337(13) 898-909.

[65] Rocken C, Shakespeare A. Pathology, diagnosis and pathogenesis of AA amyloidosis. Virchows Arch. 2002;440(2) 111-122.

[66] Murakami T, Yi S. Amyloidosis and hepatic amyloidosis. Nippon Rinsho. 1993;51(2) 453- 457.

[67] Libbey CA, Skinner M, Cohen AS. Use of abdominal fat tissue aspirate in the diagnosis. Arch Intern Med 1983;143(8) 1549-1552.

[68] Dubrey SW, Cha K, Simms RW, Skinner M, Falk RH. Electrocardiography and Doppler echocardiography in secondary (AA) amyloidosis. Am J Cardiol. 1996;77(4) 313-315.

[69] Mcalpine JC, Bancroft JD. A histological study of hyaline deposits in laryngeal, aural, and nasal polyps and their differentiation from amyloid. J Clin Pathol. 1964;17:213–219.

[70] Takahashi T, Miura H, Matsu-ura Y, Iwana S, Maruyama R, Harada T. Urine cytology of localized primary amyloidosis of the ureter: a case report. Acta Cytol. 2005;49(3) 319–322.

[71] Iijima S. Primary systemic amyloidosis: a unique case complaining of diffuse eyelid swelling and conjunctival involvement. J Dermatol. 1992;19(2) 113–118.

[72] Getz MA, Kyle RA. Secondary systemic amyloidosis. Response and survival in 64 patients. Medicine (Baltimore). 1991;70(4) 246-256.

[73] Klem PJ, Sorsa S, Happonen RP. Fine-needle aspiration biopsy from subcutaneous fat: an easy way to diagnose secondary amyloidosis. Scand J Rheumatol. 1987;16(6) 429- 431.

[74] Bogov B, Lubomirova M, and Kiperova B. Biopsy of subcutaneus fatty tissue for diagnosis of systemic amyloidosis. Hippokratia. 2008;12(4) 236–239.

[75] Kuroda T, Tanabe N, Kobayashi D, Sato H, Wada Y, Murakami S, Nakano M, Narita I. Association between clinical parameters and amyloid-positive area in gastroduodenal biopsy in reactive amyloidosis associated with rheumatoid arthritis. Rheumatol Int. 2012;32(4):933-939.

[76] Stiles KP, Yuan CM, Chung EM, Lyon RD, Lane JD, Abbott KC. Renal biopsy in high-risk patients with medical diseases of the kidney. Am J Kidney Dis. 2000;36(2) 419–433.

[77] Stiller D, Katenkamp D, Thoss K. Staining mechanism of thioflavin T with special reference to the localization of amyloid. Acta Histochem. 1972;42(2) 234–245.

[78] Nebut M, Hartmann L. Contribution of thioflavin T in the study of the early histologic lesions of experimental amyloidosis. Ann Biol Clin. 1966;24:1063–1079.

[79] Rogers DR. Screening for amyloid with the thioflavin-T fluorescent method. Am J Clin Pathol. 1965;44:59–61.

[80] Hazenberg BP, van Rijswijk MH, Piers DA, Lub-de Hooge MN, Vellenga E, Haagsma EB, Hawkins PN, Jager PL. Diagnostic performance of 123I- labeled serum amyloid P component scintigraphy in patients with amyloidosis. Am J Med. 2006;119(4) 355.e15-24.

[81] Kuroda T, Tanabe N, Kobayashi D, Wada Y, Murakami S, Nakano M, Narita I. Significant association between renal function and area of amyloid deposition in kidney biopsy specimens in reactive amyloidosis associated with rheumatoid arthritis. Rheumatol Int. 2012;32(10) 3155-3162

[82] Kuroda T, Wada Y, Kobayashi D, Murakami S, Sakai T, Hirose S, Tanabe N, Saeki T, Nakano M, Narita I. Effective anti-TNF-a therapy can induce rapid resolution and sustained decrease of gastroduodenal mucosal amyloid deposits in reactive amyloidosis associated with rheumatoid arthritis. J Rheumatol. 2009;36(11) 2409-2415.

[83] Yamada T, Okuda Y. AA amyloid quantification in biopsy samples from the stomach Ann Clin Labo Sci. 2012;42(1) 301-304.

[84] Hazenberg BP, Bijzet J, Limburg PC, Skinner M, Hawkins PN, Butrimiene I, Livneh A, Lesnyak O, Nasonov EL, Filipowicz-Sosnowska A, Gül A, Merlini G, Wiland P, Ozdogan H, Gorevic PD, Maïz HB, Benson MD, Direskeneli H, Kaarela K, Garceau D, Hauck W, Van Rijswijk MH. Diagnostic performance of amyloid A protein quantification in fat tissue of patients with clinical AA amyloidosis. Amyloid J Prot Fold Dis 2007; 14(1) 133-140.

[85] Kuroda T, Tanabe N, Harada T, Murakami S, Hasegawa H, Sakatsume M, Nakano M, Gejyo F. Long-term mortality outcome in patients with reactive amyloidosis associated with rheumatoid arthritis. Clin Rheumatol. 2006;25(4) 498-505.

[86] van Gameren II, Hazenberg BP, Bijzet J, Haagsma EB, Vellenga E, Posthumus MD, Jager PL, van Rijswijk MH. Amyloid load in fat tissue reflects disease severity and predicts survival in amyloidosis. Arthritis Care Res (Hoboken). 2010;62(3):296-301.

[87] Nakano M, Ueno M, Nishi S, Shimada H, Hasegawa H, Watanabe T, Kuroda T, Sato T, Maruyama Y, Arakawa M. Analysis of renal pathology and drug history in 158 Japanese patients with rheumatoid arthritis. Clin Nephrol. 1998;50(3) 154–160.

[88] Nagata M, Shimokama T, Harada A, Koyama A, Watanabe T. Glomerular crescents in renal amyloidosis: an epiphenomenon or distinct pathology? Pathol Int. 2001;51(3) 179-186.

[89] Nishi S, Alchi B, Imai N, Gejyo F. New advances in renal amyloidosis. Clin Exp Nephrol. 2008;12(2) 93–101.

[90] Falck HM, Törnroth T, Wegelius O. Predominantly vascular amyloid deposition in the kidney in patients with minimal or no proteinuria. Clin Nephrol. 1983; 19(3) 137-142.

[91] Uda H, Yokota A, Kobayashi K, Miyake T, Fushimi H, Maeda A, Saiki O. Two distinct clinical courses of renal involvement in rheumatoid patients with AA amyloidosis. J Rheumatol. 2006; 33(8) 1482-1487.

[92] Sen S, Sarsik B. A proposed histopathologic classification, scoring, and grading system for renal amyloidosis: standardization of renal amyloid biopsy report. Arch Pathol Lab Med. 2010;134(4):532-544.

[93] Ebert EC, Nagar M. Gastrointestinal manifestations of amyloidosis. Am J Gastroenterol. 2008;103(3) 776-787.

[94] Tada S, Iida M, Yao T, Kawakubo K, Yao T, Okada M, Fujishima M. Endoscopic features in amyloidosis of the small intestine: clinical and morphologic differences between chemical types of amyloid protein. Gastrointest Endosc. 1994;40(1) 45-50.

[95] Kuroda T, Sato H, Hasegawa H, Wada Y, Murakami S, Saeki T, Nakano M, Narita I. Fatal acute pancreatitis associated with reactive AA amyloidosis in rheumatoid arthritis with end-stage renal disease: a report of three cases. Intern Med. 2011;50(7) 739-744.

[96] Ebert EC, Hagspiel KD. Gastrointestinal and hepatic manifestations of rheumatoid arthritis. Dig Dis Sci. 2011;56(2) 295–302.

[97] Feng D, Edwards W, Oh J, Chandrasekaran K, Grogan M, Martinez M, Syed I, Hughes D, Lust J, Jaffe A, Gertz M, Klarich K. Intracardiac Thrombosis and embolism in patients with cardiac amyloidosis Circulation. 2007 ;116(21) 2420-2426.

[98] Feng D, Syed I, Martinez M, Oh J, Jaffe A, Grogan M, Edwards W, Gertz M, Klarich K. Intracardiac thrombosis and anticoagulation therapy in cardiac amyloidosis Circulation. 2009 ;119(18) 2490-2497.

[99] Hazenberg BP, van Rijswijk MH. Clinical and therapeutic aspects of AA amyloidosis. Bailliere's Clin Rheumatol. 1994; 8(3) 661-690.

[100] Lachmann HJ, Goodman HJB, Gallimore J et al. Characteristic and clinical outcome on 340 patients with systemic AA amyloidosis. In Grateau G, Kyle RA, Skinner M (eds) Amyloid and Amyloidosis:10th International Symposium on Amyloidosis. Tours, France, 2004,173–175.

[101] Kanoh T, Shimada H, Uchino H, Matsumura K. Amyloid goiter with hypothyroidism. Arch Pathol Lab Med. 1989;113(5) 542-544.

[102] Gillmore JD, Lovat LB, Persey MR, Pepys MB, Hawkins PN. Amyloid load and clinical outcome in AA amyloidosis in relation to circulating concentration of serum amyloid A protein. Lancet. 2001;358(9275) 24-29.

[103] Gottenberg JE, Merle-Vincent F, Bentaberry F, Allanore Y, Berenbaum F, Fautrel B, Combe B, Durbach A, Sibilia J, Dougados M, Mariette X. Anti-tumor necrosis factor alpha therapy in fifteen patients with AA amyloidosis secondary to inflammatory arthritides: a followup report of tolerability and efficacy. Arthritis Rheum. 2003;48(7) 2019-2024.

[104] Chevrel G, Jenvrin C, McGregor B, Miossec P. Renal type AA amyloidosis associated with rheumatoid arthritis: a cohort study showing improved survival on treatment with pulse cyclophosphamide. Rheumatology (Oxford). 2001; 40(7) 821-825.

[105] Nakamura T, Yamamura Y, Tomoda K, Tsukano M, Shono M, Baba S. Efficacy of cyclophosphamide combined with prednisolone in patients with AA amyloidosis secondary to rheumatoid arthritis. Clin Rheumatol 2003; 22(6) 371-375.

[106] Kisilevsky R, Lemieux LJ, Fraser PE, Kong X, Hultin PG, Szarek WA. Arresting amyloidosis in vivo using small-molecule anionic sulphonates or sulphates: implications for Alzheimer's disease. Nat Med. 1995;1(2) 143-148.

[107] Dember LM, Hawkins PN, Hazenberg BP, Gorevic PD, Merlini G, Butrimiene I, Livneh A, Lesnyak O, Puéchal X, Lachmann HJ, Obici L, Balshaw R, Garceau D, Hauck W, Skinner M; Eprodisate for AA Amyloidosis Trial Group. Eprodisate for the treatment of renal disease in AA amyloidosis. N Engl J Med. 2007;356(23) 2349–2360.

[108] Moriguchi M, Terai C, Koseki Y, Uesato M, Kamatani M. Renal function estimated from serum creatinine is overestimated in patients with rheumatoid arthritis because of their muscle atrophy. Mod Rheumatol. 2000;10:230–234.

[109] Sato H, Kuroda T, Tanabe N, jiro J, Wada Y, Murakami S, Sakatsume M, Nakano M, Gejyo F. Cystatin C is a sensitive marker for detecting a reduced glomerular filtration rate when assessing chronic kidney disease in patients with rheumatoid arthritis and secondary amyloidosis. Scand J Rheumatol. 2010;39(1) 33-37.

[110] Kuroda T, Tanabe N, Sato H, Ajiro J, Wada Y, Murakami S, Hasegawa H, Sakatsume M, Nakano M, Gejyo F. Outcome of patients with reactive amyloidosis associated with rheumatoid arthritis in dialysis treatment. Rheumatol Int 2006;26(12) 1147–1153.

[111] Hezemans RL, Krediet RT, Arisz L. Dialysis treatment in patients with rheumatoid arthritis. Neth J Med.1995;47(1) 6-11.

[112] Kuroda T, Tanabe N, Kobayashi D, Sato H, Wada Y, Murakami S, Sakatsume M, Nakano M, Narita I. Programmed initiation of hemodialysis for systemic amyloidosis patients associated with rheumatoid arthritis. Rheumatol Int. 2011;31(9) 1177-82.

[113] Martinez-Vea A, García C, Carreras M, Revert L, Oliver JA. End-stage renal disease in systemic amyloidosis: clinical course and outcome on dialysis. Am J Nephrol. 1990;10(4) 283-289.

[114] Heering P, Hetzel R, Grabensee B, Opelz G. Renal transplantation in secondary systemic amyloidosis. Clin Transplant. 1998;12(3) 159-164.

[115] van Rijswijk MH, Ruinen L, Donker AJ, de Blécourt JJ, Mandema E. Dimethyl sulfoxide in the treatment of AA amyloidosis. Ann N Y Acad Sci. 1983;411:67-83.

[116] Okuda Y, Takasugi K. Successful use of a humanized anti-interleukin-6 antibody, tocilizumab, to treat amyloid A amyloidosis complicating juvenile idiopathic arthritis. Arthritis Rheum. 2006;54(9) 2997–3000.

[117] Kuroda T, Otaki Y, Sato H, Fujimura T, Nakatsue T, Murakami S, Sakatsume M, Nakano M, Gejyo F. Improvement of renal function and gastrointestinal amyloidosis treated with Infliximab in a patient with AA amyloidosis associated with rheumatoid arthritis. Rheumatol Int. 2008;28(11) 1155-1159.

[118] Nakamura T, Higashi S, Tomoda K, Tsukano M, Shono M. Etanercept can induce resolution of renal deterioration in patients with amyloid A amyloidosis secondary to rheumatoid arthritis. Clin Rheumatol. 2010 ;29(12) 1395-1401.

[119] Wada Y, Kobayashi D, Murakami S, Oda M, Hanawa H, Kuroda T, Nakano M, Narita I. Cardiac AA amyloidosis in a patient with rheumatoid arthritis and systemic sclerosis – the therapeutic potential of biologic reagents. Letter. Scand J Rheumatol. 2011;40(5) 402-404.

[120] Mann DL, McMurray JJ, Packer M, Swedberg K, Borer JS, Colucci WS, Djian J, Drexler H, Feldman A, Kober L, Krum H, Liu P, Nieminen M, Tavazzi L, van Veldhuisen DJ, Waldenstrom A, Warren M, Westheim A, Zannad F, Fleming T. Targeted anticytokine therapy in patients with chronic heart failure: results of the Randomized Etanercept Worldwide Evaluation (RENEWAL). Circulation. 2004;109(13) 1594-1602.

[121] Sato H, Sakai T, Sugaya T, Otaki Y, Aoki K, Ishii K, Horizono H, Otani H, Abe A, Yamada N, Ishikawa H, Nakazono K, Murasawa A, Gejyo F. Tocilizumab dramatically ameliorated life-threatening diarrhea due to secondary amyloidosis associated with rheumatoid arthritis. Clin Rheumatol. 2009;28(9) 1113-1116.

[122] Migita K, Koga T, Komori A, Torigoshi T, Maeda Y, Izumi Y, Sato J, Jiuchi Y, Miyashita T, Yamasaki S, Kawakami A, Nakamura M, Motokawa S, Ishibashi H. Influence of Janus kinase inhibition on interleukin 6-mediated induction of acute-phase serum amyloid A in rheumatoid synovium. J Rheumatol. 2011;38(11) 2309-2317.

[123] Narváez J, Hernández MV, Ruiz JM, Vaquero CG, Juanola X, Nollaa JM. Rituximab therapy for AA-amyloidosis secondary to rheumatoid arthritis. Joint Bone Spine. 2011;78(1) 101-103.

[124] Yeo W, Johnson PJ. Diagnosis, prevention and management of hepatitis B virus reactivation during anticancer therapy. Hepatology 2006;43(2) 209-220.

[125] Hui CK, Cheung WW, Zhang HY, Au WY, Yueng YH, Leung AY, Leung N, Luk JM, Lie AK, Kwong YL, Liang R, Lau GK. Kinetics and risk of de novo hepatitis B infection in HBsAg- negative patients undergoing cytotoxic chemotherapy. Gastroenterology. 2006;131(1) 59-68.

[126] Kuroda T, Kobayashi D, Sato H, et al. Effect of etanercept and entecavil in a patient with rheumatoid arthritis who is a hepatitis B carrier: A review of the literature. Rheumatol Int. 2012;32(4) 1059-1063.

[127] Kishida D, Okuda Y, Onishi M, Takebayashi M, Matoba K, Jouyama K, Yamada A, Sawada N, Mokuda S, Takasugi K. Successful tocilizumab treatment in a patient with adult-onset Still's disease complicated by chronic active hepatitis B and amyloid A amyloidosis. Mod Rheumatol. 2011;21(2) 215-218.

[128] van Gameren II, Hazenberg BP, Bijzet J, Haagsma EB, Vellenga E, Posthumus MD, Jager PL, van Rijswijk MH. Amyloid load in fat tissue reflects disease severity and predicts survival in amyloidosis. Artritis Care Res (Hoboken). 2010;62(3) 296-301.

[129] Suzuki A, Ohosone Y, Obana M, Mita S, Matsuoka Y, Irimajiri S, Fukuda J. Cause of death in 81 autopsied patients with rheumatoid arthritis. J Rheumatol. 1994;21(1) 33–36.

[130] Joss N, McLaughlin K, Simpson K, Boulton-Jones JM. Presentation, survival and prognostic markers in AA amyloidosis. QJM. 2000;93(8) 535–542.

[131] Mori S, Sugimoto M. Pneumocystis jirovecii infection: an emerging threat to patients with rheumatoid arthritis. Rheumatology (Oxford). 2012 Sep 22, doi:10.1093/rheumatology/kes244.

[132] Bergesio F, Ciciani AM, Manganaro M, Palladini G, Santostefano M, Brugnano R, Di Palma AM, Gallo M, Rosati A, Tosi PL, Salvadori M; Immunopathology Group of the Italian Society of Nephrology. Renal involvement in systemic amyloidosis: an Italian collaborative study on survival and renal outcome. Nephrol Dial Transplant. 2008;23(3) 941-951.

[133] Bollée G, Guery B, Joly D, Snanoudj R, Terrier B, Allouache M, Mercadal L, Peraldi MN, Viron B, Fumeron C, Elie C, Fakhouri F. Presentation and outcome of patients with systemic amyloidosis undergoing dialysis. Clin J Am Soc Nephrol. 2008;3(2) 375-381.

[134] Shah KB, Inoue Y, Mehra MR. Amyloidosis and the heart. Arch Intern Med 2006; 166(17) 1805-1813.

[135] Falk RH. Diagnosis and management of the cardiac amyloidoses. Circulation. 2005; 112(13) 2047-2060.

Chapter 10

# Therapeutic Strategies in Amyloid A Amyloidosis Secondary to Rheumatoid Arthritis

Tadashi Nakamura

Additional information is available at the end of the chapter

http://dx.doi.org/10.5772/53801

## 1. Introduction

Amyloidosis is a disorder of protein conformation and metabolism that results in the deposition of insoluble amyloid fibrils in tissues, which causes organ dysfunction; systemic amyloidosis is characterized by failure of multiple organs and the presence of amyloid precursor protein in the serum [1-3]. Reactive amyloid A (AA) amyloidosis is one of the most severe complications of several chronic disorders, particularly rheumatoid arthritis (RA) [4], and indeed, most patients with reactive AA amyloidosis have an underlying rheumatic disease. An extra-articular complication of RA, AA amyloidosis is a serious, potentially life-threatening disorder caused by deposition in organs of AA amyloid fibrils, which derive from the circulatory acute-phase reactant, serum amyloid A protein (SAA) [5]. AA amyloidosis secondary to RA is thus one of the intractable conditions found in patients with collagen vascular diseases and is an uncommon yet important complication of RA [6]. However, the actual pathological mechanisms that are responsible for the relationship between SAA and AA amyloidosis have not been fully elucidated.

With new biological therapies, both treatment and understanding of the roles of cytokines and inflammatory cellular events in RA have seen considerable progress. Biologics are recommended for patients with RA who have a suboptimal response or an intolerance to traditional disease-modifying anti-rheumatic drugs (DMARDs), such as methotrexate (MTX). Early diagnosis and rapidly subsequent treatment are essential because patients with advanced disease can't usually undergo intensive therapy. Specific treatment of AA amyloidosis caused by RA aims to stop SAA production. Cytotoxics such as chlorambucil and cyclophosphamide (CYC) and biologics such as anti-tumor necrosis factor (TNF)$\alpha$ inhibitors and anti-interleukin (IL)-6 receptor antibody are reportedly useful for both RA and AA amyloidosis [7, 8]. By the way, the genetic predisposition allele SAA1.3, one of SAA1 gene polymorphism, can serve not only as a risk factor for the association of AA amyloidosis, but also as a poor prognostic factor in Japanese RA patients [9]. Both the association of AA amyloidosis arising early in the RA disease course and symptomatic variety and severity were found in amyloidotic patients carrying SAA1.3 allele. Etanercept (ETN) for patients with AA amyloidosis secondary to RA, who carry SAA1.3 allele, showed the amelioration of rheumatoid inflammation, including marked reduction of SAA, improvement of proteinuria and creatinine clearance [10], that would demonstrate efficacy and safety even in patients undergone on hemodialysis [11]. These lead us to the notion of clinical significance of SAA1.3 allele in the clinical strategy of Japanese RA patients.

This article will discuss on therapeutic strategies from the point of biologics view on RA treatment in relation to AA amyloidosis secondary to RA based on our reports and literature reviews.

## 2. Significance of SAA1.3 allele genotype in Japanese RA patients with AA amyloidosis

It was reported that the frequency of SAA1.3 allele was markedly increased in AA amyloidosis in Japanese RA patients (Fig. 1), suggesting that this allele was a risk factor for AA amyloidosis secondary to RA [12]. That is, SAA1.3 allele has been reported to be associated with increased risk of AA amyloidosis and SAA1.1 with decreased risk [13], while SAA1.1 was revealed to be a risk factor for developing AA amyloidosis in the Caucasian population [14]. We calculated the hazard ratio in the presence or absence of SAA1.3/1.3 homozygosity as a survival parameter after the onset of RA. By means of Cox proportional hazard survival analysis, carrying with SAA1.3/1.3 homozygosity was statistically significant for survival ($P$=0.015) with hazard ratio of 2.101 (95% CI: 1.157 - 3.812). Also, the Kaplan-Meier curve showed a significant difference during observation from diagnosis of RA (Fig. 2). The mean survival period of the all patients with and without SAA 1.3/1.3 was 6.52±6.18 years and 13.8±8.47 years, with 43.8% and 71.6% surviving for 10 years, respectively. The SAA1.3 allele, particularly homozygosity for SAA1.3, was a univariate predictor of survival. The presenting factors which adversely influenced clinical outcome after diagnosis of AA amyloidosis were age ($P$=0.001), raised serum creatinine (Crea) concentration ($P=2.14 \times 10^{-5}$), lowered serum albumin (Alb) concentration ($P$=0.001), and presence of SAA1.3/1.3 ($P$=0.035). While, after diagnosis of RA, age of RA onset ($P=2.95 \times 10^{-4}$) and presence of renal involvement ($P$=0.011) were extracted as survival parameter. The serum Crea value of >2.5mg/dl upon diagnosis of AA amyloidosis was closely related with poorer survival, when compared with a serum Crea value of ≦2.5mg/dl by Kaplan-Meier technique ($P$=0.013 with log-rank statistic) (Fig. 3). The presence of cardiac involvement was likely to be a risk factor to survival ($P$=0.062). These results have revealed the significance of SAA1.3 allele genotype in Japanese RA patients with AA amyloidosis when we follow-up such patients in daily practice [15, 16]. However, we just need more studies about the large prospective trials to prove the usefulness of SAA1.3 allele genotype.

http://dx.doi.org/10.5772/53801

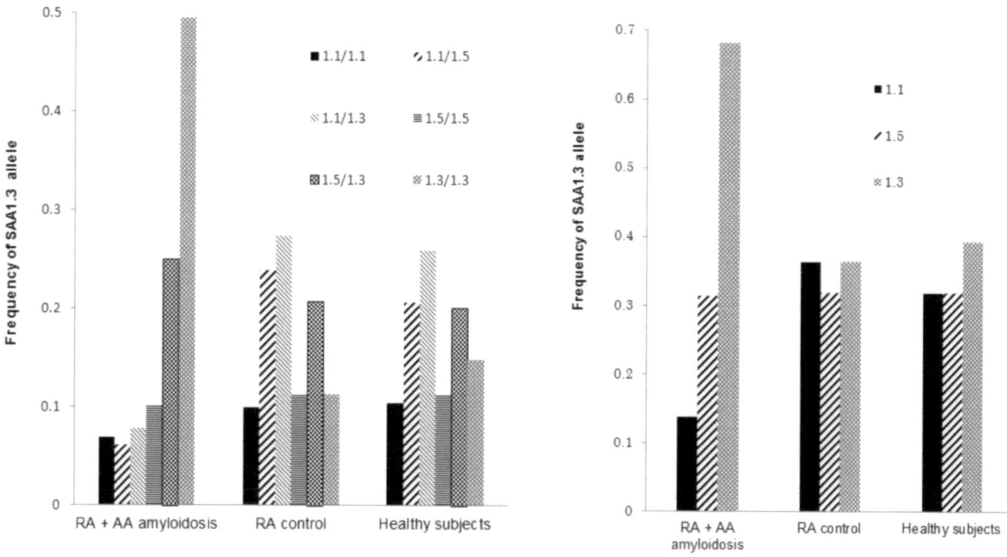


**Figure 1.** SAA1.3 allele frequency and AA amyloidosis in Japanese RA patients. SAA1.3 allele is associated with increased risk of AA amyloidosis in Japanese RA patients. Figures are courtesy of Satoshi Baba, MD and modified from Reference No. 12.

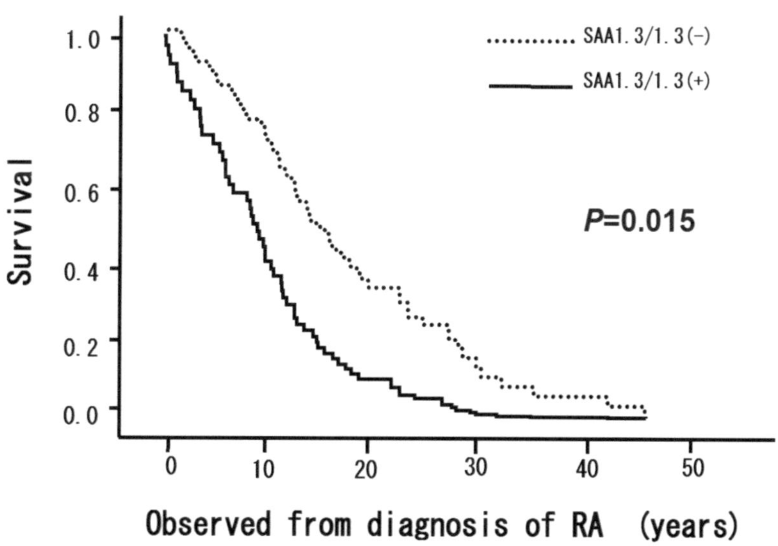


**Figure 2.** Kaplan-Meier survival curve in RA disease course for RA patients with (continuous line) and without (dotted line) SAA1.3/1.3 (P=0.015, log-rank test) from Reference No. 9.

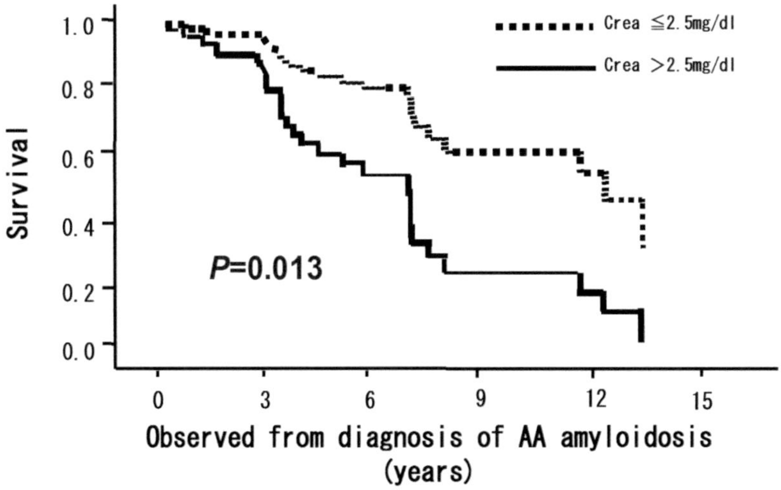


**Figure 3.** Kaplan-Meier survival curve after diagnosis of AA amyloidosis for patients with serum creatinine >2.5mg /dl (continuous line) and serum creatinine ≦2.5mg/dl (dotted line) (P=0.013, log-rank test) from Reference No. 9.

## 3. Fundamental thoughts for therapies

According to the information on the studies using radiolabelled human serum amyloid component P (SAP) as a specific quantitative *in vivo* scintigraphic tracer for monitoring of systemic AA amyloidosis [17], treatments those effectively suppress production of SAA halt the progressive accumulation of AA amyloid deposits and, in many cases, they are associated with AA amyloid regression, improved organ function and survival [18, 19]. AA amyloid deposits are evidently turning over, their net size reflecting the balance of deposition and regression [20]. Therefore, AA amyloid deposits may regress at a low rate over a period of years and exist in a sate of dynamic turnover. The usual clinical impression of inexorable progression of AA amyloidosis actually reflects the progressive and usually incurable nature of the underlying primary condition, which is complicated by AA amyloidosis. However, new and aggressive approaches to therapy, such as cytotoxic anti-inflammatory drugs and biologic agents in chronic rheumatic inflammation, will lead to impressive AA amyloid regression and prolonged survival. Unfortunately these treatments do not always work and there are many difficult cases in those approaches are neither possible now nor likely to become feasible in future. In view of clinical significance of AA amyloidosis, there is an urgent need to facilitate studies into this complication. Early diagnosis and intervention are essential for RA, however, few specific features are useful for diagnosis of RA and its diagnosis is often difficult in daily RA practice. Reduction of SAA load is currently the most rational approach thereby arresting further deposition [21]. It is not exactly known why some patients develop a progressive AA amyloidosis while others do not, although latent deposits may be present. While there is startling variation in the frequency of AA amyloidosis worldwide, differences also exist for AA amyloidosis complicating RA [22]. The reasons, however, for

http://dx.doi.org/10.5772/53801

the marked geographic differences are unclear. The difference in the frequency of AA amyloidosis among different races, and the fact that AA amyloidosis is not consistently related to the length and severity of chronic inflammation suggests that AA amyloidosis may be, at least in part, influenced by genetic factors [23-25].

## 4. Treatments of AA amyloidosis secondary to RA

The principal aim in treating RA patients with AA amyloidosis is to switch off SAA production by controlling the RA inflammatory process. Anti-inflammatory treatment must be empirical but, as in all patients with AA amyloidosis, should be guided by frequent assessment of SAA concentrations in view of reported correlations between survival and this measure. Treatment of AA amyloidosis secondary to RA may involve the following strategies as outlined in Table 1 [26].

| | |
|---|---|
| **Prevention** | (1)Be careful not to raise AA amyloidosis |
| | (2)Keep the serum levels of SAA[3]less than 10 μg/ml |
| | (3)Control tightly rheumatoid inflammatory responses |
| | (4)Follow-up RA patients carrying SAA1.3 allele carefully |
| **Diagnosis** | (1)Do not underestimate proteinuria |
| | (2)Evaluate renal function by the levels of eGFR[4], cystatin C, and Ccr[5] |
| | (3)Watch GI[6] tract symptoms |
| | (4)Detect AA amyloid fibrils with organ biopsy like GI tracts, labia, and abdominal subcutaneous fat |
| | (5)Require renal biopsy in cases with proteinuria or renal dysfunction in RA patients |
| **Therapy:** | (1)Control acute-phase responses to suppress the synthesis of SAA |
| | (2)Control RA disease activity tightly |
| | (i) Do not lose window of opportunity |
| | (ii) Control RA disease tightly according to T2T[7] recommendations even in patients undergoing HD[8] |
| | (iii) Choose MTX[9] plus biologics in cases uncontrollable from early phase |
| | (iv) Challenge new biologics and signal transduction inhibitors |
| | (3)Steroid, codeine phosphate, lactate bacteriae, and especially octreotide for refractory diarrhea |
| | (4)Stand on the notion of deposited AA amyloid fibrils existing in a state of dynamic turnover |

[1]AA:amyloid A, [2]RA:rheumatoid arthritis, [3]SAA:serum amyloid A protein, [4]eGFR: estimated glomerular filtration rate, [5]Ccr:creatinine clearance, [6]GI:gastrointestine, [7] T2T: treat RA to target, [8] HD:hemodialysis,[9]MTX:methotrexate

**Table 1.** Clinical strategies in the management of AA[1] amyloidosis secondary to RA[2]

### 4.1. Suppression of SAA production

For AA amyloidosis in patients with RA, treatment has centered on using cytotoxic agents and is shifting to biologics recently. Although case reports and studies of small series of patients showed that these agents can reverse nephrotic syndrome and even lead to complete resolution of proteinuria, anticytokine agents have recently been proposed as therapeutic options. Traditional management of AA amyloidosis has been to target RA disease to process behind the inflammation. Although there is no evidence that DMARDs have a specific effect on amyloidogenesis and AA amyloidosis in RA [27, 28], there have been encouraging reports evaluating alkylating agents as beneficial in clinical trials in RA patients with AA amyloidosis [29-33]. Treatments in AA amyloidosis secondary to RA including immunosuppressants, biologics, and other supportive therapies will be discussed as follows.

#### *4.1.1. Immunosuppressants*

It is suggested that the use of immunosuppressive agents can improve prognosis [34], and CYC was superior to MTX in the management of RA patients with AA amyloidosis [9]. As regards MTX and CYC treatments, we observed differences of both serum C-reactive protein (CRP) and Crea concentrations. That is, we subtracted the CRP- and/or Crea-value at initiation from the CRP- and/or Crea-value at endpoint of corresponding to each treatment. The each deducted value was dotted in Fig. 4. It was clear that more CYC treatments resided within minus area than MTX treatments. CRP improved 1.23±1.67 (mg/dl) in CYC treatments with statistical significance ($P<0.001$). We reported the possibility that CYC would be more effective predominantly in patients with SAA1.3/1.3 homozygosity than heterozygosity, suggesting of CYC treatment-susceptible factor as SAA1.3/1.3 homozygosity [35]. Concerning immunosuppressants, whether specific therapies were warranted and were superior to previously reported regimens should be elucidated. The strategy of these treatments focuses on tight control of underlying RA disease activity [28]. Requirements include diagnosis of RA as early as possible and treatment with DMARDs, including MTX as the anchor drug. Achieving low disease activity via DMARDs in the early disease course has a strong positive outcome on disease progression. However, although MTX is the most common and effective drug for RA, management of patients with AA amyloidosis secondary to RA and renal involvement is too complex to limit the discussion on MTX.

For signal transduction, IL-6 binds to membrane-bound IL-6 receptor gp80 [36], and then the IL-6-gp80 dimer interacts with gp130. Formation of gp130-containing complexes leads to activation of Janus kinases (JAKs), which stimulates signal transducers and activators of transcription (STATs) [37]. Certain evidence suggests that STAT3 is the key transcription factor responsible for IL-6 activation of SAA gene transcription [38]. Therefore, the function of JAK inhibition in the IL-6 signaling pathway will be one target of RA treatments. Suppressing IL-6-mediated proinflammatory signaling pathways via JAK inhibitors may be a novel anti-inflammatory therapeutic strategy for RA and AA amyloidosis. Another agent, tacrolimus, may inhibit T-cell function in pathogenesis of AA amyloidosis. The function of JAK inhibition in the IL-6 signaling pathway will be one target of RA treatments [39, 40].

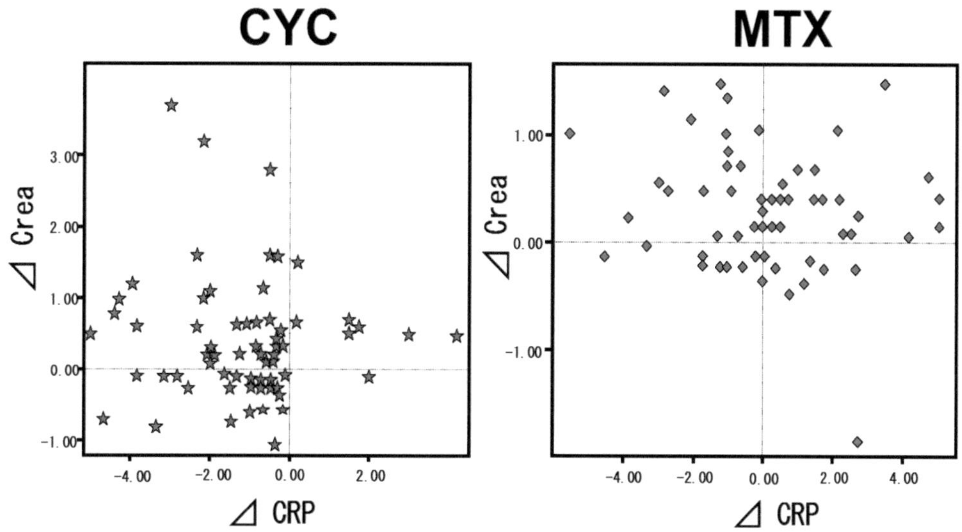


**Figure 4.** Differences between CYC and MTX treatments for RA patients with AA amyloidosis. The detected value (placed in figures) was calculated by subtracting the starting value of CRP and/or serum creatinine from the endpoint value in each treatment from Reference No. 9.

*4.1.2. Biologics*

In RA treatment, tight control of RA is emphasized to obtain clinical remission or lower disease activity; this control is possible through periodic evaluations of RA disease activity and aggressive pursuit of other more effective treatments [41-43]. Anti-proinflammatory cytokine therapy is expected to show efficacy against both systemic and local inflammation mediated by macrophage differentiation or activation in glomeruli, such as in renal AA amyloidosis secondary to RA [44].

Infliximab (IFX) and ETN, both TNF$\alpha$ antagonists, can reduce serum SAA levels in RA patients with AA amyloidosis, which improves rheumatoid inflammation, reduces swollen and tender joint counts, lowers or normalizes proteinuria, and ameliorates renal function [45-48]. Also, these agents showed amelioration in renal function for AA amyloidosis secondary to RA (Table 2) [10]. Despite the small number of series of patients with AA amyloidosis secondary to RA who had ETN treatment, this drug did benefit both RA inflammation and AA amyloidosis, as measured via the surrogate markers, disease activity score (DAS)28-erythrocyte sedimentation rate (ESR), CRP, SAA, and proteinuria, in SAA1.3 allele-carrying RA patients (Fig. 5, Table 3). Further, Crea levels significantly improved in patients with mild RA disease and renal dysfunction (Table 4). This result suggests that the earlier the intervention with biologics, the better the outcome for patients. ETN alone may therefore be efficacious, without MTX [49-53].

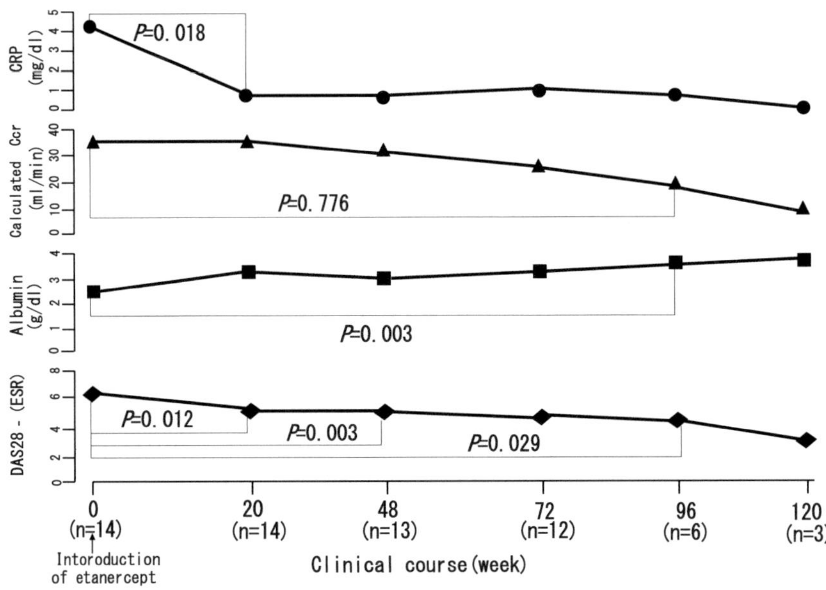


**Figure 5.** Chronological changes among surrogate markers following etanercept treatment. Ccr: creatinine clearance, CRP: C-reactive protein, DAS: disease activity score, n: number of patients treated with etanercept in the designated observation periods. CRP decreased dramatically by 20 weeks (P=0.018) and DAS28-ESR improved to low values significantly following the treatment of etanercept. Although serum and calculated Ccr are coincided to be renal function markers, only serum albumin showed stastical significance between 0 and 96 weeks ( P=0.003), whereas the calculated creatinine clearance fell gradually 0 and 96 weeks (P=0.776).

| Case/Age/Sex | Duration (years) | | Biologics | Proteinuria (g/day) | | Serum Crea (mM/L) | | Observation Periods (months) |
|---|---|---|---|---|---|---|---|---|
| | RA | AA amyloidosis | | Initial | Last | Initial | Last | |
| 1/70/F | 18 | 1 | IFX | 2 | 6 | 93 | 130 | 3 |
| 2/59/F | 13 | 4 | ETN | 1.2 | 0.2 | 398 | 425 | 12 |
| 3/59/F | 13 | 4 | ETN | 1.2 | 0.72 | 229 | 246 | 7 |
| 4/37/M | 22 | 2 | IFX | 3 | 0.9 | 134 | 145 | 17 |

Quoted and modified from Reference No. 47. Data are represented as renal functions between the initial- and last-vist following biologics treatment. RA: rheumatoid arthritis, AA: amyloid A, Crea: levels of creatinine, IFX: infliximab, ETN: etanercept.

**Table 2.** Effect of TNF alpha blockers on renal AA amyloidosis secondary to RA.

http://dx.doi.org/10.5772/53801

| Parameter | Initial-visit | Last-visit | P-value |
|---|---|---|---|
| **RA inflammation** | | | |
| DAS28-ESR | 5.99±0.69 | 2.99±0.15 | <0.01 |
| CRP(mg/dl) | 4.68±0.87 | 0.48±0.29 | <0.01 |
| **AA amyloidosis** | | | |
| SAA(μg/ml) | 250±129 | 26±15 | <0.01 |
| Proteinuria(g/day) | 2.24±0.81 | 0.57±0.41 | <0.01 |
| Serum creatinine(mg/dl) | 2.54±1.38 | 2.50±2.21 | 0.896 |

The values of DAS28=ESR, CRP, SAA, and proteinuria between the initial visit (before etanercept) and the last treatment (the index time) with etanercept. All improved with statistical significance. In contrast, the serum creatinine did not change statistically. RA: rheumatoid arthritis, DAS: disease activity score, ESR: erythrocyte sedimentation rate, CRP: C-reactive protein, AA: amyloid A, SAA: serum amyloid A protein, *serum levels. Quoted and modified from Reference No. 10.

**Table 3.** Surrogate markers between initial- and last-visit following treatment with etanercept

| Less than 2.0(mg/dl) (n=6) | | More than 2.0(mg/dl) (n=8) | |
|---|---|---|---|
| Initial-visit (mg/dl) | Last-visit (mg/dl) | Initial-visit (mg/dl) | Last-visit (mg/dl) |
| 1.37±0.49 | 1.07±0.59 | 3.43±1.14 | 3.56±2.39 |
| * | | ** | |

*P=0.021,**not significant

Although Table 3 shows that the change in serum creatinine value was not statistically significant, when using a cutoff value as less than 2.0 mg/dl at the initial-visit, it was demonstrated that the creatinine value improved significantly at the last-visit. Quoted and modified from Reference No. 10.

**Table 4.** Changes in the values of serum creatinine statifying by 2.0(mg/dl) at the commencement of etanercept

Tocilizumab (TCZ), an IL-6 receptor antagonist, can demonstrate excellent suppression of SAA levels and may have potential as the first candidate of the therapeutic agent for AA amyloidosis [7]. Circulating SAA normally reflects changes in CRP, and levels of both acute-phase reactants usually increase simultaneously, but some differences can occur. SAA and CRP seem to be partly influenced by different cytokines. IL-6-blocking therapy has shown promise in normalizing serum SAA levels in RA patients. Moreover, blocking IL-6 alone, but not IL-1 or TNF$\alpha$, completely prevented SAA mRNA expression in human hepatocytes during triple cytokine stimulation [54, 55]. Some reports with promising effect on AA amyloidosis secondary to RA may suggest a possibility of usefulness of this agent [56, 57]. Our case with end-stage renal disease due to AA amyloidosis secondary to RA showed validity of TCZ usage which is reaching to sustain normal SAA levels with successive treatment for 4 years (Fig. 6). In this case due to loss of joint function in advanced RA stage, in spite of lower and limited quality of life, both CRP and SAA are keeping within normal limits, those may lead to decreasing proteinuria. It is needed to clarify the dissociation between inflammatory rheumatoid activity and destructed articular function under current RA therapeutic strategies using biologics like "disconnect" phenomenon [58].

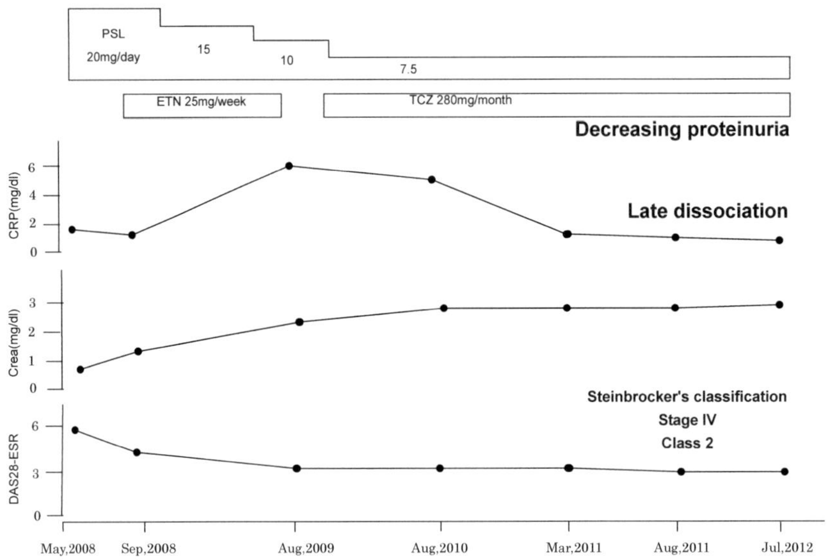


**Figure 6.** Effect of tocilizumab on AA amyloidosis secondary to RA. DAS28-ESR showed gradually regressed with the association of CRP, however, levels of serum creatinine increased leading to end-stage renal disease. TCZ had an effect on both proteinuria and rheumatoid inflammation, nevertheless, this case showed late dissociation between rheumatoid inflammation and joint functional activity. TCZ: tocilizumab, ETN: etanercept, PSL: prednisolone, Crea: serum creatinine, CRP: C-reactive protein.

T lymphocyte costimulation is a key point in the regulation of immune tolerance, immune response, and autoimmunity. T lymphocyte activation does not take place upon the simple engagement of T cell receptor; a second signal is needed to fully stimulate T lymphocytes. There are a variety of molecules that can act as costimulators, and among these cluster of differentiation (CD)28/CD80 signaling plays a crucial role in modulating T lymphocyte response. Cytotoxic T lymphocyte antigen-4 (CTLA4) is a physiologic antagonist of CD28, and abatacept (ABT), a synthetic analogue of CTLA4, has recently been approved to treat RA. A 70-year-old Japanese woman had been suffering from RA for 28 years with Steinbrocker's Stage IV and functional Class 2. She was biopsy-confirmed as AA amyloidosis carried with SAA1.3/1.5 allele genotype. ABT was initiated from January 2011 and her clinical course was shown in Fig. 7. The histopathological findings from upper gastrointestinal (GI) biopsy between before and after 1 year from the commencement of ABT revealed a disappearance of AA amyloid fibril deposition (Fig. 8-A, -B). The changes in markers on cytokines and lymphocyte expression might suggest an effect of ABT from the points of immunological aspect in the case (Table 5). These results would show effectiveness of this agent on both RA and AA amyloidosis, with being required further elucidations. In experimental mouse models of AA amyloidosis, blocking T lymphocytes function by the calcinulin inhibitor showed that

http://dx.doi.org/10.5772/53801

tacrolims inhibited AA amyloid fibril deposits in a dose-dependent manner without influencing SAA concentrations. Also, the locality of CD4+ T lymphocytes in the spleen was partially identical to AA amyloid fibril deposits histologically, suggesting the role of T lymphocytes in the pathogenesis of AA amyloidosis [39].

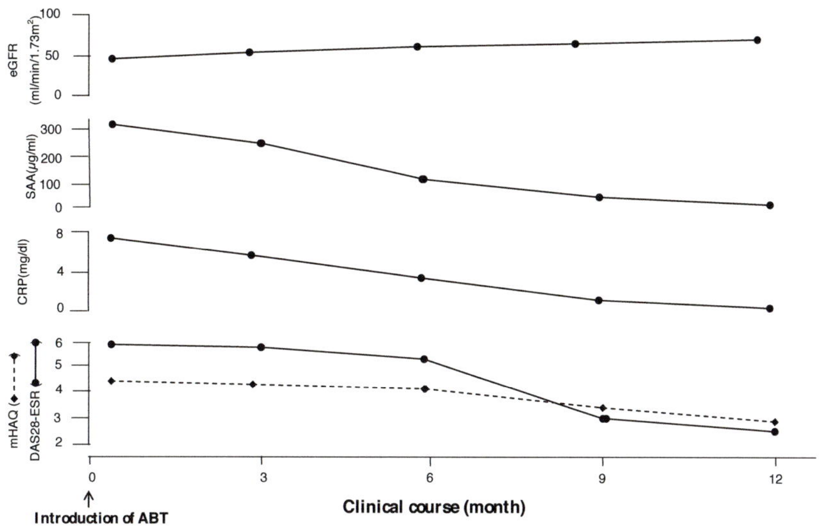


**Figure 7.** Effect of abatacept on AA amyloidosis secondary to RA. Inflammatory markers, CRP and SAA, decreased gradually, and renal dysfunction ameliorated with the treatment of abatacept. ABT: abatacept, eGFR: estimated glomerular filtration rate, SAA: serum amyloid A protein, CRP: C-reactive protein, mHAQ: modified health assessment questionnaire, DAS: disease activity score, ESR: erythrocyte sedimentation rate.

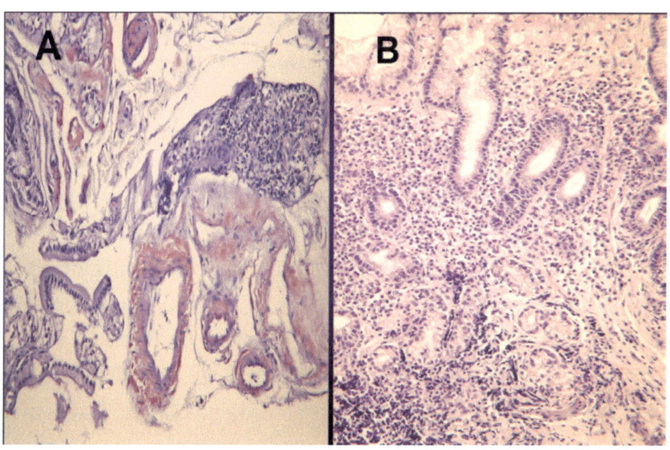


**Figure 8.** Histological changes before (A) the treatment with abatacept and after (B) one year in the disease course. Amorphous deposits were detected in the specimen from upper gastrointestinal biopsy with Congo Red staining (A). Those disappeared with abatacept treatment after one year (B).

| Parameter | Baseline | Clinical course (month) | | | | |
|---|---|---|---|---|---|---|
| | (n=14) | 0 | 3 | 6 | 9 | 12 |
| IL-6 (pg/ml) | 11.2±12.9 | 107 | 40.4 | 24.8 | 7.6 | 1.7 |
| TNFα (pg/ml) | 1.04±0.36 | 2.2 | 1.4 | 1.3 | 1.1 | 1.1 |
| IL-2 (U/ml) | <0.8 | <0.8 | <0.8 | <0.8 | <0.8 | <0.8 |
| CD4+/CD8+ | 1.30±0.58 | 2.04 | 1.63 | 1.54 | 1.72 | 1.77 |
| CD4+CD25++FoxP3+ reg T cells gated on | | | | | | |
| Lymphocytes (%) | 1.60±0.85 | 4.8 | 2.6 | 2.1 | 2.4 | 2.4 |
| CD4+ T lymphocytes (%) | 4.79±1.60 | 9 | 5.4 | 4.8 | 5.2 | 5.1 |

Baseline values were determined and expressed by mean ± S.D. of 14 RA patients, matched by disease duration and disease severity to this case. IL-6: interleukin-6, TNFa: tumor necrosis factor alpha, IL-2: interleukin -2, reg T: regulatory T lymphocyte.

**Table 5.** Changes in cytokines and regulatory T lymphocyte expression after abatacept treatment

Rituximab (RTX), an anti-CD20 monoclonal antibody, was efficacious for patients with severe active RA who have exhibited an inadequate response to one or more TNF$\alpha$ inhibitors [59]. Also, this agent was administered alone in two RA patients and in combination with MTX in other two RA cases with histologic confirmation of AA amyloidosis. The four patients showed a significant clinical improvement of the articular symptoms and marked reduction of the acute phase-reactants. Renal function remained stable in all patients and proteinuria improved in two, worsened in one, and remained stable in the fourth with few adverse effects [60].

Clinical trials are warranted to assess the long-term safety and efficacy of biological treatments and their impacts on the survival of RA patients with AA amyloidosis.

### *4.1.3. Corticosteroids*

The effect of corticosteroid treatment on AA amyloidosis is still controversial. Corticosteroids are capable of reducing the magnitude of the acute phase reaction including the synthesis of CRP and SAA. In human hepatocyte cultures a stimulating effect of corticosteroids was seen on SAA but not on CRP production [61, 62]. Although corticosteroid therapy suppresses both CRP and SAA levels in longitudinal studies of patients with RA, the effect is somewhat more pronounced for CRP than for SAA [63]. Monitoring of SAA instead of CRP levels would be advisable particularly if corticosteroids are being used. It seems reasonable to treat patients with AA amyloidosis secondary to RA using cytostatic drugs either alone or in combination with prednisolone [64-66]. As the effect of cytostatics may take weeks or months to appear, it is recommended to give steroids additionally in order to ensure an immediate reduction of the acute phase response and in particular the synthesis of SAA. Low-dose prednisolone inclusion in a MTX-based tight control strategy for early RA would be effective, thus could be improved for AA amyloidosis secondary to RA [67].

### 4.2. Inhibition of AA amyloid fibril deposits

Eprodisate, a small sulfonated molecule with structural similarity to heparan sulfate, which can cause regression of amyloidosis by destabilizing the glycoasaminoglycan backbone of amyloid deposits, delayed progression of renal disease associated with AA amyloidosis. In a trial for AA amyloidosis, eprodisate had a beneficial effect on the rate of deterioration of renal function but no effect on urinary protein excretion [68]. Because eprodisate did not affect SAA levels and preserved kidney function but had no effect on proteinuria, the interesting possibility that it is the precursors of mature amyloid fibrils are responsible for proteinuria in amyloidosis would raise. In the light of higher effects of biologics on AA amyloidosis secondary to RA, the usefulness of eprodisate seems to be inferior to that of biologic under the biologics era.

### 4.3. Removal of deposited AA amyloid fibrils

The normal plasma protein SAP binds to all types of amyloid fibrils and contributes to amyloidosis pathogenesis [69]. A pyrrolidine carboxylic acid derivative, which is a competitive inhibitor of SAP binding to amyloid fibrils, can intervere in this process and affect SAP levels. This compound cross-linked and dimerized SAP molecules, which led to extremely rapid clearance by the liver, and thus produced marked depletion of circulating human SAP. Therefore, this drug action removed SAP from human amyloid deposits in tissues and may have a favorable effect on amyloidosis [70].

Another compound, dimethyl sulfoxide (DMSO), is a hydrogen-bond disrupter, cell-differentiating agent, hydroxyl radical scavenger, cryoprotectant, and solubilizing agent that is used as a compound for preparation of samples for electron microscopy, as an intracellular low-density lipoprotein-derived cholesterol-mobilizing antidote to extravasation of vesicant anticancer agents, and as a topical analgesic. A notable DMSO side effect is garlic-like breath odor and taste in the mouth because of pulmonary excretion of a small amount of DMSO as dimethyl sulfide [71]. Oral DMSO was effective against AA amyloidosis, especially GI involvement and early renal dysfunction [72], but using it would not likely be feasible in current clinical practice.

### 4.4. Treatment of organ failure

The predominant feature of AA amyloidosis is proteinuria with or without renal failure. If conservative treatment of renal failure is not sufficient, renal replacement therapy including renal transplantation, continuous ambulatory peritoneal dialysis, or hemodialysis (HD) should be considered. Even in RA patients with AA amyloidosis who undergo HD, anti-TNF$\alpha$ blockers can demonstrate efficacy [11, 73]. HD reportedly had no effect on plasma ETN concentration, and ETN pharmacokinetics in patients undergoing HD for chronic renal failure were similar to those with normal renal function [74]. Administration of ETN to HD patients would therefore appear reasonable. Renal replacement therapy is discussed in Table 6.

**Renal transplantation**

- Immonen K, et al: J Rheumatol 2008; 35: 1334-8
    - 30 cases in 332 RA patients with AA amyloidosis
    - Median survival: 2.11 years

**Peritoneal dialysis/Hemodialysis (HD)**

- Bergesio F, et al: Nephrol Dial Transplant 2008; 23: 941-51
    - Prognosis: 17 months
- Kuroda T, et al: Reference No. 73
    - 96.9 person-year followup: 42 patients died
    - 50% survival from the initiation of HD: 251 days
    - Ccr was superior to Crea, Advisable planned initiation of HD
- Nakamura T, et al: Reference No. 11
    - 51.8 months Dialysis with ETN 27.8 months Use
    - Amelioration of DAS28-ESR, CRP, mHAQ, and ESR

RA: rheumatoid arthritis, AA: amyloid A, HD: hemodialysis, Ccr: creatinine clearance, Crea: serum levels of creatinine, ETN: etanercept, DAS: disease activity score, ESR: erythrocyte sedimentation rate, CRP: C-reactive protein, mHAQ: modified health assessment questionnaire.

**Table 6.** Renal replacement therapy in AA amyloidosis secondary to RA

## 5. Comparison of effectiveness between biologic and alkylating agent

We previously showed that the genetic predisposition allele SAA1.3 was not only a univariate predictor of survival but also a risk factor for association of AA amyloidosis with RA in Japanese patients [9], and in view of our earlier reports on the efficacy of ETN [10, 48] and CYC [35, 64] given alone for AA amyloidosis secondary to RA, we compared the effectiveness of ETN and CYC, and we assessed biomarkers and analyzed the effect of SAA1.3 allele on these treatments [75].

### 5.1. Patients and methods

This retrospective cohort study compared effectiveness of CYC and ETN for RA patients with AA amyloidosis who were homozygous for the SAA1.3 allele or other polymorphisms. Sixty-two RA patients received CYC and 24 did ETN; all had biopsy-confirmed AA amyloidosis. The presence of AA amyloid deposits was confirmed histologically via positive Congo Red staining, potassium permanganate susceptibility, and green birefringence seen by polarization microscopy after Congo Red staining, as well as immunohistochemical analysis using anti-AA antibody and anti-immunoglobulin light-chain (AL) antibody to differentiate AL amyloidosis.

Patients with RA had been treated with non-steroidal anti-inflammatory drugs (NSAIDs), prednisolone, DMARDs, and immunosuppressive agents but were often refractory to these agents. Although CYC had been unallowable medico-legally in Japanese governmental health insurance system and we were able to use CYC for RA treatment from August 2010 in Japan, we finally used CYC and investigated its efficacy for enrolled patients until December 2004.

Age, sex, and duration of RA and AA amyloidosis were recorded, as were changes in laboratory indices and clinical evaluations of disease activity included CRP, SAA, ESR, rheumatoid factor (RF), serum Alb, Crea, 24-hour proteinuria, and eGFR. Use of DMARDs, immunosuppressants, or PSL from the time of RA onset to the index time was noted. We chose CRP as an indicator of rheumatoid inflammation and Alb as an indicator of severity of AA amyloidosis [76]. Because renal dysfunction is the most common symptom in AA amyloidosis secondary to RA, we selected Crea and eGFR to assess treatment effectiveness. We calculated eGFRs via the nomogram for modification of diet reported in a Japanese renal disease study (index 0.741) using Crea measured by using an enzymatic method [77]. We also obtained information on drugs including DMARDs, NSAIDs, angiotensin-converting enzyme inhibitors, and angiotensin II receptor blockers. We recorded clinical symptoms and arthritis activity for each time point. We carefully checked adverse effects of immunosuppressants, *e.g.* infection risks, myelosuppression, haemorrhagic cystitis, and carcinogenesis.

We monitored biomarker levels and compared initial (before treatment) and last (after treatment) values. We used statistical analysis to assess effects of the SAA1.3 allele on therapies. We determined the onset of RA by reviewing of charts after AA amyloidosis diagnosis had been confirmed. Clinical symptoms at presentation were the main reason for physicians to obtain tissue biopsies to demonstrate AA amyloid deposits. We estimated survival curves via the Kaplan-Maier technique; we analyzed statistical differences between two curves by the log-rank test. We used Cox proportional hazards models to assess effects of treatments on eGFR and 24-hour proteinuria, with risk of death as the endpoint. We used two-way repeated-measures analysis of ANOVA to simultaneously estimate effects of SAA1.3 or treatments on individual changes in biomarkers. In the model, individual change was defined as within-subjects factors; categorical groups, i.e. polymorphisms of the SAA1.3 allele and treatments, were defined as between-subjects factors. To determine the factor affecting individual change, a combined factor (within and between) was defined as interaction. We evaluated significant effects of these factors via ANOVA. We determined significant interaction of effects of groups (SAA1.3 or treatments) on changes in individual markers. Findings were statistically significant at $P<0.05$. We used SPSS Statistics 17.0, Base and Advanced (SPSS Inc, Chicago, IL, USA) for statistical analyses.

### 5.2. Results

Table 7 provides patients' clinical characteristics and laboratory findings. Despite treatments being administered during different periods, clinical and laboratory findings of both groups were quite similar at the start of each treatment, except for the SAA1.3 genotype and duration AA amyloidosis since diagnosis ($P$=0.015 and $P$<0.001, respectively). With regard to biomarkers indicating renal dysfunction, ETN had worse kidney damage than did CYC. During the study, patients died in each treatment group at the almost same rate. In the CYC group, congestive heart failure and infectious pneumonia occurred frequently. Patients given ETN had a lower rate of congestive heart failure as cause of death, suggesting of the possibility of an inhibitory effect on progressive heart failure.

Years since RA onset and years since diagnosis of AA amyloidosis were significantly different for SAA1.3 homozygosity *vs* other genotypes (15.6±7.8 *vs* 21.4±9.9, $P$=0.046, and 7.44±4.9 *vs* 9.7±4.5, $P$=0.016, respectively). Comparison of CRP, Alb, eGFR, and Crea for both groups at initial and final observations, disregarding SAA1.3 allele polymorphisms, showed that ETN reduced serum CRP levels and increased serum Alb levels more than did CYC (ETN *vs* CYC: CRP: from 4.7±0.8 to 0.5±0.3 mg/dl *vs* from 4.0±1.6 to 2.8±1.2 mg/dl, $P$<0.01; Alb: from 2.6±0.4 to 3.5±0.4 g/dl *vs* from 2.8±0.3 to 2.8±0.5 g/dl, $P$<0.01, respectively). Thus, ETN significantly improved serum CRP and Alb levels and was clearly more effective than CYC. CRP and Alb interactions with polymorphism (homozygous for SAA1.3 or other polymorphisms) showed no significance ($P$=0.777 and $P$=0.715, respectively), but CRP and Alb interactions with treatment (ETN or CYC) demonstrated significant results (both $P$<0.01). Within-subject analysis showed that treatments improved eGFR: ETN: from 21.8±18.9 to 24.9±18.7 ml/min/1.73m$^2$ *vs* CYC: from 29.3±12.7 to 18.6±9.3 ml/min/1.73m$^2$, $P$=0.035, with ETN's effect on eGFR being significant ($P$=0.032). ETN increased eGFR, thus improving the decreased renal function caused by AA amyloidosis, more than did CYC (Fig. 9A), but this effect was not related to SAA1.3 allele polymorphisms (Fig. 9B). Neither treatment affected Crea levels. SAA1.3 allele did not affect treatment in both groups of patients, as evidenced by interactions of SAA1.3 allele with CRP, Alb, eGFR, and Crea ($P$=0.777, $P$=0.715, $P$=0.465, and $P$=0.228, respectively).

Because ETN was more effective than CYC, according to CRP, Alb, and eGFR measures, we calculated the hazard ratio between ETN and CYC as a survival parameter. According to Cox proportional hazards survival analysis, ETN significantly improved survival ($P$=0.025). Also, the Kaplan-Meier curves showed a significant difference between ETN and CYC (Fig. 10). The hazard ratio for ETN evidenced significant results for the risk of death endpoint (eGFR: $P$=0.024 and 24-hour proteinuria: $P$=0.025, respectively) but CYC did not (Table 8).

| | | | CYC (n=62)[2] | ETN (n=24)[3] | P-value[4] |
|---|---|---|---|---|---|
| I. | Sex, Male/Female, n | | 12/50 | 4/20 | 1.000 |
| | SAA1.3 allele, Homozygout/Others, n | | 22/40 | 16/8 | 0.015 |
| | Months since RA onset (mean) | | 176.0 (111.0) | 195.3 (88.3) | 0.447 |
| | Months since diagnosis of AA amyloidosis (mean) | | 22.9(41.7) | 67.5 (42.5) | <0.001 |
| | Months of treatment (mean) | | 38.0 (27.4) | 34.0 (23.1) | 0.526 |
| | Steinbrocker's classification[5] | | | | |
| | Stage | II,III,IV, n | 5/18/39 | 3/7/14 | |
| | Class | 2/3/4, n | 38/18/6 | 14/7/3 | |
| II | MTX therapy (yes/no), n | | 31/31 | 15/9 | 0.297 |
| | PSL dosage (mg/day, mean) | | 9.91(5.88) | 7.97 (4.96) | 0.516 |
| III | CRP (mg/dl, mean) | | 3.99 (1.72) | 3.89 (1.97) | 0.820 |
| | SAA (µg/ml, mean) | | 294.8 (166.0) | 327.0 (223.4) | 0.467 |
| | eGFR (ml/min/1.73 ㎡, mean) | | 29.2 (23.9) | 31.2 (20.6) | 0.714 |
| | Crea(mg/dl, mean) | | 2.04 (0.95) | 2.23 (1.27) | 0.465 |
| | 24-Hour urinary protein (g, mean) | | 1.53 (0.84) | 2.09 (1.27) | 0.020 |
| | Serum Alb (g/dl, mean) | | 2.92 (0.32) | 3.04 (0.68) | 0.128 |
| | RF (U/ml, mean) | | 237.8 (262.1) | 200.8 (154.3) | 0.519 |
| IV | Cause of death, n (%) | | n=26 (41.9) | n=8 (33.3) | 0.464 |
| | Infectious pneumonia | | 6 | 3 | |
| | Sepsis | | 2 | | |
| | GI ulcer/bleeding | | 3 | | |
| | Interstitial pneumonia | | 4 | 1 | |
| | Myocardial infarction | | 2 | | |
| | Congestive heart failure | | 7 | 2 | |
| | Renal failure | | 1 | 1 | |
| | Malignancy | | | 1 | |
| | Unknown | | 1 | | |

[1] Baseline data were at the initiation of each treatment. All patients, except those who died, were followed from January 1995 to December 2010. Last observations were made in December 2004 for the CYC group and December 2010 for the ETN group. Vales are represented by mean (S.D.) unless otherwise noted. Causes of death of patients who died during the study, and these causes were most closely related to their death. [2]CYC was given until December, 2004. Thirty-six alive [8 males, 28 females; mean (S.D.) age = 65.7 (10.8) years] and 26 dead [3 males, 23 females; mean (S.D.) age = 71.9 (8.5) years]. CYC was treated according to the level of 24-h Ccr: Ccr≧80 (ml/min): 100 (mg/day), 60≦Ccr < 80 (ml/min): 75 (mg/day), 40≦Ccr < 60 (ml/min): 40 (mg/day), 10≦Ccr < 20 (ml/min): 25 (mg/day), Ccr < 10 (ml/min): 20 (mg /day). [3]ETN was until December, 2010. Sixteen alive [3 males, 13 females; mean (S.D.) age = 64.2 (8.5) years] and 8 dead [1 male, 7 females; mean (S.D.) age = 66.0 (7.8) years]. [4]Student's-*t* analysis was performed to compare CYC and ETN, with $P < 0.05$ indicating a significant result. [5]Stenbrocher'scalassification according to JAMA 1949; 140: 659-62. Quoted from Reference No. 75.

**Table 7.** Clinical characteristics and laboratory findings of patients[1]

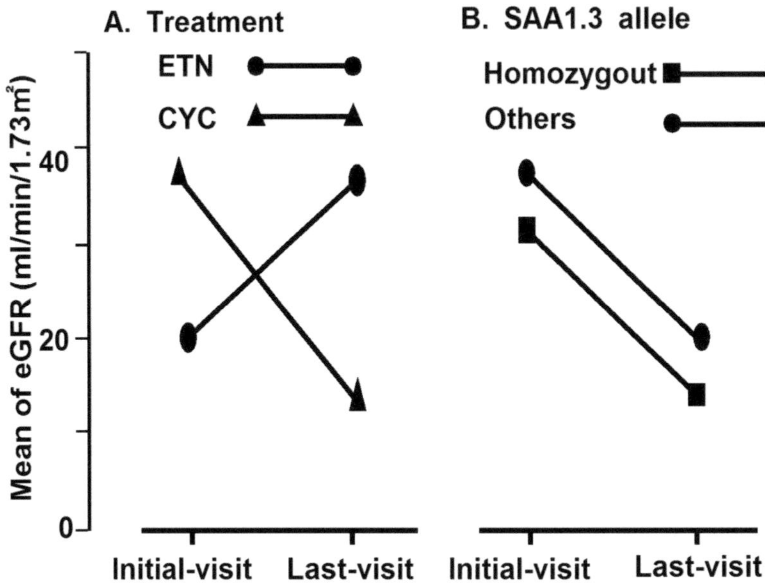


**Figure 9.** A) Changes in eGFR between initial- and last-visit as an effect of treatment (ETN or CYC). (B) Changes in eGFR between initial- and last-visit as an effect of SAA1.3 allele genotype (homozygosity or other polymorphisms). Quoted and modified from Reference No. 75.

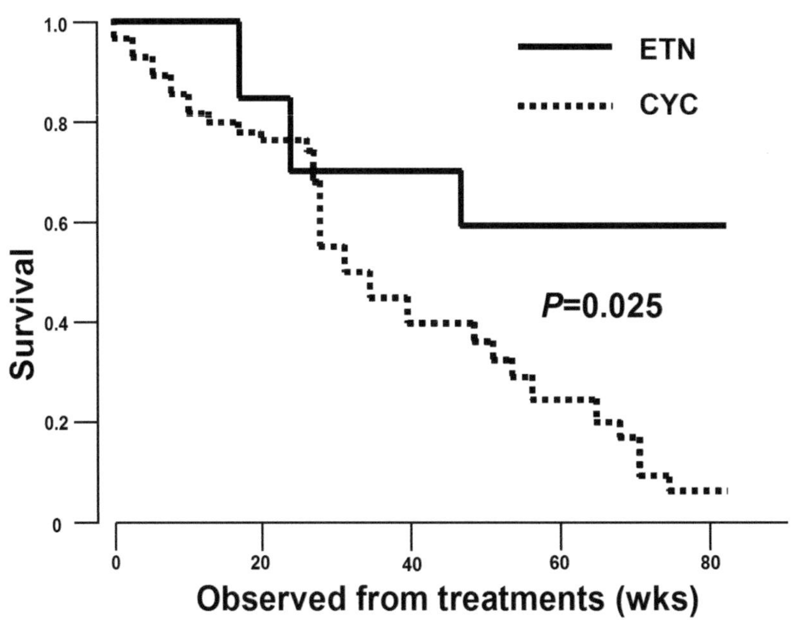


**Figure 10.** Kaplan-Meier survival curves after treatment with ETN (continuous line) and CYC (dotted line; P=0.025, log-rank test). Quoted and modified from Reference No. 75.

| | eGFR | | 24-Hour proteinuria | |
|---|---|---|---|---|
| | Hazard ratio (95% confidence interval) | P-value | Hazard ratio (95% confidence interval) | P-value |
| ETN | 0.949 (0.907-0.993) | 0.024 | 1.779 (1.074-2.946) | 0.025 |
| CYC | 0.951 (0.894-1.012) | 0.110 | 1.161 (0.542-2.488) | 0.701 |

Hazard ratio for each treatment using the Cox proportional hazards models to assess effect of treatments on the risk of death as the endpoint, being determined by two variables, eGFR and 24-h proteinuria. Quoted and modified from Reference No. 75. ETN: etanercept, CYC: cyclophosphamide, eGFR: estimated glomerular filtration rate.

**Table 8.** Hazard ratio for each treatment

### 5.3. Discussion

The goal of AA amyloidosis therapy is control of the underlying disorder. Treatment suppressing inflammatory activity reduces circulatory levels of SAA, an acute-phase reactant. In AA amyloidosis secondary to RA, treatment has focused on using cytotoxic drugs such as CYC and chlorambucil [29, 32] and more recently on TNF$\alpha$ inhibitors and IL-6 receptor antibody [45,56]. Before the advent of biologics, encouraging reports of alkylating agents as benefiting RA patients with AA amyloidosis were published. The rationale of this treatment seems to be similar to autologous stem cell transplantation, which generates new self-tolerant lymphocytes after alkylating agent treatment by eliminating self-reactive lymphocytes [78]. In the light of the reported superiority of CYC compared with MTX for managing RA patients with AA amyloidosis [9], using alkylating agents may improve AA amyloidosis. Cytotoxic drugs and cytokine inhibitors affect AA amyloid deposits by suppressing SAA production. Also, anti-TNF$\alpha$ therapies, by inhibiting expression of receptors of advanced glycation end-products (RAGE), may reduce interactions between AA amyloid fibrils and RAGE and thereby prevent AA-mediated cell toxicity [79, 80]. Thus, our findings that ETN had greater effects on AA amyloidosis secondary to RA than did CYC was not unexpected, and early therapeutic intervention in RA may avoid the complication of AA amyloidosis by controlling rheumatoid disease activity [26].

In Japan, use of MTX to treat with RA patients was permitted in 1999, the maximum dose being 8 mg/week, until February 2011; use of ETN was allowed in 2005. In our study the time from diagnosis of AA amyloidosis was shorter for the CYC group than the ETN group (Table 8), but treatment strategies and DMARDs used were the same, except for the use of biologics. Although MTX is now considered an anchor drug for RA treatment, it was used infrequently for AA amyloidosis patients because of its renal damage. No significant differences between groups in MTX therapy were found (Table 7). The recovery of Alb biosynthesis, improved acute-phase response, and ameliorated eGFR are all demonstrable endpoints, and we suggest that Alb reflects the severity of AA amyloidosis. We found that the different therapies rather than SAA1.3 allele polymorphism influenced changes in CRP and Alb. Also, eGFR may reflect diminished renal blood flow, and only ETN improved eGFR, thus indicating better renal function and greater efficacy of ETN than CYC (Fig. 9A). We found no evidence linking SAA1.3 allele to treatment efficacy (Fig. 9B).

## 6. Conclusion

Although significant advances have been made in understanding of the pathology, pathogenesis, and clinical treatment of AA amyloidosis secondary to RA, the disease is still an important complication that warrants further investigation. The SAA1.3 allele serves not only as a risk factor for AA amyloidosis but also as a factor related to poor prognosis and shortened survival in Japanese patients with RA, and understanding both disorders would benefit from investigation of the SAA1.3 allele. AA amyloidosis secondary to RA is now clearly influenced by many variables, and clinical pictures differ among patients. The pathological process in RA patients with AA amyloidosis seems to be more complicated and subtle than previously realized. Clarification of the formation and degeneration or turnover of AA amyloid fibrils and elucidation of the biological contributions of SAA in health and disease are indispensable prerequisites to the management of AA amyloidosis secondary to RA. By employing with the newly developed therapies, AA amyloidosis secondary to RA will already become both treatable and curable disease. Further, genetic predisposition, SAA1.3 allele genotype, would serve one of personalized medicines to make AA amyloidosis secondary to RA a preventable disease.

## Acknowledgements

The author would like to thank his colleagues Shin-ya Hirata, MD, PhD, Hirokazu Takaoka, MD, Syu-ichi Higashi, MD, PhD, Hironori Kudoh, MD, PhD, Kunihiko Tomoda, MD, PhD, Michishi Tsukano, MD, PhD, Satoshi Baba, MD, PhD, and Masahiro Shono, MD, PhD, for their collaborations and contributions to this work. This work was supported in part by a Grant-in-Aid for scientific research from the Japanese Ministry of Health, Labor, and Welfare and the Amyloidosis Research Committee for Intractable Diseases, Epochal Diagnosis, and Treatment in Japan.

## Author details

Tadashi Nakamura

Address all correspondence to: nakamura@k-shinto.or.jp

Section of Clinical Rheumatology, Kumamoto Shinto General Hospital and Graduate School of Medical Sciences, Kumamoto University, Japan

The author has declared no conflicts of interest.

http://dx.doi.org/10.5772/53801

## References

[1] Westermark GT, Westermark P: Serum amyloid A and protein AA: molecular mechanisms of a transmissible amyloidosis. FEBS Lett 2009; 583: 2685-90.

[2] Westermark P, Lundmark K, Westermark GT: Fibrils from designed non- amyloid-related synthetic peptides induce AA-amyloidosis during inflammation in an animal model. PLoS One 2009; 4: e6041.

[3] Larsson A, Malmstrom S, Westermark P: Signs of cross-seeding: aortic medin amyloid as a trigger for protein AA deposition. Amyloid 2011; 18: 229-34.

[4] Obici L, Raimondi S, Lavatell F, Bellotti V, Merlini G: Susceptibility to AA amyloidosis in rheumatic diseases: a critical overview. Arthritis Rheum (Arthritis Care Res) 2009; 61: 1435-40.

[5] Koivuniemi R, Paimela L, Suomalainen R, Leirisalo-Repo M: Amyloidosis as a cause of death in patients with rheumatoid arthritis. Clin Exp Rheumatol 2008; 26: 408-13.

[6] Nakamura T: Amyloid A amyloidosis secondary to rheumatoid arthritis: an uncommon yet important complication. Curr Rheumatol Rev 2007; 3: 231-41.

[7] Okuda Y, Takasugi K: Successful use of a humanized anti-interleukin-6 receptor antibody, tocilizumab, to treat amyloid A amyloidosis complicating juvenile idiopathic arthritis. Arthritis Rheum 2006; 54: 2997-3000.

[8] Kuroda T, Wada Y, Kobayashi D, Murakami S, Sakai T, Hirose S, et al : Effective anti-TNF-alpha therapy can induce rapid resolution and sustained decrease of gastrointestinal mucosal amyloid deposits in reactive amyloidosis associated with rheumatoid arthritis. J Rheumatol 2009; 36: 2409-15.

[9] Nakamura T, Higashi S, Tomoda K, Tsukano M, Baba S, Shono M: Significance of SAA1.3 allele genotype in Japanese patients with amyloidosis secondary to rheumatoid arthritis. Rheumatology (Oxford) 2006; 45: 43-9.

[10] Nakamura T, Higashi S, Tomoda K, Tsukano M, Shono M: Etanercept can induce resolution of renal deterioration in patients with amyloid A amyloidosis secondary to rheumatoid arthritis. Clin Rheumatol 2010; 29: 1395-401.

[11] Nakamura T, Higashi S, Tomoda K, Tsukano M, Arizono K, Nakamura T: Etanercept treatment in patients with rheumatoid arthritis on dialysis. Rheumatol Int 2010; 30: 1527-8.

[12] Baba S, Masago SA, Takahashi T, Kasama T, Sugimura H, Tsugane S, et al: A novel allelic variant of serum amyloid A, SAA1$\gamma$: genomic evidence, evolution, frequency, and implication as a risk factor for reactive systemic AA-amyloidosis. Hum Mol Genet 1995; 4: 1083-7.

[13] Moriguchi M, Terai C, Kosei Y, Uesato M, Nakajima A, Inada S, et al: Influence of genotypes at SAA1 and SAA2 loci on the development and the length of latent peri-

od of secondary AA-amyloidosis in patients with rheumatoid arthritis. Hum Genet 1999; 105: 360-6.

[14] Booth DR, Booth SE, Gillmore JD, Hawkins PN, Pepys MB: SAA1 alleles as risk factors in reactive systemic AA amyloidosis. Amyloid 1998; 5: 262-5.

[15] Nakamura T, Tomoda K,, Tsukano M,, Yamamura Y, Baba S: Gustatory sweating due to autonomic neuropathy in a patient with amyloidosis secondary to rheumatoid arthritis. Mod Rheumatol 2004; 14: 498-501.

[16] Nakamura T, Yamamura Y, Tomoda K, Tsukano M, Baba S: Massive hematuria due to bladder amyloidosis in patients with rheumatoid arthritis: three case reports. Clin Exp Rheumatol 2003; 21: 673-4.

[17] Hawkins PN, Pepys MB: Imaging amyloidosis with radiolabelled SAP. Eur J Nucl Med 1995; 22: 595-9.

[18] Tennent GA, Lovat LB, Pepys MB: Serum amyloid P component prevents proteolysis of the amyloid fibrils of Alzheimer's disease and systemic amyloidosis. Proc Natl Acad Sci USA 1995; 92: 4299-303.

[19] Hawkins PN: The diagnosis, natural history and treatment of amyloidosis. The Goulstonian Lecture 1995. J R Coll Physicians Lond 1997; 31: 552-60.

[20] Pepys MB: Science and serendipity. Clin Med 2007; 7: 562-78.

[21] Gillmore JD, Lovat LB, Persey MR, Pepys MB, Hawkins PN: Amyloid load and clinical outcome in AA amyloidosis in relation to circulating concentration of serum amyloid A protein. Lancet 2001; 358: 24-9.

[22] Wakhlu A, Krisnani N, Hissatia P, Aggarwal A, Misra R: Prevalence of secondary amyloidosis in Asian north Indian patients with rheumatoid arthritis. J Rheumatol 2003; 30: 948-51.

[23] Laiho K, Tiitinen S, Kaarela K, Helin H, Isomaki H: Secondary amyloidosis has decreased in patients with inflammatory joint disease in Finland. Clin Rheumatol 1999; 18: 122-3.

[24] Kaipiainen-Seppanen O, Myllykangas-Luosujarvi R, Lampainen E, Ikaheimo R: Intensive treatment of rheumatoid arthritis reduces need for dialysis due to secondary amyloidosis. Scand J Rheumatol 2000; 29: 232-5.

[25] Hanzenberg BPC, van Rijswijk MH:. Where has secondary amyloidosis gone? Ann Rheum Dis 2000; 59: 577-9.

[26] Nakamura T: Clinical strategies for amyloid A amyloidosis secondary to rheumatoid arthritis. Mod Rheumatol 2008; 18: 109-18.

[27] David J, Vouyiouka O, Ansell BM, Hall A, Woo P: Amyloidosis in juvenile chronic arthritis: a morbidity and mortality study. Clin Exp Rheumatol 1993; 2: 85-90.

[28] Nakamura T: Amyloid A amyloidosis secondary to rheumatoid arthritis: pathophysiology and treatment. Clin Exp Rheumatol 2011; 29: 850-7.

[29] Keysser G, Keysser C, Keysser M: Treatment of refractory rheumatoid arthritis with low-dose cyclophosphamide. Long-term follow-up of 108 patients. Z Rheumatol 1998; 57: 101-7.

[30] Berglund K, Keller C, Thysell H: Alkylating cytostatic treatment in renal amyloidosis secondary to rheumatoid arthritis. Ann Rheum Dis 1987; 46: 757-62.

[31] Ahlmen M, Ahlmen J, Svalander C, Bucht H: Cytotoxic drug treatment of reactive amyloidosis in rheumatoid arthritis with special reference to renal insufficiency. Clin Rheumatol 1987; 6: 27-38.

[32] Berglund K, Thysell H, Keller C: Results, principles and pitfalls in the management of renal AA-amyloidosis: a 10-21 year followup of 16 patients with rheumatic disease treated with alkylating cytostatics. J Rheumatol 1993; 20: 2051-7.

[33] Chevrel G, Jenvrin C, McGregor B, Miossec P: Renal type AA amyloidosis associated with rheumatoid arthritis: a cohort study showing improved survival on treatment with pulse cyclophosphamide. Rheumatology (Oxford) 2001; 40: 821-5.

[34] Shapiro DL, Spiera H: Regression of the nephritic syndrome in rheumatoid arthritis and amyloidosis treated with azathioprine. A case report. Arthritis Rheum 1995; 38: 1851-4.

[35] Nakamura T, Yamamura Y, Tomoda K, Tsukano M, Shono M, Baba S: Efficacy of cyclophosphamide combined with prednisolone in patients with AA amyloidosis secondary to rheumatoid arthritis. Clin Rheumatol 2003; 22: 371-5.

[36] Kishimoto T, Akira S, Taga T: IL-6 receptor and mechanism of signal transduction. Int J Immunopharmacol 1992; 14: 431-8.

[37] Hirano T, Ishihara K, Hibi M: Roles of STAT3 in mediating the cell growth, differentiation and survival signals relayed through the IL-6 family of cytokine receptors. Oncogene 2000; 19: 2548-56.

[38] Hagihara K, Nishikawa T, Sugamata Y, Song J, Isobe T, Taga T, et al: Essential role of STAT3 in cytokine-driven NF-kappaB-mediated serum amyloid A gene expression. Gene Cells 2005; 10: 1051-63.

[39] Ueda M, Ando Y, Nakamura M, Yamashita T, Himeno S, Kim J, et al: FK506 inhibits murine AA amyloidosis: possible involvement of T cells in amyloidogenesis. J Rheumatol 2006; 33: 2260-70.

[40] Kogina K, Shoda H, Yamaguchi Y, Tsuno NH, Takahashi K, Fujio K, et al: Tacrolimus differentially regulates the proliferation of conventional and regulatory $CD4^+$ T cells. Mol Cells 2009; 28: 125-30.

[41] Pettersson T, Konttinen YT, Maury CPJ: Treatment strategies for amyloid A amyloidosis. Expert Opin Pharmacother 2008; 9: 2117-28.

[42] Dember LM: Modern treatment of amyloidosis: unresolved questions. J Am Soc Nephrol 2009; 20: 469-72.

[43] Perfetto F, Moggi-Pignone A, Livi R, Tempestini A, Bergesio F, Matucci-Cerinic M: Systemic amyloidosis: a challenge for the rheumatologist. Nat Rev Rheumatol 2010; 6: 417-29.

[44] Masutani K, Nagata M, Ikeda H, Takeda K, Katafuchi R, Hirakata H, et al: Glomerular crescent formation in renal amyloidosis. A clinicopathological study and demonstration of upregulated cell-mediated immunity. Clin Nephrol 2008; 70: 464-74.

[45] Kuroda T, Ootaki Y, Sato H, Fujimura T, Nakatsue T, Murakami S, et al: A case of AA amyloidosis associated with rheumatoid arthritis effectively treated with infliximab. Rheumatol Int 2008; 28: 1155-9.

[46] Elkayam O, Hawkins PN, Lachmann H, Yaron M, Caspi D: Rapid and complete resolution of proteinuria due to renal amyloidosis in a patient with rheumatoid arthritis treated with infliximab. Arthritis Rheum 2002; 46: 2571-3..

[47] Gottenberg JE, Merle-Vincent F, Bentaberry F, Allanore Y, Berenbaum F, Fautrel B, et al: Anti-tumor necrosis factor alpha therapy in fifteen patients with AA amyloidosis secondary to inflammatory arthritides: a followup report of tolerability and efficacy. Arthritis Rheum 2003; 48: 2019-24.

[48] Nakamura T, Higashi S, Tomoda K, Tsukano M, Baba S: Efficacy of eternercept in patients with AA amyloidosis secondary to rheumatoid arthritis. Clin Exp Rheumatol 2007; 25: 518-22.

[49] Ishii W, Kishida D, Suzuki A, Shimojima Y, Matsuda M, Hoshii Y, et al: A case with rheumatoid arthritis and systemic reactive AA amyloidosis showing rapid regression of amyloid deposition on gastroduadenal mucosa after a combination therapy of corticosteroid and etanercept. Rheumatol Int 2011; 31; 247-50.

[50] Smith GR, Tymms KE, Falk M: Etanercept treatment of renal amylopidosis complaining rheumatoid arthritis. Intern Med 2004; 34: 570-2.

[51] Fernandes-Nebro A, Torero E, Ortiz-Santamaria V, Castro MC, Olive A, et al: Treatment of rheumatic inflammatory disease in 25 patients with secondary amyloidosis using tumor necrosis factor alpha antagonists. Am J Med 2003; 115: 589-90.

[52] Roque R, Ramiro S, Corderio A, Goncalves P, Canas SD, Santos M: Development of amyloidosis in patients with rheumatoid arthritis under TNF-blocking agents. Clin Rheumatol 2011; 30: 869-70.

[53] Nobre CA, Callado MRM, Rodriges CEM, de Menezes DB, Vieira WP : Anti-TNF therapy in renal amyloidosis in refractory rheumatoid arthritis: a new therapeutic perspective. Bras J Rheumatol 2010; 50: 205-10.

[54] Nishimoto N, Yoshizaki K, Miyasaka N, Yamamoto K, Kawai S, Takeuchi T, et al: Treatment of rheumatoid arthritis with humanized anti-interleukin-6 receptor anti-

body: a multicenter, double-blind, placebo-controlled trial. Arthritis Rheum 2004; 50: 1761-9.

[55] Hagiwara K, Nishikawa T, Isobe T, Song J, Sugamata Y, Yoshizaki K: Il-6 plays a critical role in the synergistic induction of human serum amyloid A (SAA) gene when stimulated with proinflammatory cytokines as analyzed with an SAA isoform real-time quantitative RT-PCR assay system. Biochem Biophys Res Commun 2004; 314: 363-9.

[56] Hattori Y, Ubara Y, Simida K, Hiramatsu R, Hasegawa E, Yamanouchi M, et al: Tocilizumab improves cardiac disease in a hemodialysis patient with AA amyloidosis secondary to rheumatoid arthritis. Amyloid 2012; 19: 37-40.

[57] Nishida S, Hagihara K, Shima Y, Kawai M, Kuwahara Y, Arimitsu J, et al: Rapid improvement of AA amyloidosis with humanized anti-interleukin 6 receptor antibody treatment. Ann Rheum Dis 2009; 68: 1235-6.

[58] Landewe R, van der Heijde D, Klareskog L, van Vollenhoven R, Fatenejad S: Disconnect between inflammation and joint destruction after treatment with etanercept plus methotrexate: results from the trial of etanercept and methotrexate with radiographic and patient outcomes. Arthritis Rheum 2006; 54: 3119-25.

[59] Rubbert-Roth A, Finckh A: Treatment options in patients with rheumatoid arthritis failing initial TNF inhibitor therapy: a critical review. Arthritis Res Ther 2009; 11(Suppl. 1): S1.

[60] Narvaez J, Hernandes MV, Ruiz JM, Vaqueero CG, Juanola X, Nollaa JM: Rituximab therapy for AA-amyloidosis secondary to rheumatoid arthritis. Joint Bone Spine 2011; 78: 98-101.

[61] Smith JW, McDonald TL: Production of serum amyloid A and C-reactive protein by HepG2 cells stimulated with combinations of cytokines or monocyte conditioned media: the effects of prednisolone. Clin Exp Immunol 1992; 90: 293-9.

[62] Migita K, Yamasaki K, Shibatomi H, Ida H, Kita M, Kawakami A, et al: Impaired degradation of serum amyloid A (SAA) protein by cytokine-stimulated monocytes. Clin Exp Immunol 2001; 123: 408-11.

[63] Nakamura T, Baba S, Yamamura Y, Tsuruta T, Matsubara S, Tomoda K, et al: Combined treatment with cyclophosphamide and prednisolone is effective for secondary amyloidosis with SAA1γ/γ genotype in a patient with rheumatoid arthritis. Mod Rheumatol 2000; 10: 160-4.

[64] Nakamura T, Yamamura Y, Tomoda K, Tsukano M, Shono M, Baba S: Efficacy of cyclophosphamide combined with prednisolone in patients with AA amyloidosis secondary to rheumatoid arthritis. Clin Rheumatol 2003; 22: 371-5.

[65] Matsuda M, Morita H, Ikeda S: Long-term follow-up of systemic reactive AA amyloidosis secondary to rheumatoid arthritis: successful treatment with intermediate-dose corticosteroid. Intern Med 2002; 41: 403-7.

[66] Fushimi T, Takahashi Y, Kashima Y, Fukushima K, Ishii W, Kaneko K, et al: Severe protein losing enteropathy with intractable diarrhea due to systemic AA amyloidosis, successfully treated with corticosteroid and octreotide. Amyloid 2005; 12: 48-53.

[67] Bakker M, Jacobs JWG, Welsing PMJ, Verstappen SMM, Tekstra J, Ton E, et al: Low-dose prednisolone inclusion in a methotrexate-based, tight control strategy for early rheumatoid arthritis. A randomized trial. Ann Intern Med 2012; 156: 326-39.

[68] Dember LM, Hawkins PN, Hazenberg BP, Gorevic PD, Merlini G, Butrimiene I, et al: Eprodisate for the treatment of renal disease in AA amyloidosis. N Engl J Med 2007; 356: 2349-60.

[69] Noborn F, O'Callaghan P, Hermansson E, Zharng X, Ancsin JB, Damas AM, et al: Heparan sulfate/heparin promotes transthyretin fibrillization through selective binding to a basic motif in the protein. Proc Natl Acad Sci USA 2011; 108: 5584-9.

[70] Pepys MB, Herbert J, Hutchinson L, Tennent GA, Lachmann HJ, Gallimore JR, et al: Targeted pharmacological depletion of serum amyloid P component for treatment of human amyloidosis. Nature 2002; 417: 254-9.

[71] Santos NC, Figueria-Coelho J, Martins-Silva J, Saldanha C: Multidisciplinary utilization of dimethyl sulfoxide: pharmacological, cellular, and molecular aspects. Biochem Pharmacol 2003; 65: 1035-41.

[72] Amemori S, Iwakiri R, Endo H, Ootani A, Ogata S, Noda T, et al: Oral dimethyl sulfoxide for systemic amyloid A amyloidosis complication in chronic inflammatory disease: a retrospective patient chart review. J Gastroenterol 2006; 41: 444-9.

[73] Kuroda T, Tanabe N, Sato H, Ajiro J, Wada Y, Murakami S, et al: Outcome of patients with reactive amyloidosis associated with rheumatoid arthritis in dialysis treatment. Rheumatol Int 2006; 26: 1147-53.

[74] Don BR, Spin G, Nestorov I, Hutmacher M, Rose A, Kaysen GA: The pharmacokinetics of etanercept in patients with end-stage renal disease on haemodialysis. J Pharm Pharmacol 2005; 57: 1407-13.

[75] Nakamura T, Higashi S, Tomoda K, Tsukano M, Shono M: Effectiveness of etanercept vs cyclophosphamide as treatment for patients with amylopid A amyloidosis secondary to rheumatoid arthritis. Rheumatology (Oxford) 2012; 51: 2064-9.

[76] Maury CPJ, Teppo A-M: Mechanism of reduced amyloid-A-degrading activity in serum of patients with secondary amyloidosis. Lancet 1982; 2: 234-7.

[77] Matsuo S, Imai E, Horio M, Yasuda Y, Tomita K, Nitta K, et al: Revised equations for estimated GFR from serum creatinine in Japan. Am J Kidney Dis 2009; 53: 982-92.

[78] Shapiro DL, Spiera H: Regression of the nephrotic syndrome in rheumatoid arthritis and amyloidosis treated with azathioprine. A case report. Arthritis Rheum 1995; 38: 1851-4.

[79] Tanaka N, Yonekura H, Yamagishi S, Fujimori H, Yamamoto Y, Yamamoto H: The receptor for advanced glycation end products is induced by the glycation products themselves and tumor necrosis factor-α through nuclear factor kB, and 17β-estradiol through Sp-1 in human vascular endothelial cells. J Biol Chem 2000; 33: 25781-90.

[80] Okamoto M, Katagiri Y, Kiire A, Momohara S, Kamatani M: Serum amyloid A activates nuclear factor kB in rheumatoid synovial fibroblasts through binding to receptor of advanced glycation end-products. J Rheumatol 2008; 35: 752-6.